MASTERING MEDICAL LANGUAGE

MASTERING MEDICAL LANGUAGE

Anthony L. Spatola

Camden County College, Blackwood, New Jersey

Prentice-Hall, Inc., Englewood Cliffs, New Jersey 07632

Library of Congress Cataloging in Publication Data

Spatola, Anthony L.
    Mastering medical language.

    Includes index.
    1. Medicine—Terminology. I. Title
R123.S64   610'.14   81-10539
ISBN 0-13-560151-7 (pbk.)   AACR2

Anatomical illustrations are taken from William F. Evans,
Anatomy and Physiology, Second Edition, © 1976. Reprinted
by permission of Prentice-Hall, Inc., Englewood Cliffs,
New Jersey

Printed in the United States of America

10 9 8 7 6 5 4 3

Editorial/production supervision and interior design
        by Zita de Schauensee
Manufacturing buyer: John Hall

Prentice-Hall International, Inc., *London*
Prentice-Hall of Australia Pty. Limited, *Sydney*
Prentice-Hall of Canada, Ltd., *Toronto*
Prentice-Hall of India Private Limited, *New Delhi*
Prentice-Hall of Japan, Inc., *Tokyo*
Prentice-Hall of Southeast Asia Pte. Ltd., *Singapore*
Whitehall Books Limited, Wellington, *New Zealand*

Contents

To the Teacher   xi

To the Student   xiii

1   BASIC ELEMENTS OF MEDICAL WORDS   1

The base form   *1*
The combining vowel   *3*
Prefixes and suffixes   *4*
Basic patterns   *6*
Order of combining elements   *7*
Competing forms   *8*
Review of basic concepts   *9*
Exercises   *9*
Answers to text exercises   *13*
Answers to exercises   *14*

2   SUFFIXES   16

Exercises   *20*
Answers to exercises   *24*

3   PREFIXES   25

Exercises   *28*
Answers to exercises   *34*

4   PRONUNCIATION, SPELLING, AND FORMATION OF PLURALS   36

Pronunciation   *36*
Spelling   *39*
Formation of plurals   *42*
Exercises   *43*
Answers to exercises   *46*

5   ANATOMY OF THE CELL; COMMON MEDICAL EXPRESSIONS   48

Anatomy of the cell   *48*
Common medical expressions   *52*
Exercises   *53*
Answers to exercises   *57*

6   BODY REGIONS, DIRECTIONS, NUMBERS, AND COLORS   59

Major body regions   *59*
Body cavities   *61*
Directional terms   *63*
Terms for body movements   *63*
Body planes   *64*
Surface anatomy   *64*
Numbers and colors   *67*
Exercises   *68*
Answers to exercises   *74*

7   THE SKIN   76

Combining forms   *76*
Anatomy of the skin   *78*
Appendages of the skin   *78*
Effects of aging on the skin   *80*
Clinical and pathological conditions   *81*
Exercises   *84*
Answers to exercises   *91*

8   THE MUSCULOSKELETAL SYSTEM   93

Combining forms   *93*
Anatomy of the skeleton   *97*
The joints   *110*
The muscles   *110*

Contents

Clinical and pathological conditions   *111*
Exercises   *113*
Answers to exercises   *122*

9   THE NERVOUS SYSTEM   125

Combining forms   *125*
The neuron and its function   *127*
Divisions of the nervous system   *130*
Clinical and pathological conditions   *142*
Exercises   *143*
Answers to exercises   *153*

10   THE SPECIAL SENSES   155

Combining forms: Sight   *155*
Sight   *156*
Clinical and pathological conditions   *161*
Taste and smell   *163*
Exercises: The eye   *164*
Combining forms: Hearing   *169*
Hearing   *170*
Clinical and pathological conditions   *172*
Exercises: The ear   *173*
Answers to exercises: The eye   *176*
Answers to exercises: The ear   *178*

11   CARDIOVASCULAR SYSTEM; BLOOD AND LYMPH   179

Combining forms   *179*
Anatomy of the heart   *183*
Heartbeat and cardiac cycle   *185*
Reflexes influencing heart rate   *186*
The blood vessels   *186*
Fetal circulation   *187*
Arterial and venous blood pressures   *190*
The composition of blood   *191*
Blood typing   *195*
Blood buffers   *196*
The lymphatic system   *196*
Clinical and pathological conditions   *199*
Exercises   *204*
Answers to exercises   *214*

12 THE RESPIRATORY SYSTEM 217

Combining forms *217*
Anatomy of the respiratory system *219*
Breathing *222*
Pulmonary function tests *223*
Vocal mechanism *224*
Clinical and pathological conditions *224*
Exercises *228*
Answers to exercises *233*

13 THE DIGESTIVE SYSTEM 235

Combining forms *235*
Anatomy of the digestive system *240*
The peritoneum *244*
The teeth *244*
Clinical and pathological conditions *245*
Exercises *248*
Answers to exercises *257*

14 THE URINARY SYSTEM 259

Combining forms *259*
Anatomy of the urinary system *260*
The mechanism of micturition *262*
The formation of urine *264*
Clinical and pathological conditions *265*
Exercises *267*
Answers to exercises *271*

15 THE REPRODUCTIVE SYSTEMS 273

Combining forms *273*
The male reproductive system *277*
The female reproductive system *279*
Gestation *281*
Childbirth *282*
The mammary glands *283*
Clinical and pathological conditions *283*
Exercises *288*
Answers to exercises *297*

16   THE ENDOCRINE SYSTEM   299

Combining forms   *299*
The pituitary gland   *300*
The thyroid gland   *302*
The parathyroid glands   *303*
The adrenal glands   *303*
The pancreas   *303*
The gonads   *304*
Other hormone-producing organs   *304*
Clinical and pathological conditions   *305*
Exercises   *307*
Answers to exercises   *313*

17   PHARMACOLOGY   315

Combining forms   *315*
Drug nomenclature and standards   *316*
The effects of drugs   *317*
Drug preparations   *318*
Administration of medication   *318*
Drug groups   *319*
Antibiotics   *322*
Vitamins and minerals   *322*
Abbreviations used in prescription writing   *324*
Exercises   *325*
Answers to exercises   *331*

18   ONCOLOGY   333

Combining forms   *333*
Types of tumors   *334*
Etiology of cancer   *335*
Diagnosis of cancer   *337*
Treatment   *338*
Exercises   *339*
Answers to exercises   *345*

19   RADIOLOGY AND SURGERY   348

Combining forms   *348*
Radiology   *350*
Surgery   *353*
Exercises   *364*
Answers to exercises   *371*

20 MENTAL ILLNESS   374

Combining forms   *374*
Exercises   *378*
Answers to exercises   *382*

APPENDIX 1:   Additional bases, suffixes, and prefixes   385

APPENDIX 2:   Medical abbreviations   390

APPENDIX 3:   Drugs   396

APPENDIX 4:   Review exercises   410

Review unit 1   *410*
Review unit 2   *427*
Review unit 3   *442*
Review unit 4   *454*
Review unit 5   *465*

Index of Combining Forms   477

General Index   484

To the Teacher

Along with the traditional premedical and nursing students there has been an impressive growth in the number of students in the various allied health professions. This is especially noticeable in the community colleges where students are prepared for such occupations as nursing, dental assistant, laboratory technician, medical secretary, and various hospital, office, and support personnel. These students find mastering medical terminology a formidable task and frequently settle for learning "just enough to get by." This textbook has been written to serve the needs not only of the traditional students of medical terminology but of these students as well. Because the career objectives and the training of both groups of students are so varied, the author of this text has tried to steer a middle course between the vocabulary versus scientific content approaches to the teaching of medical terminology. The anatomy, physiology, and pathology contained in this text are presented so that students will have at least a basic knowledge of the body systems and diseases, and will see many medical words in context. How much a student is required to master should be based on the objectives of the course and the needs of the student, both of which vary from institution to institution. The teacher may emphasize one or several aspects of medical language according to his or her objectives and training.

Several features distinguish this book from other textbooks and, the author believes, make it an outstanding text. There is a comprehensive introduction to the language of medicine; the textbook was developed from classroom experience; spelling and pronunciation are stressed throughout; in addition to the commonly used vocabulary, terms that are often limited to more "bookish" writing are included; the vocabulary is presented in logical sequence and is drawn from both anatomy and pathology; the content is supported by numerous and meaningful exercises; and there are many clear and pertinent illustrations.

The first four chapters present the "mechanics" of medical language. Chapter 1 begins with a step-by-step analysis of the basic components of medical words by first presenting these elements in English words. From the same English words medical terms are then formed. At each step the student participates by completing the brief exercises. The *patterns* illustrate the various combinations of the combining elements and demonstrate the logical formulation of medical words. Problems arising from incorrectly combining the elements of medical words are illustrated with clear and effective examples. *Duplication* and the *types of duplicates*, always a source of students' questions, are given a brief but thorough explanation. The exercises at the end of the chapter provide the student with extensive and meaningful reinforcement. Many of the words are already familiar to the student.

Chapters 2 and 3 give an extensive list of the most commonly occurring suffixes and prefixes and supporting exercises. Chapter 4 emphasizes spelling and pronunciation, an emphasis that is long overdue. Beginning with Chapter 4, all combining forms and medical words are given with their pronunciation.

The rest of the book deals primarily with the combining forms for each of the body systems. Each chapter presents: (1) a list of combining forms, (2) the anatomy of the system, (3) clinical and pathological conditions, and (4) exercises. Any combining form or medical word presented for the first time is followed by its pronunciation, and several illustrations of its use are included in each chapter. Without omitting the pertinent anatomical and pathological detail, the text is short enough for a one-semester course.

Haddonfield, New Jersey   Anthony L. Spatola

To the Student

When you come across medical words, your first reaction may be that these words are mind-boggling. The forms, the sounds, and the very length of these words seem to place them beyond comprehension. Don't despair! Medical terminology is a language. It can be analyzed and studied like any other language.

This text is organized so that you will first learn the "mechanics" or what you might call the grammar of the language of medicine. After you have mastered the basics, learning the vocabulary of your new language will be relatively simple. The vocabulary has been arranged so that you are not memorizing meaningless lists; on the contrary, you will be given a context for understanding each new entry. Although it is not necessary to master anatomy and pathology to learn medical terminology, a general understanding of both will help you to remember much of the medical vocabulary that you learn. Also, the terminology becomes more interesting when it is anchored in anatomy and pathology.

Throughout this course your goals should be:

To become familiar with the system on which the language of medicine is built;

To master the combining forms so that you can both recognize and build medical words;

To pay close attention to the spelling and pronunciation of medical words;

To have a general knowledge of the anatomy, and the clinical and pathological conditions for each system. (Your teacher may or may not require that you learn anatomy and pathology.)

A.L.S.

1 Basic Elements of Medical Words

The study of medical terminology is the study of the parts that make up medical words and the building of both a general vocabulary and a vocabulary for each of the body systems. Few linguistic concepts need be understood before you can analyze the terms themselves. Most medical words are made from a combination of the following elements: the part of the word that we shall call the BASE because it contains the most fundamental meaning of that word, prefixes and suffixes, and vowels that join all these parts.

THE BASE FORM

The BASE* of a medical word is that word structure that is capable of combining with another base or a suffix to form a medical word that has meaning. The word base is what is left after all added elements are removed. This reduced part of the word contains its most fundamental meaning. The examples in the table illustrate how words are reduced to their bases.

Word	Separation of affixes	Base	Meaning
epigraphic	epi/graph/ic	graph	write
atrophy	a/troph/y	troph	nourish
homogenous	hom/o/gen/ous	gen	produce
interjection	inter/jec/tion	jec	throw
hysterical	hyster/ical	hyster	uterus
linguist	lingu/ist	lingu	tongue
ductile	duct/ile	duc(t)	lead
poetic	poet/ic	poe(t)	make

Notice how the prefixes and suffixes alter the meaning of these bases. The base GRAPH

*Sometimes called a root or a stem.

has the meaning of WRITE. When we add a prefix and a suffix to the base, we change its original meaning.

EPI	GRAPH	IC
on	write	pertaining to

EPIGRAPHIC means "pertaining to the writing" (on buildings and monuments). In the medical word ELECTROENCEPHALOGRAPH we can recognize the word GRAPH as one of the bases that form the word. We can divide the word into its parts in the following manner.

ELECTR/O/EN/CEPHAL/O/GRAPH
electrical   in   head   write
impulses

In medical language electroencephalograph refers to an instrument that records the electrical impulses of the brain.

Let's analyze the other examples on our list and use the bases to make medical terms.

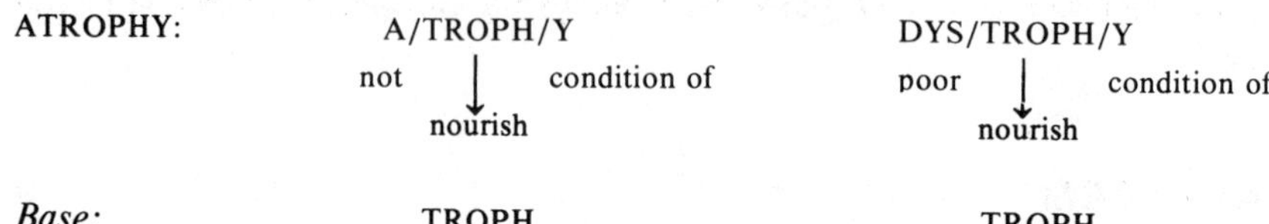

ATROPHY:

A/TROPH/Y
not — condition of
nourish

DYS/TROPH/Y
poor — condition of
nourish

Base: TROPH   TROPH

Meaning: Both are medical terms. Atrophy refers to the physical deterioration due to a lack of nourishment. (Atrophy is most commonly used to refer to a decrease in tissue size resulting from a reduction of the number and/or size of cells.) Dystrophy refers to a physical deterioration due to poor or insufficient nourishment.

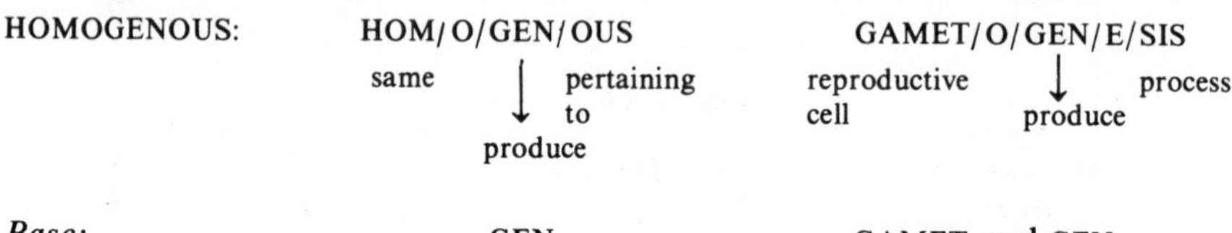

HOMOGENOUS:

HOM/O/GEN/OUS
same — pertaining to
produce

GAMET/O/GEN/E/SIS
reproductive cell — process
produce

Base: GEN   GAMET and GEN

Meaning: Homogenous means producing something that is the same—that is, something uniform in its parts or structure. Gametogenesis refers to the process of producing male and female reproductive cells.

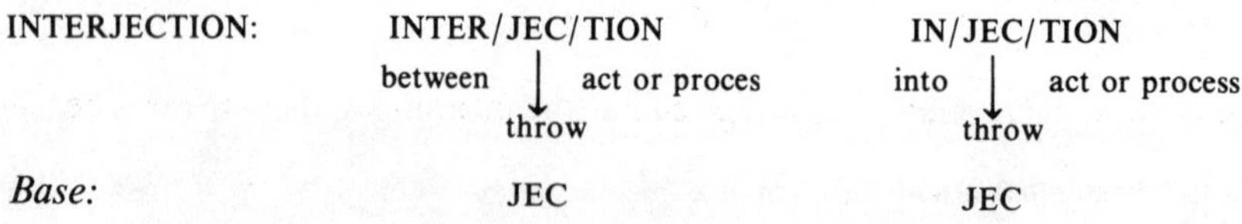

INTERJECTION:

INTER/JEC/TION
between — act or proces
throw

IN/JEC/TION
into — act or process
throw

Base: JEC   JEC

Meaning: Interjection refers to an exclamatory word in a sentence. An injection is the process of putting a liquid into the body by means of a hypodermic syringe.

HYSTERICAL:	HYSTER/IC/AL	HYSTER/EC/TOM/Y
	uterus pertaining to	uterus out cut process
Base:	HYSTER	HYSTER

Meaning: A person who is hysterical is one lacking emotional control. The ancient Greeks believed that hysteria was a disturbance of the uterus. Hysterectomy refers to the surgical procedure for removing the uterus.

LINGUIST:	LINGU/IST	SUB/LINGU/AL
	tongue one who specializes in	under ↓ pertaining to / tongue
Base:	LINGU	LINGU

Meaning: A linguist is one who specializes in the science that deals with language. Sublingual refers to the area under the tongue.

DUCTILE:	DUCT/ILE	OV/I/DUCT
	lead capable of	egg lead
Base:	DUC (T)	OV and DUC (T)

Meaning: What is ductile is capable of being led. An oviduct is a tube that leads the egg from the ovary to the uterus.

POETIC:	POET/IC	THROMB/O/POIE/SIS
	make pertaining to	clots make process
Base:	POE (T)	THROMB and POE (T)

Meaning: The poet is one who makes or creates. Thrombopoiesis refers to the formation of blood clots.

THE COMBINING VOWEL

When two bases are combined or a suffix is added to a base, if no vowel occurs at the junction of the two forms, a vowel called the COMBINING VOWEL is added (Ex: THROMB/O/POIESIS; /O/ is the combining vowel). Usually the combining vowel is O. The combining vowel O has been used so extensively that it has replaced other combining vowels (I, E, A) in many medical words. As a result, O is the most commonly occurring combining vowel. I is the second most common combining vowel. We call a base with a combining vowel a combining form. For example, HEMATO (HEMAT+O) and GASTRO (GASTR +O) are combining forms. Here are some examples of common English words that use O as a combining vowel. Using a dictionary, give their meanings by analyzing their parts.

GE/O/GRAPH/Y...

METR/O/POLIS ....

ORTH/O/DOX ....

MON/O/TON/OUS ....

ANTH/O/LOG/Y ....

Do the same for the following medical terms.

LOB/O/TOM/Y ....

OPT/O/METR/IST ....

UR/O/LOG/Y ....

HYDR/O/THERAP/Y ....

AUR/I/SCOP/E ....

CENT/I/GRAD/E ....

CORN/I/FAC/TION ....

MILL/I/METER ....

PELV/I/METER ....

VENTR/I/DUCT ....

Notice that in the last six medical terms I is used as the combining vowel.

PREFIXES AND SUFFIXES

PREFIXES are placed before a word to alter the basic meaning of the word. SUFFIXES appear at the end of the word and, in a sense, function like prefixes. Suffixes, however, not only alter the meaning of a word, but they also determine the various word functions, such as part of speech or whether the word is singular or plural. We will deal with prefixes and suffixes in great detail in Chapters 2 and 3. For now let us look at how they affect the word base in general.

We have a word base CARDI, meaning heart. Notice how the addition of a prefix and suffix alter the basic meaning.

PERI/CARDI/O/TOM/Y

around   heart   cut   process

Translated, pericardiotomy means the process of making an incision into the pericardium, the sac that encloses the heart. Notice that when we translated the medical word into an English phrase, we translated the suffix first. In translating medical terms, we frequently begin with the suffix and then end with the beginning of the term.

PERI/CARDI/O/TOM/Y
3   4   2 1

NEPHR/O/TOM/Y   NEPHR means kidney
3   2 1

NEPHR/O/PATH/Y   PATH means disease
3   2 1

but in   NEPHR O LITH   LITH means stone
            1   2

The term NEPHROLITH has two base forms *without* any suffix.

In the medical terms given below divide each word into its parts, number the order of translating the parts, and translate the entire term. Use a dictionary for any unfamiliar terms.

                         3   2 1

NEPHROGRAPHY   nephr/o/graph/y   process of recording the kidney (x ray)

ANTIFUNGAL ....

PROPHYLACTIC ....

HYPERTROPHIC ....

INTRAVENOUS ....

ECTOPIA ....

PERIODONTIST ....

ESOPHAGOJEJUNOSTOMY ....

BASIC PATTERNS

Recognizing the elements of medical words and how these elements combine to form words will enable you to reduce a word correctly into its parts and also to form many new words. All medical terms begin with a BASE and build from it. Theoretically almost any number of elements can be added to the base.

Pattern 1	*Base*	*Nothing added*
	CARIES	decay
	MENSES	menstrual cycle

Pattern 2 *Base + Combining vowel + Suffix*

THERM/O/METER instrument to measure heat

Base + Suffix

HEPAT/ITIS inflammation of the liver

Pattern 3 *Base + Combining vowel + Base*

TROPH/O/BLAST a group of undifferentiated cells that will channel nourishment to the fetus

Base + Base

SIAL/ADEN a salivary gland

Pattern 4 *Base + Base + Suffix*

ENTER/ADEN/ITIS inflammation of intestinal glands

Base + Combining vowel + Base + Suffix

LABI/O/DENT/AL pertaining to the lips and teeth

With this pattern you can join a number of bases and combining vowels to a suffix.

OT/O/RHIN/O/LARYNG/O/LOG/IST one who specializes in the study and treatment of the ears, nose, and throat

Pattern 5 *Prefix + Base + Combining vowel + Suffix*

DYS/MEN/O/RHE/A painful menstruation

Prefix + Base + Suffix

EPI/GASTR/IC pertaining to the region over the pit of the stomach

Pattern 6   *Prefix+ Base+ Combining vowel+ Base+ Suffix*

    SUB/MICR/O/SCOP/IC   pertaining to that which is too small to be seen under the microscope

Pattern 7   *Prefix+ Prefix+ Base+ Combining vowel+ Suffix*

    CONTRA/IN/DIC/A/TION   that which indicates the inappropriateness of some form of treatment

    Prefix+ Prefix+ Base+ Suffix

    SUB/PERI/OSTE/AL   under the tissue that covers the bone

Pattern 8   *Prefix+ Suffix*

    PARA/CENTESIS   surgical puncture of a cavity in order to drain it

ORDER OF COMBINING ELEMENTS

The order in which you combine the various elements that form medical terms is extremely important. If you change the order of the elements within a word, you will either create a form that is not used—and hence is meaningless—or you will make a different word. HEMOSTAT refers to something that checks or arrests the flow of blood. STATOHEM, if used, could mean stopping blood; however, it is not used. Here are two more examples.

PODAGRA means a painful seizure of the foot.

AGROPOD is an unused and thus meaningless form.

LITHOTRIPSY refers to the crushing of a stonelike deposit.

TRIPSOLITH, like agropod, is not used.

Notice how the following terms have different meanings simply because we have switched the order of the bases within the words.

BLASTOCYTE   an undifferentiated embryonic cell

CYTOBLAST   an obsolete word meaning the cell nucleus

PHAGOCYTE   a cell that destroys microorganisms or harmful cells

CYTOPHAGY   the destruction of cells by other cells

COMPETING FORMS

One characteristic of medical language is duplication. The use of both Greek and Latin as sources for word bases and the ease of word formation have resulted in a significant number of duplicate forms. We call these duplicates COMPETING FORMS. There are three types of competing forms: (a) those that have the same base but different combining vowels, (b) two forms of the same base, and (c) two bases—one Greek, one Latin—with the same meaning.

Duplicates from the same Greek or Latin base present no problem because they are easily recognizable. The examples below illustrate the first type of duplicate: forms that differ only in their combining vowel.

BRONCH/I/AL	BRONCH/O/PNEUMON/IA
OV/I/DUCT	OV/O/PLASM
SPERM/I/CIDE	SPERM/O/LY/TIC
PELV/I/METR/Y	PELV/O/SCOP/Y

The second type of duplicate, as we said, is the result of drawing from two forms of the same base. For example, in the words HEMORRHAGE and HEMATOLOGY the bases HEM and HEMAT (blood) are simply different forms of the same base.* In the list below, each set of words contains competing bases of the second type. Using a dictionary, provide meanings for each term.

HEM/O/RRHAG/E .... HEMAT/O/LOG/Y ....

IR/O/TOM/Y .... IRID/O/MALAC/IA ....

MEGA/COCC/US .... MEGAL/O/CEPHAL/Y ....

GANGLI/EC/TOM/Y .... GANGLION/EC/TOM/Y ....

SPERM/I/CID/E .... SPERMAT/O/CID/AL ....

STEAR/RHE/A .... STEAT/O/LY/SIS ....

Because medical language draws on both Greek and Latin for its vocabulary, a number of medical terms have a Greek or Latin synonym. As a result, we have two words—one from Greek, the other from Latin—to denote the same object, process, condition, or function. Study the following examples.

*HEM is the root form, HEMAT the stem form.

Latin	Greek	Meaning
DENT/IST	ODONT/O/LOG/IST	tooth
LACRIM/AL	DACRY/O/CYST	tear
OR/AL	STOMAT/O/PATH/Y	mouth
VAGIN/ITIS	COLP/ITIS	vagina

Using a dictionary, give the meanings for these terms.

DENTIST ....   ODONTOLOGIST ....

LACRIMAL ....   DACRYOCYST ....

ORAL ....   STOMATOPATHY ....

VAGINITIS ....   COLPITIS ....

REVIEW OF BASIC CONCEPTS

1. Define the following terms and provide an example for each.
   (a) Base
   (b) Combining vowel
   (c) Combining form
   (d) Prefix
   (e) Suffix

2. In medical language we have two words that mean *pertaining to the tongue:* LINGUAL and GLOSSAL. Why do both terms occur? What is the significance of this occurrence?

3. In what ways does the suffix affect the manner in which you translate medical terms?

EXERCISES

I. Below are some medical terms that you should already know. After looking them up in the dictionary, underline the base forms and then give the meanings for the bases and the terms themselves. *Example:*

DYSPEPSIA digestion ....   indigestion ....

1. HYPOCHONDRIAC ....

2. SEBACEOUS ....

3. BENIGN ....

4. THERAPEUTIC ....

5. ANTIDOTE ....

  6. HYDROPHOBIA ....

  7. BIOPSY ....

  8. PODIATRIST ....

  9. CORPUSCLE ....

10. EPIDEMIC ....

11. PEDIATRICS ....

12. ANEMIA ....

13. DYSTROPHY ....

14. ASTRINGENT ....

15. MICROBE ....

16. OSTEOPATH ....

17. HEMOPHILIA ....

18. ENDOCRINE ....

19. GERMICIDE ....

20. ORTHODONTIST ....

21. DERMATOLOGIST ....

22. TOXIC ....

23. MYOPIA ....

24. HOMOGENOUS ....

25. NEUROLOGY ....

    II. In the following list mark off by slashes the word components; then give the meaning of the word. Use a dictionary for any unfamiliar terms. *Example:*

HYDROPHOBIA   hydr/o/phob/ia   abnormal fear of water
....

1. OSTEOPATH ....

2. TONSILLECTOMY ....

3. DENTIFRICE ....

4. MEGALOMANIA...

5. ERYTHROCYTOPENIA ....

6. ATROPHY ....

7. INJECTION ....

8. HEMATOLOGIST ....

9. ARTHROSCLEROSIS ....

10. LARYNGITIS ....

11. ENDOCRINOLOGY ....

12. CARDIOMEGALY ....

13. STETHOSCOPE ....

14. CALCIFICATION ....

15. ANEMIC ....

16. THERMAL ....

17. ENCEPHALITIS ....

18. EUPHORIA ....

19. ACROPHOBIA ....

20. GERIATRICS ....

21. DYSENTERY ....

22. GASTROSCOPY ....

23. OPHTHALMOLOGY ....

24. ANESTHESIA ....

25. ALBUMINURIA ....

III. Combine the following elements to make medical terms. *Example:*

HYSTER EC TOM Y ....hysterectomy...........surgical removal of the uterus

1. ARTHR TOM E ....

2. GLYC PHIL IA ....

3. PERI CARDI ITIS ....

4. OSTE MALAC IA ....

5. HYDR CEPHAL IC ....

6. MILL METER ....

7. CLAUSTR PHOB IA ....

8. SPLEN MEGAL Y ....

9. ANDR GEN ....

10. SUB LINGU AL ....

11. GLAUC OMA ....

12. HEMAT CRIT ....

13. ELECTR CARDI GRAPH ....

14. MAST EC TOM Y ....

15. ESOPHAG GASTR SCOP Y ....

ANSWERS TO TEXT EXERCISES

Page 4

1. ge: earth, graph: write, y: process: the process of describing the earth's surface
2. metr: mother, polis: city: the main city of a region
3. orth: straight/correct, dox: opinion/view: holding the correct viewpoint
4. mon: one, ton: sound, ous: pertaining to: pertaining to that which lacks variety of sound, tone, pitch, etc.
5. anth: flower/pick of the crop, log: study, y: process of: the process of studying the best of something
6. lob: lobe of the brain, tom: cut, y: process: the process of making an incision into the lobes of the brain
7. opt: sight, metr: measure, ist: one who: one who measures sight
8. ur: urine, log: study, y: process: examining and testing of urine
9. hydr: water, therap: treat/heal, y: process: the process of using water as a treatment
10. aur: ear, scop: examine, e: instrument: instrument to examine the ear
11. cent: hundred, grade: step/degree: divided into a hundred degrees
12. corn: horny/hard-surfaced, fac: make, tion: action: the action of making hard-surfaced
13. mil: thousand, meter: measure: to measure by the thousandth
14. pelv: pelvis, meter: instrument to measure: instrument to measure the pelvis
15. ventr: belly, duct: lead: that which leads to the belly

Page 5

1.   2   3   1
anti/fung/al,   pertaining to that which acts against fungus
2.   2   3   1
pro/phylact/ic,   pertaining to that which protects against disease
3.   2   3   1
hyper/troph/ic,   pertaining to the abnormal growth of tissue
4.   2   3   1
intra/ven/ous,   within a vein
5.   2 3 1
ec/top/ia,   abnormal placement
6.   2   3   1
peri/odont/ist,   one who specializes in the treatment of the tissue surrounding a tooth
7.   2   3   2 1
esophag/o/jejun/o/stom/y,   the process of making an opening between the esophagus and the jejunum

Page 8

1. hemorrhage: flow of blood (from a ruptured blood vessel)
hematology: science dealing with blood and blood diseases
2. irotomy: incision of the iris of the eye
iridomalacia: softening of the iris of the eye
3. megacoccus: large, spherical bacteria
megalocephaly: abnormal increase in the size of the head

4. **gangliectomy** and **ganglionectomy**: excision of a ganglion (a mass of nerves)
5. **spermicide**: a substance that destroys sperm
   spermatocidal: pertaining to a substance that destroys sperm
6. **stearrhea**: discharge of fat, oily secretion
   steatolysis: breakdown of fat

Page 9

1. dentist: one who specializes in the treatment of teeth
   odontologist: one who specializes in the treatment of teeth
2. lacrimal: pertaining to tears
   dacryocyst: tear sac
3. oral: pertaining to the mouth
   stomatopathy: diseased condition of the mouth
4. vaginitis and colpitis: inflammation of the vagina

ANSWERS TO EXERCISES

I.

1. hypochondriac, cartilage, refers to someone who is abnormally concerned about his health, so named because the hypochondrium was thought to be the source of this affliction
2. sebaceous, oily secretion, pertaining to the oily secretion of the sebaceous glands
3. benign, favorable, as opposed to malignant
4. therapeutic, treatment, pertaining to healing
5. antidote, give, that which is given to counteract a poison
6. hydrophobia, water, fear, abnormal fear of water: rabies
7. bi/opsy, life, look, diagnostic examination of living tissue
8. pod/iatrist, foot, healing, pertaining to the treatment of foot disorders
9. corpuscle, body, any small body—for example, a red blood cell
10. epidemic, people, rapid spread of a disease
11. ped/iatrics, child, healing, pertaining to the treatment of children and children's diseases
12. anemia, blood, blood deficiency
13. dystrophy, nourish, faulty nutrition
14. astringent, contract, that which causes a contraction
15. microbe, small, life, minute living organism
16. osteopath, bone, disease, one who treats diseases and ailments by manipulation of the bones
17. hemophilia, blood, affinity, abnormal affinity for blood
18. endocrine, secrete, pertaining to internal secretion
19. germicide, germ, killing, an agent that destroys harmful microorganisms
20. orthodontist, straight, tooth, one who specializes in correcting irregularities of the teeth
21. dermatologist, skin, study, one who specializes in the study of the skin and the treatment of its diseases
22. toxic, poison, poisonous
23. my/opia, shut, eye, nearsightedness

24. <u>homogen</u>ous, same, kind, uniform
25. <u>neurolog</u>y, sinew, study, the study of the nervous system and the treatment of its disorders

II.

1. oste/o/path,   one who treats diseases and ailments by manipulating the bones
2. tonsill/ec/tom/y,   excision of the tonsils
3. dent/i/fric/e,   a substance used to clean teeth
4. megal/o/man/ia,   mental disorder characterized by delusions of greatness
5. erythr/o/cyt/o/pen/ia,   deficiency of red blood cells
6. a/troph/y,   a wasting away due to a lack of nourishment
7. in/jec/tion,   process of introducing fluids into the body by means of a hypodermic syringe
8. hemat/o/log/ist,   one who studies the blood and its disorders
9. arthr/o/scler/o/sis,   abnormal stiffening or hardening of the joints
10. laryng/itis,   inflammation of the larynx
11. endo/crin/o/log/y,   study of the internal secretion glands
12. cardi/o/megal/y,   enlargement of the heart
13. steth/o/scop/e,   instrument used to listen to the heart, lungs, and other internal organs
14. calc/i/fic/a/tion,   deposit of calcium salts in the tissue
15. an/em/ic,   pertaining to a blood deficiency
16. therm/al,   pertaining to heat
17. en/cephal/itis,   inflammation of the brain
18. eu/phor/ia,   a feeling of well-being (abnormal)
19. acr/o/phob/ia,   abnormal fear of heights
20. ger/iact/rics,   pertaining to the treatment of diseases and ailments associated with old age
21. dys/enter/y,   lower intestinal disorder
22. gastr/o/scop/y,   examination of the stomach
23. ophthalm/o/log/y,   study of the eye and treatment of its diseases
24. an/esthes/ia,   abnormal lack of feeling
25. albumin/ur/ia,   abnormal presence of albumin in the urine

III.

1. arthrotome, instrument for cutting a joint
2. glycophilia, abnormal affinity for sugar
3. pericarditis, inflammation of the sac that encloses the heart
4. osteomalacia, softening of the bones
5. hydrocephalic, pertaining to an accumulation of fluid in the cranium
6. millimeter, measuring in thousandths
7. claustrophobia, abnormal fear of being in an enclosed place
8. splenomegaly, enlargement of the spleen
9. androgen, male sex hormone
10. sublingual, under the tongue
11. glaucoma, disease of the eye characterized by internal swelling
12. hematocrit, determination of blood: the determination of erythrocytes present in whole blood by means of a centrifuge
13. electrocardiograph, instrument for recording the electrical impulses of the heart
14. mastectomy, excision of a breast
15. esophagogastroscopy, examination of the esophagus and stomach

2 Suffixes

A suffix is added to the end of a word base to change the meaning of the base or to make the base a noun, verb, adjective, and so forth. In either case, a new word is formed.

Base	Suffix	New word
DENT (tooth)	AL (pertaining to)	DENTAL (pertaining to the teeth)
GASTR (stomach)	IC (pertaining to)	GASTRIC (pertaining to the stomach)
PHARMAC (drug)	IST (one who specializes in)	PHARMACIST (one who specializes in drugs)
CARDI (heart)	LOGY (study of)	CARDIOLOGY (the study of the heart and its disorders)

In medical language there are two types of suffixes: simple and compound. Simple suffixes are those suffixes that have nothing added to them (e.g., -ic as in HEPATIC, pertaining to the liver). Compound suffixes, however, are usually formed by joining a base and a simple suffix. For instance, we can join the base LOG and the suffix Y to make the compound suffix LOGY, which means THE ACT or PROCESS OF STUDYING (or just THE STUDY OF). Thus HISTOLOGY (HIST/O/LOG/Y) is the study of the various tissues that make up living organisms. Another compound suffix TOMY means THE PROCESS OF CUTTING INTO something, or INCISION. A NEPHROTOMY (NEPHR/O/TOM/Y) is an incision of the kidney. The compound suffix ECTOMY is the combination of a prefix (EC), a base (TOM), and a suffix (Y). It means the PROCESS OF CUTTING OUT, or EXCISION. A TONSILLECTOMY (TONSILL/EC/TOM/Y) is the cutting out of the tonsils. Here is a list of simple suffixes.

Suffix	*Meaning*	*Example*
-ia	condition	ANEMIA (AN/EM/IA), a condition characterized by a blood deficiency
-y	condition, act, process	SPLENOMEGALY (SPLEN/O/MEGAL/Y), enlargement of the spleen HEPATOTOMY (HEPAT/O/TOM/Y), the process of cutting into the liver
-e	an instrument	OPHTHALMOSCOPE (OPHTHALM/O/SCOP/E), an instrument for examining the interior of the eye

(The suffix -e can also function as just a noun marker; an ERYTHROCYTE is a red blood cell.)

Suffix	*Meaning*	*Example*
-itis	inflammation	HEPATITIS (HEPAT/ITIS), inflammation of the liver
-ist	one who specializes in	DERMATOLOGIST (DERMAT/O/LOG/IST), one who specializes in the treatment of the skin and its diseases
-or (er)	refers to a doer, either a person or thing	INCISOR (IN/CIS/OR), a tooth that cuts into
-osis	condition, usually abnormal or pathological	SCLEROSIS (SCLER/OSIS), abnormal hardening
-oma	swelling, tumor	SARCOMA (SARC/OMA), fleshy tumor
-ism	a condition, usually the result of a prior condition	EMBOLISM (EM/BOL/ISM), the movement of a mass or object within the vascular system to a site where it obstructs the flow of blood
-(i)um	refers to a part in relation to a whole, related to	PERICARDIUM (PERI/CARDI/UM), belonging to the area around the heart, the sac that encloses the heart EPIGASTRIUM (EPI/GASTR/IUM), that portion of the abdomen over the stomach

The preceding suffixes are called noun-forming suffixes because they make nouns when they combine with word bases.

Here is a list of simple suffixes that combine with word bases to form adjectives.

Suffix	*Meaning*	*Example*
-ac	pertaining to	CARDIAC (CARDI/AC), pertaining to the heart
-al	pertaining to	BRONCHIAL (BRONCH/I/AL), pertaining to the bronchus
-ar	pertaining to	TONSILLAR (TONSILL/AR), pertaining to the tonsils

Suffix	*Meaning*	*Example*
-ic	pertaining to	HEPATIC (HEPAT/IC), pertaining to the liver
-eal	pertaining to	ESOPHAGEAL (ESOPHAG/EAL), pertaining to the esophagus
-ary	pertaining to	CILIARY (CILI/ARY), pertaining to the cilia, the eyelashes

(-ary can also function as a noun-forming suffix: OVARY (OV/ARY), the female reproductive gland where ova are formed; CAPILLARY (CAPILL/ARY), minute or hairlike blood vessel.)

Suffix	*Meaning*	*Example*
-ous	pertaining to	MUCOUS (MUC/OUS), pertaining to mucous, also containing mucus
	containing	FIBROUS (FIBR/OUS), containing or composed of fiber
	secreting	SEBACEOUS (SEB/ACE/OUS), containing or secreting sebum
-oid	resembling, -like	CYSTOID (CYST/OID), resembling a sac, saclike

There are many compound suffixes—that is, suffixes made from a word base and a simple suffix. They, along with their meanings, will become obvious as you work through the text. For now here is a list of the most common compound suffixes.

Suffix	*Meaning*	*Example*
-algia	pain	ARTHRALGIA (ARTHR/ALGIA), pain in a joint
-ectasia or ectasis	stretching, dilatation	NEPHRECTASIA (NEPHR/ECTASIA), dilatation of the renal pelvis
-emia	blood condition	LEUKEMIA (LEUK/EMIA), condition of the blood in which the white blood cells reproduce uncontrollably
-malacia	softening	OSTEOMALACIA (OSTE/O/MALACIA), softening of the bones
-meter	instrument for measuring	THERMOMETER (THERM/O/METER), instrument for measuring heat
-metry	measurement	PELVIMETRY (PELV/I/METRY), measurement of the pelvic structure
-odynia	pain	CARDIODYNIA (CARDI/ODYNIA), pain in the heart region
-penia	deficiency, lack	LEUKOCYTOPENIA (LEUK/O/CYT/O/PENIA), deficiency of white blood cells
-plegia	stroke, paralysis	THERMOPLEGIA (THERM/O/PLEGIA), heat or sunstroke
-(o)rrhea	flow, discharge	DIARRHEA (DIA/RRHEA), watery stools produced by the rapid flow of feces through the intestine

Suffix	*Meaning*	*Example*
	(Pronunciation and spelling of -rrhea are easier if you add the combining vowel to the suffix when it appears alone.)	
-(o)rrhagia	excessive flow	GASTRORRHAGIA (GASTR/O/RRHAGIA), hemorrhage from the stomach
-uria	urine condition	HEMATURIA (HEMAT/URIA), presence of blood in the urine
-iatry or -iatrics	healing, frequently refers to a branch of medicine	PODIATRY (POD/IATRY), that branch of medicine that treats foot ailments
-graphy -graph -gram	process of recording that which records the record itself	ELECTROCARDIOGRAPHY (ELECTR/O/CARDI/O/GRAPHY), process of recording the electrical impulses of the heart
-logy	act or process of studying	PHARMACOLOGY PHARMAC/O/LOGY), the study of drugs and their application
-logist	one who studies and treats	UROLOGIST (UR/O/LOGIST), one who specializes in that branch of medicine dealing with the urinary system and its diseases
-lysis	dissolution decomposition destruction	HEMOLYSIS (HEM/O/LYSIS), destruction of blood cells, causing the release of hemoglobin
-pathy	disease, diseased condition	OPHTHALMOPATHY (OPHTHALM/O/PATHY), any disorder of the eye
-pexy	a fixing or setting firmly in place by suturing	HEPATOPEXY (HEPAT/O/PEXY), the attaching of a displaced liver to the abdominal wall
-plasty	surgical reshaping or repair	OSTEOPLASTY (OSTE/O/PLASTY), surgical reshaping of the bones
-(o)rrhaphy	suturing, process of suturing	HERNIORRHAPHY (HERNI/O/RRHAPHY), the surgical repair of a hernia by suturing the abdominal wall
-scopy	examination, process of examining visually	CYSTOSCOPY (CYST/O/SCOPY), visual examination of the bladder by means of a cystoscope
-tomy	incision, process of cutting into	CRANIOTOMY (CRANI/O/TOMY), incision of the skull
-ectomy	excision, process of cutting out	APPENDECTOMY (APPEND/ECTOMY), excision of the appendix
-(o)stomy	process of making an opening into or a connection between	GASTROSTOMY (GASTR/O/STOMY), making an opening into the stomach
		ANASTOMOSIS is another way of indicating a connection between two structures.

Suffix	Meaning	Example
-cyte	noun marker referring to a cell	LEUKOCYTE (LEUK/O/CYTE), white blood cell
-blast	a cell that is undifferentiated, primitive, embryonic	HEMOCYTOBLAST (HEM/O/CYT/O/BLAST), an immature blood cell
-cele	hernia, herniation	THYROCELE (THYR/O/CELE), herniation of the thyroid, goiter
-scope	instrument for viewing	OPHTHALMOSCOPE (OPHTHALM/O/SCOPE), instrument for examining the interior of the eye
-tome	instrument for cutting	ARTHROTOME (ARTHR/O/TOME), instrument for cutting a joint
-centesis	surgical puncture to withdraw fluid	AMNIOCENTESIS (AMNI/O/CENTESIS), puncture of the amniotic sac to obtain amniotic fluid
-clysis	washing, introduction of fluid for the purpose of irrigation	BRONCHOCLYSIS (BRONCH/O/CLYSIS), introduction of a fluid into the bronchus to irrigate it
-ptosis	a falling, the dropping or sagging of an organ	NEPHROPTOSIS (NEPHR/O/PTOSIS), a downward dropping or displacement of a kidney
-(o)rrhexis	rupture	HEPATORRHEXIS (HEPAT/O/RRHEXIS), rupture of the liver
-sclerosis	a hardening	ARTERIOSCLEROSIS (ARTERI/O/SCLEROSIS), hardening of the arteries (their thickening and loss of elasticity)
-stasis	arresting, halting, maintaining a constant level	BACTERIOSTASIS (BACTERI/O/STASIS), halting the growth of bacteria
-stenosis	a narrowing, a stricture	ARTERIOSTENOSIS (ARTERI/O/STENOSIS), constriction of an artery

EXERCISES

I. Add suffixes to the following bases* according to the phrases in parentheses. *Example:*

DENT (pertaining to) .... dental ....

1. DERMAT (abnormal condition) ....

2. CONGENIT (pertaining to) ....

*You may use the index for any unfamiliar bases.

3. DYSTROPH (condition of) ....

4. ADEN (resembling) ....

5. ENCEPHAL (tumor of) ....

6. PHOB (condition) ....

7. GASTR (inflammation of) ....

8. ILI (pertaining to) ....

9. THERAPEUT (pertaining to) ....

10. ASPIRAT (that which) ....

11. GERMICID (that which) ....

12. SEP (condition of) ....

13. LARYNG (pertaining to) ....

14. DENT (one who specializes in) ....

15. OCUL (pertaining to) ....

    II. Divide the following medical words into their parts and give their meanings. *Example:*

ARTHRITIS   arthr/itis   inflammation of the joints
....

1. HEMATOLOGIST ....

2. MENORRHAGIA (MENSES—menstruation) ....

....

3. HEPATOSCOPY ....

4. ERYTHROCYTE (ERYTHR/O—red)

....

5. AMNIORRHEXIS (AMNI/O—amniotic sac)

....

6. LARYNGOCENTESIS ....

7. BRONCHOSTENOSIS ....

8. SPLENALGIA ....

9. PSYCHIATRY ....

10. DERMATOPLASTY ....

11. DERMOLYSIS ....

12. GASTRECTASIA ....

13. NEPHROGRAM ....

14. CARDIOPATHY ....

15. HEMOSTASIS ....

16. SPLENORRHAPHY ....

17. CARDIOPTOSIS ....

18. GLYCEMIA ....

19. LARYNGOPLEGIA ....

20. HYSTEROPEXY ....

21. GASTRECTOMY ....

22. GASTROSTOMY ....

23. GASTROTOMY ....

24. ENCEPHALOCELE ....

25. NEUROMALACIA ....

26. BRONCHOCLYSIS ....

27. GLOSSODYNIA ....

28. DERMATOSCLEROSIS ....

29. THROMBOCYTOPENIA ....

30. ALBUMINURIA ....

    III. Put the following phrases into medical language. *Example:*

excision of the tonsils .... tonsillectomy ....

1. pain in the stomach ....

2. inflammation of the kidney ....

3. pertaining to a muscle ....

4. containing membrane ....

5. an instrument for cutting the cranium ....

6. suturing of the stomach ....

7. the record made by recording the electrical impulses of the brain ....

    ....

8. abnormal or diseased condition of a joint ....

9. surgical creation of an opening into the bronchus ....

10. resembling fiber ....

11. (visual) examination of the larynx ....

12. a heart specialist ....

13. watery discharge (HYDR/O—water) ....

14. enlargement of the liver ....

15. destruction of nerve tissues ....

ANSWERS TO EXERCISES

I.

1. DERMAT<u>OSIS</u>;   2. CONGENIT<u>AL</u>;   3. DYSTROPH<u>Y</u>;   4. ADEN<u>OID</u>;
5. ENCEPHAL<u>OMA</u>;   6. PHOB<u>IA</u>;   7. GASTR<u>ITIS</u>;   8. ILI<u>AC</u>;
9. THERAPEUT<u>IC</u>;   10. ASPIRAT<u>OR</u>;   11. GERMICID<u>E</u>;   12. SEP<u>SIS</u>;
13. LARYNG<u>EAL</u>;   14. DENT<u>IST</u>;   15. OCUL<u>AR</u>.

II.

1. HEMAT/O/LOGIST,   one who specializes in the study of the blood and its diseases
2. MEN/O/RRHAGIA,   excessive menstrual flow
3. HEPAT/O/SCOPY,   examination of the liver
4. ERYTHR/O/CYTE,   red blood cell
5. AMNI/O/RRHEXIS,   rupture of the amniotic sac
6. LARYNG/O/CENTESIS,   surgical puncture of the larynx to drain it
7. BRONCH/O/STENOSIS,   stricture of the bronchial tube
8. SPLEN/ALGIA,   pain in the spleen
9. PSYCH/IATRY,   the branch of medicine that treats disorders of the mind
10. DERMAT/O/PLASTY,   surgical repair of the skin
11. DERM/O/LYSIS,   destruction of the skin
12. GASTR/ECTASIA,   stretching of the stomach
13. NEPHR/O/GRAM,   an x ray of the kidney
14. CARDI/O/PATHY,   diseased condition of the heart
15. HEM/O/STASIS,   halting the escape of blood
16. SPLEN/O/RRHAPHY,   suture of the spleen
17. CARDI/O/PTOSIS,   downward sagging or displacement of the heart
18. GLYC/EMIA,   sugar in the blood
19. LARYNG/O/PLEGIA,   paralysis of the larynx
20. HYSTER/O/PEXY,   a surgical setting in place of the uterus
21. GASTR/ECTOMY,   excision of all or part of the stomach
22. GASTR/O/STOMY,   creation of an opening into the stomach
23. GASTR/O/TOMY,   incision of the stomach
24. ENCEPHAL/O/CELE,   herniation of brain tissue
25. NEUR/O/MALACIA,   softening of the nerves
26. BRONCH/O/CLYSIS,   irrigation of the bronchus
27. GLOSS/ODYNIA,   pain in the tongue
28. DERMAT/O/SCLEROSIS,   hardening of the skin
29. THROMB/O/CYT/O/PENIA,   deficiency of clotting cells in the blood
30. ALBUMIN/URIA,   presence of albumin in the urine

III.

1. GASTRALGIA;   2. NEPHRITIS;   3. MUSCULAR;   4. MEMBRANOUS;
5. CRANIOTOME;   6. GASTRORRHAPHY;   7. ELECTROENCEPHALOGRAM;
8. ARTHROSIS;   9. BRONCHOSTOMY;   10. FIBROID;
11. LARYNGOSCOPY;   12. CARDIOLOGIST;   13. HYDRORRHEA;
14. HEPATOMEGALY;   15. NEUROLYSIS.

3 Prefixes

A prefix is added before a word base and, like a suffix, changes the meaning of that base.

Base	Base + suffix	Prefix + base + suffix
DERM	DERMIC (pertaining to the skin)	HYPODERMIC (beneath the skin, an injection beneath the skin)
SEPT	SEPTIC (producing or resulting from decay)	ANTISEPTIC (checking or halting decay)
KINES	KINESIS (motion)	DYSKINESIA (difficulty of movement)
ODONT	ODONTITIS (inflammation of a tooth)	PERIODONTITIS (inflammation of the tissue around a tooth)

Here is a table of the most commonly occurring prefixes.

Prefix	Meaning	Example
a-, an-	without	AMORPHOUS (having no definite form, shapeless)
ab-	from, away from	ABARTICULAR (away from a joint)
ad-	to, toward, near	ADRENAL (REN-kidney, near the kidney)
ana-	up, back again	ANABOLISM (the metaBOLic phase in which the cells synthesize)
ante-	before	ANTEFLEXION (FLEX-bending, bending an organ so that its top is brought forward)
anti-	against	ANTIDOTE (DOT-give, an agent that is given to counteract a poison)
auto-	self	AUTOTROPHIC (self-nourishing)

Prefix	Meaning	Example
bi(n, s)-	two, double	BICEPS (CEP or CAP-head, a muscle having two heads)
circum-	around	CIRCUMDUCTION (the circular movement of a limb)
co(n)-	with, together	COCARCINOGENESIS (CARCIN-cancer, development of cancer in cells that are favorable to its growth)
contra-	against	CONTRACEPTIVE (against or preventing conception)
de-	from	DEOXIDATION (removal of oxygen from a substance)
di-	twice, double	DIARTHRIC (pertaining to or affecting two joints)
dia-	through	DIATHERMY (THERM-heat, healing through the application of heat)
dis-	apart, free from, separate	DISLOCATION (LOC-place, separation of a bone from a joint)
dys-	bad, painful, difficult	DYSENTERY (ENTER—small intestine, painful condition of the small intestine, lower intestinal infection)
ecto-	outside, outer	ECTODERM (outer layer of cells in an embryo)
en-	in, within	ENCEPHALIC (CEPHAL-head, pertaining to the brain)
endo-	inside, inner	ENDOCRINE (KRIN-secrete, pertaining to those glands that secrete internally)
epi-	over, upon, on	EPIGASTRIUM (the upper abdominal region over the stomach)
eu-	good, well, normal	EUPHORIA (PHOR-carry, bear, feeling, a feeling of well-being)
ex-	out of, from	EXCISION (CIS- cut, removal by cutting)
extra-	outside of, beyond	EXTRACORPOREAL (CORP-body, pertaining to that which is outside the body)
hemi-	half	HEMIPARALYSIS (paralysis of only one side of the body)
hyper-	above, excessive	HYPERGLYCEMIA (GLYC-sugar, glucose, excess of sugar in the blood)
hypo-	under, less than normal	HYPOGLYCEMIA (a less than normal amount of sugar in the blood)

Prefix	Meaning	Example
in-	in, into	INGESTION (GEST-carry, the taking of food into the digestive tract)
in-	not	INCOAGULABILITY (the inability to coagulate)
infra-	below, lower	INFRACOSTAL (COST-rib, below a rib)
inter-	between	INTERVENTRICULAR (VENTRICUL-a hollow or cavity, situated between the ventricles of the heart)
intra-	within	INTRAVENOUS (VEN-vein, within a vein)
para-	beside, alongside, abnormal	PARANEPHRIC (situated alongside the kidney)
per-	through	PERORAL (done or administered through the mouth)
peri-	around	PERIHEPATITIS (inflammation of the tissues around the liver)
post-	after, behind	POSTNASAL (NAS-nose, behind the nose)
pre-	before, in front of	PREMOLAR (before the molar teeth)
pro-	before, in front of	PROGNOSIS (GNO-know, prediction of the outcome of a disease)
pros-	to, near, in addition to	PROSTHETICS (THET-put, place, the replacing of missing or defective body parts with artificial parts)
semi-	half	SEMISYNTHETIC (artificially produced in part)
sub-	under	SUBCUTANEOUS (CUT-skin, under the skin)
super-	above, over	SUPERLACTATION (oversecretion of milk)
supra-	above, over	SUPRACRANIAL (CRANI-skull, located above the cranium)
syn-	with, together	SYNAPSE (APS or T- join, junction between two neurons)
trans-	across, through, over	TRANSABDOMINAL (across the abdomen)

Because Greek and Latin prefixes with the same meaning are used to form medical words, it is not uncommon to find two words having the same meaning but different prefixes. For example, HYPODERMIC and SUBDERMIC both mean *under the skin*. BICEPHALOUS and DICEPHALOUS mean *having two heads*. The phrase, *the oversecretion of milk*, can be expressed in medical language either by HYPERLACTA-

TION or by SUPERLACTATION. Again, as we said in Chapter 1, two words can have the same meaning.

	Greek	*Latin*	
	HYPODERMIC	SUBCUTANEOUS	under the skin
	PERINEPHRIC	CIRCUMRENAL	located around the kidney

As you study the medical vocabulary, try to remember the combinations of prefixes and bases that are most frequently used. Avoid forming new words that may be understood by others but are not found in medical dictionaries. Look at the following medical words and notice how easily synonyms that are not used can be formed.

Medical word	*Unused synonym*
EXTRAVAGINAL	ECTOCOLPIC
PERIODONTAL	CIRCUMDENTAL

A base may have two prefixes added to it, both changing its meaning.

HEMIHYPERTROPHY   excessive growth of one side of the body

ANTIANTIBODY   a substance that acts against an antibody

CONTRAINDICATION   a condition that prevents the use of a particular drug

EXERCISES

I.   Divide each example on the list of prefixes (page 25) into its parts.
Example: AMORPHOUS

A/MORPH/OUS
....

1. ....
2. ....
3. ....
4. ....
5. ....
6. ....
7. ....
8. ....
9. ....
10. ....
11. ....
12. ....
13. ....
14. ....
15. ....
16. ....

17. ....   **18.** ....

19. ....   **20.** ....

21. ....   **22.** ....

23. ....   **24.** ....

25. ....   **26.** ....

27. ....   **28.** ....

29. ....   **30.** ....

31. ....   **32.** ....

33. ....   **34.** ....

35. ....   **36.** ....

37. ....   **38.** ....

39. ....   **40.** ....

41. ....   **42.** ....

43. ....

II. Choose the meaning that most closely translates the prefix.

1. anti-
   (a) before
   (b) against
   (c) after
   (d) again

2. a-
   (a) toward
   (b) up
   (c) apart from
   (d) without

3. circum-
   (a) with
   (b) against
   (c) around
   (d) none of the above

4. dys-
   (a) painful
   (b) separate
   (c) through
   (d) from

5. en-
   (a) outer
   (b) over
   (c) within
   (d) well

6. epi-
   (a) over
   (b) in
   (c) out of
   (d) none of the above

7. hemi-
    (a) above
    (b) excessive
    (c) beyond
    (d) half

8. hyper-
    (a) excessive
    (b) insufficient
    (c) outside
    (d) lack of

9. intra-
    (a) near
    (b) within
    (c) alongside
    (d) around

10. para-
    (a) within
    (b) around
    (c) outside of
    (d) beside

11. pros-
    (a) to, in addition to
    (b) before, in front of
    (c) beyond, abnormal
    (d) after, behind

12. sub-
    (a) alongside
    (b) near
    (c) under
    (d) behind

13. syn-
    (a) with
    (b) near
    (c) across
    (d) above

14. trans-
    (a) above
    (b) under
    (c) alongside
    (d) across

15. per-
    (a) across
    (b) behind
    (c) through
    (d) near

III.   Match those prefixes that have the same meaning.

contra-	hypo-	endo-	an-	super-
pre-	di-	sub-	bi-	circum-
pros-	anti-	ecto-	semi-	co(n)-
intra-	a-	en-	in-	extra-
hemi-	pro-	dia-	super-	supra-
syn-	ad-	peri-	per-	hyper-

1. . . . .

2. . . . .

3. . . . .

4. . . . .

5. . . . .

6. . . . .

7. . . . .

8. . . . .

9. . . . .   10. . . . .

11. . . . .   12. . . . .

13. . . . .   14. . . . .

15. . . . .

IV. Divide the following medical words into their parts and translate them into English phrases. *Example:*

HYPODERMIC   . . . . hypo/derm/ic . . . . under the skin . . . .

1. HEMICYSTECTOMY   . . . .

2. ADNASAL   . . . .

3. PREANESTHETIC   . . . .

4. INTRAERYTHROCYTIC   . . . .

5. AUTOKINETIC   . . . .

6. ENDOCOLPITIS   . . . .

7. ANESTHESIA   . . . .

8. PARA-APPENDICITIS   . . . .

9. SYNALGIA   . . . .

10. ANTIFUNGAL   . . . .

11. EXTRASPINAL   . . . .

12. DIGLOSSIA   . . . .

13. INFRACARDIAC   . . . .

14. PROPTOSIS   . . . .

15. ABORAL   . . . .

16. BINUCLEAR ....

17. HYPERACIDITY ....

18. SUPERALBUMINOSIS ....

19. PERIODONTAL ....

20. SEMIPTOSIS ....

21. ANTENATAL ....

22. DYSMENORRHEA ....

23. PERACIDITY* ....

24. HYPOKINESIA ....

25. INTERLABIAL ....

V. Make medical terms from the following phrases.

1. difficulty of movement ....

2. excess of blood ....

3. (situated) beside the liver ....

4. (situated) above a kidney ....

5. free from bacteria ....

6. to deprive of or take out calcium ....

7. process of cutting up ....

8. (situated) outside the liver ....

9. within the skin ....

10. inflammation of tissue around the bladder ....

*Sometimes prefixes like per-, in- don't change the meaning of bases to which they are attached but serve only to reinforce or intensify that original meaning.

11.   deviating from the normal   ....

12.   counteracting agents that destroy (red) blood (cells)   ....

      ....

13.   that which frees from infection   ....

14.   (situated) below the nose   ....

15.   under the mucous membrane   ....

16.   excision of half (or part) of the tongue   ....

17.   that which counteracts an acid   ....

18.   process of (treating) through heat   ....

19.   within the larynx   ....

20.   inflammation of the tissue on the bladder   ....

21.   examination of the underpart of the pharynx   ....

      ....

22.   having two feet   ....

23.   between the muscles   ....

24.   (occurring) after a hemorrhage   ....

25.   disease of the ectodermal tissues   ....

ANSWERS TO EXERCISES

I.

1. ab/articul/ar;   2. ad/ren/al;   3. ana/bol/ism;   4. ante/flex/ion;
5. anti/dot/e;   6. auto/troph/ic;   7. bi/ceps;   8. circum/duc/tion;
9. co/carcin/o/gen/e/sis;   10. contra/cept/ive;   11. de/oxid/a/tion;
12. di/arthr/ic;   13. dia/therm/y;   14. dis/loc/a/tion;   15. dys/enter/y;
16. ecto/derm;   17. en/cephal/ic;   18. endo/crin/e;   19. epi/gastr/ium;
20. eu/phor/ia;   21. ex/cis/ion;   22. extra/corpor/eal;   23. hemi/para/ly/sis;

24. hyper/glyc/emia;   25. hypo/glyc/emia;   26. in/ges/tion;
27. in/co/agul/ability;   28. infra/cost/al;   29. inter/ventricu/lar;
30. intra/ven/ous;   31. para/nephr/ic;   32. per/or/al;   33. peri/hepat/itis;
34. post/nas/al;   35. pre/mol/ar;   36. pro/gno/sis;   37. pros/thet/ics;
38. semi/syn/thet/ic;   39. sub/cut/ane/ous;   40. super/lact/a/tion;
41. supra/crani/al;   42. syn/aps/e;   43. trans/ab/domin/al.

II.

1. (b);   2. (d);   3. (c);   4. (a);   5. (c);   6. (a);   7. (d);   8. (a);
9. (b);   10. (d);   11. (a);   12. (c);   13. (a);   14. (d);   15. (c).

III.

a-, an-;   anti, contra-;   di, bi-;   hyper-, super- (supra-);
hypo-, sub-;   hemi, semi-;   peri-, circum-;   per-, dia-;
syn-, co(n)-;   en-, in-;   ecto, extra-;   intra-, endo-;
pre-, pro-;   super-, supra- (hyper-);   pros-, ad-.

IV.

1. hemi/cyst /ectomy,   excision of half or part of the bladder
2. ad/nas/al,   near the nose
3. pre/an/esthet/ic,   (administered or occurring) before anesthesia
4. intra/erythr/o/cyt/ic.   (occurring or situated) within red blood cells
5. auto/kinet/ic,   pertaining to a self or voluntary motion
6. endo/colp/itis,   inflammation (of the mucous membrane) within the vagina
7. an/esthes/ia,   the loss of feeling or sensation
8. para/appendic/itis,   inflammation of the appendix
9. syn/alg/ia,   with pain: pain produced in one area as the result of stimuli in another area
10. anti/fung/al,   halting or checking the growth of fungus
11. extra/spin/al,   outside the spine
12. di/gloss/ia,   a double tongue
13. infra/cardi/ac,   below the heart
14. pro/ptosis,   the sagging forward of an organ
15. ab/or/al,   (situated) away from the mouth
16. bi/nucle/ar,   having two nuclei
17. hyper/acid/ity,   excessive acidity
18. super/albumin/osis,   abnormal increase of albumin
19. peri/odont/al,   pertaining to the tissue around a tooth
20. semi/ptosis,   the downward sagging of half or part of an organ
21. ante/nat/al,   (occurring) before birth
22. dys/men/o/rrhea,   painful menstrual flow
23. per/acid/ity,   excessive acidity
24. hypo/kines/ia,   less than normal motion
25. inter/labi/al,   between the lips

V.

1. dyskinesia;   2. hyperemia;   3. parahepatic;   4. suprarenal;
5. abacterial;   6. decalcify;   7. anatomy;   8. extrahepatic;
9. intradermal;   10. pericystitis;   11. abnormal;   12. antihemolytic;
13. disinfectant;   14. infranasal;   15. submucous;   16. hemiglossectomy;
17. antiacid;   18. diathermy;   19. endolaryngeal;   20. epicystitis;
21. hypopharyngoscopy;   22. biped;   23. intermuscular;
24. posthemorrhagic;   25. ectodermosis.

4 Pronunciation, Spelling, and Formation of Plurals

PRONUNCIATION

Beginning with this chapter, new bases and their examples will be followed by a pronunciation guide. Whenever you learn a new base, practice the pronunciation guide. Ask your teacher to pronounce each new entry. Discuss any words that you find difficult to pronounce.

Medical words are pronounced like English words. Avoid using any Latinized pronunciation. The following consonants frequently cause confusion in pronunciation.

C before a, o, u sounds is pronounced like the C in Car.
Example: CARDIAC (kar′de-ak*)

C before e or i sounds is pronounced like the s in See.
Example: CYSTIC (sis′tik)

G before a, o, u sounds is pronounced like the g in Gun.
Example: GONAD (go′nad)

G before e or i sounds is pronounced like the g in Gene.
Example: GINGIVITIS (jin-ji-vy′tis)

CH is pronounced like the ch in CHord.
Example: CHROMATOLYSIS (kro″ma-tol′i-sis*)

Initial PS has an S sound: elsewhere it sounds like the ps in hiPS.
Examples: PSYCHIATRY (sy-ky′a-tre), PSYCHANOPSIA (si-kan-op′se-a)

Initial X has a Z sound; elsewhere it sounds like the x in waX.
Examples: XANTHEMIA (zan-the′me-a), AXILLA (aks-il′a)

*The stress mark ′ indicates primary or main stress, the mark ″ secondary or weak stress.

Accent is the placing of stress on a syllable. There are two accents: primary and secondary. The primary accent is given to the syllable that has the strongest stress (marked ′). The secondary accent is placed on syllables that are stressed but not as strongly as the syllable with the primary accent (secondary accent is marked by two lines ″). A word can have several secondary accents but only one primary accent. Syllables without accent marks receive no stress: CHROMATOLYSIS (kro″ma-tol′i-sis), the a and both i's are unstressed.

Two factors determine where the main stress of a word will occur.

1. Generally medical words follow the Latin system of accent, which is as follows.
   (a) The stress is never on the last syllable.
   (b) The main stress is on the second-to-the-last syllable if it is long.
   (c) The main stress is on the third-to-the-last syllable if the second-to-the-last syllable is short.

   Examples: HEMOPOIESIS (he″mo-poy-e′sis), e is long.
   NEPHRITIS (nef-ry′tis), i is long.
   PLACENTOID (pla-sen′toid), e is long because it is followed by two consonants.

2. The second-to-last syllable is sometimes shortened so that the main stress is moved up or the accent of the base persists:

   Examples: AB′DOMEN for ABDO′MEN
   GIN′GIVA for GINGI′VA
   DUO′DENAL for DUODE′NAL (both are used)
   SAPH′ENOUS for SAPHE′NOUS (both are used)
   LITH′OTRIPSY ⎱
   OS′TEOCLAST ⎰ accent of the base persists

Each word below contains sounds that may be difficult to pronounce correctly. Cover the pronunciation guide and pronounce each word aloud. MARK the primary stress of each word.

1. P<u>SY</u>CHOLOGY — sy-kol′o-je
2. O<u>X</u>YGEN — ok′si-jen
3. STIMUL<u>I</u> — stim′you-lie
4. R<u>OE</u>NTGEN — rent′jen, unit of measurement of the exposure dose of x or γ radiation
5. <u>CH</u>YME — kym′, a mixture of partly digested food and digestive secretions
6. SUBLIN<u>GU</u>AL — sub-ling′-wal
7. NEUROS<u>ES</u> — new-roe′sez, disorders of the thought process unrelated to any structural disease
8. SE<u>PS</u>IS — sep′sis, putrefaction, toxins produced by decaying
9. <u>CH</u>EMOTHERAPY — kee″mo-ther′a-pe

10. AN<u>EU</u>RYSM   an'you-rizm, abnormal extension of a blood vessel
11. A<u>PH</u>THA   af'tha, small ulcer on the mucous membrane of the mouth
12. DEMEN<u>TI</u>A   dee-men'she-a, insanity
13. GL<u>AU</u>COMA   glaw-ko'ma, diseased condition of the eye as a result of pressure within the eye
14. <u>CE</u>CUM   se'kum, a blind pouch that forms the first portion of the large intestine
15. <u>G</u>ASTRIC   gas'tric
16. DYSTRO<u>PHY</u>   dis'tro-fe
17. <u>JE</u>JUNUM   je-jou'num, second portion of the small intestine
18. <u>G</u>ENUS   jee'nus, biological classification: family, genus, species
19. <u>X</u>ERODERMA   zer-o-der'ma, dryness of the skin
20. <u>P</u>NEUMONIA   new-moan'ya, disease of the lungs
21. PHARMAC<u>EU</u>TICAL   far-ma-sou'ti-kal
22. CON<u>J</u>UNCTIVA   kon-junk-tie'va, mucous membrane that lines the eyelids
23. <u>CH</u>EILOPLASTY   ky'lo-plast-te, surgical restructuring of the lips
24. VA<u>CC</u>INE   vak-seen', a suspension of infectious microorganisms given to establish resistance to an infectious disease
25. SUB<u>C</u>UTANEOUS   sub-ku-tay'ne-us

Remember that when you form a word from prefixes, suffixes, and bases, the stress and word division (syllabification) may differ from the stress and word division of the simple forms. Avoid pronouncing medical words according to their elements.

BRONCH/O+PATHY become BRONCHOPATHY, pronounced bron-kop'a-the, NOT bron'ko-pa-the.

ANDR/O (male)+GEN+OUS become ANDROGENOUS, pronounced an-droj'e-nus, NOT an'dro-jen-us.

CHIR/O (hand)+POD (foot)+IST become CHIROPODIST, pronounced ky-rop'o-dist*, NOT ky'ro-pod'ist.

CYST+ITIS become CYSTITIS, pronounced sis-tie'tis, NOT sist'eye-tis.

PROCT (anus and rectum)+ALG+IA become PROCTALGIA, pronounced prok-tal'je-a, NOT prokt'al-je-a.

HEMAT/O+LY+SIS become HEMATOLYSIS, pronounced hem-a-tol'i-sis, NOT he-ma'to-li-sis.

MICR/O+TOMY become MICROTOMY, pronounced my-krot'o-me, NOT my'kro-toe-me.

*Frequently pronounced she-rop'o-dist.

SPELLING

Misspelled words, like mispronounced words, are embarrassing and erode the confidence that members of your profession have in you. Some mispellings can cause confusion: Do you mean *aboral* or *adoral?* Most of the time, however, misspellings are annoying and a sign of a careless and unprofessional attitude. Correct spelling begins with the close observation of how a word is formed. Whenever you learn a new medical word, do the following steps.

1. Learn the meaning of the word and how it is formed.

    PERIOSTEOEDEMA (per-e-os-te-o-e-dee′ma), a swelling of the membrane surrounding a bone PERI/OSTE/O/EDEMA

2. Isolate any new forms and practice their spelling.

    EDEMA, a swelling

3. Go back to the entire word and look for any parts whose spelling you are uncertain of. For example, you may tend to spell the base OSTE/O with an i, OSTI/O, or omit the h from words like op<u>h</u>thalmology and dip<u>h</u>theria.

4. As you go through the new list of medical words, add those whose spelling you find difficult to master to your list of frequently misspelled words. Review this list frequently and try to eliminate from it as many words as possible.

Sound changes, when two or more elements combine, are frequently a source of spelling problems. Study the following changes in the formation of new words; they will help you to avoid some common misspellings.

Combining Form and Name of Object

Sometimes the combining form and the name that represents that object differ in spelling.

Name	*Combining form*
PHARYNX (far′inks)	PHARYNG/EAL (far-in′jee-al)
THORAX (thō′raks)	THORAC/OPATHY (tho-ra-kop′a-the)
CARTILAGE (kar′ti-lij)	CARTILAGEN/OUS (kar-ti-laj′i-nus)
FEMUR (fee′mur)	FEMOR/AL (fem′or-al)

Attraction

The attraction of one consonantal sound to another is called *assimilation* (ad- to, simil- like, a- combining vowel, tion- process). Assimilation is the representation in both spelling and pronunciation of a sound change.

APPENDECTOMY (ap-en-dek'toe-me) from AD (to), PEND (hang), ECTOMY (cut out)

APPROXIMAL (a-proks'i-mal) from AD/PROXIM (near)/AL

AFFUSION (a-fu'zhun) from AD/FUS (pour)/ION

COLLAPSE from CON (with, together)/LAPSE (fall)/E

COMPRESS from CON/PRESS

IMMISCIBLE (i-mis'i-bul) from IN (not)/MISC (mix)/IBLE

SYMBIOSIS (sim-by-o'sis) from SYN (with)/BI (life)/OSIS

Silent Letters

When letters are not sounded in a word, they are easily omitted in spelling. Initial P and G and H after R and C are silent letters.

PSORIASIS (so-ry'a-sis, inflammation of the skin characterized by red patches and scaling)

PTOSIS (toe'sis, the falling or sagging of an organ or part of it)

GNATHITIS (nath-ēye'tis, GNATH/O, jaw)

RHINAL (ry'nal, RHIN/O, nose)

RHICNOSIS (rik-nō'sis, RHICN/O, wrinkle)

Shortened Forms

In some instances, usage over a period of time has caused a vowel or a consonant, or both, to be omitted from a word because either pronunciation becomes easier or the retention of that sound seems repetitious. Here are some examples.

APPENDECTOMY for APPENDICECTOMY

POLYDONTIA (pol-e-dun'she-a) for POLYODONTIA (having many teeth)

MEGASTRIA (me-gas'tre-a) for MEGAGASTRIA (enlargement of the stomach)

HYPALGIA (hi-pal'ge-a) for HYPOALGIA (reduced sensitivity to pain)

ANTACID (an-ta'sid) for ANTIACID (counteracting an acid)

URINALYSIS (your-i-nal'i-sis) for URINANALYSIS (analysis of the urine)

NEVER shorten a word unless you have seen the shortened form in print several times. Sometimes shortened forms become so popular that their original forms fall into disuse.

FLU (flu) from INFLUENZA (in-flu-en'za, an infectious disease)

LEUKOPENIA (lou-ko-pee'ne-a) from LEUKOCYTOPENIA (lack of white blood cells)

POLIO from POLIOMYELITIS (pol-e-o-my-el-eye'tis, inflammation of the gray matter of the spinal cord)

BICEPS (by'seps) from MUSCULUS BICEPS (mus'ku-lus by-seps)

Similarity of Sound

There are a few words that sound alike (homophones) but have different spellings and meanings.

ILEAC (il'e-ak, pertaining to the ileum, a portion of the small intestine)

ILIAC (il'e-ak, pertaining to the ilium, a portion of the hipbone)

CEROUS (ser'us, containing wax)

SEROUS (ser'us, pertaining to or containing serum)

CYTOLOGY (sy-tol'o-je, study of cells)

SITOLOGY (sy-tol'o-je, the study of nutrition, SIT/O, food)

Misspellings resulting from sound confusion can become a careless habit. Avoid them. For example,

ANTeBIOTIC for ANTIBIOTIC

HEMiPHILIA for HEMOPHILIA

AbORAL for ADORAL

HYPerGLYCEMIA for HYPOGLYCEMIA

Hyphenation

When a prefix or base is joined to a base that begins with the same vowel with which the prefix or base ends, a hyphen is used. For example,

MULTI-INFECTION

PARA-APPENDICITIS

SALPINGO-OOPHOROCELE (sal-ping-o-o-of'or-o-seel,* herniation of the ovary and fallopian tube)

There is a tendency, however, to omit the hyphen:

MICROORGANISM

FORMATION OF PLURALS

The plural forms of medical words are based on the classification that they were given in Latin and Greek. It is becoming increasingly acceptable, however, to make the plurals of many words with an s (ampullas instead of ampullae).
    Here is a table of the more frequently occurring plural endings.

Plural ending	*Words that form their plural in this way*
-ae (pronounced as a long i, as in hi or long e)	AMPULLA (am-pul'la), pl. ampullae, a saclike extension of a canal or a duct
	CORONA (ko-ro'na), pl. coronae, any crownlike structure
	VERTEBRA (ver'te-bra), pl. vertebrae, any one of the bony portions of the spinal column
-i (pronounced as a long i)	BRONCHUS (bron'kus), pl. bronchi, one of the two large branches of the trachea, the windpipe
	CAPILLUS (ka-pil-us), pl. capilli, a hair, something as fine as a hair
	FUNGUS (fun'gus), pl. fungi (fun'jī), a fungus
	OMPHALOS (om'fal-os), pl. omphali, the navel
-era	GENUS (jee'nus) pl. genera, biological classification: family, genus, species
-ora	STERCUS (ster'kus), pl. stercora, feces, stools
-es (pronounced -ēz)	GONAD (go'nad), pl. gonades, sex glands
	TESTIS (tes'tis), pl. testes, male gonad
	DIAGNOSIS (di-ag-no'sis), pl. diagnoses, determination of the cause and nature of an individual's disease or illness
-es	PSYCHOSIS (sy-ko'sis), pl. psychoses, severe mental disorder
	EPIDIDYMIS (ep-e-did'e-mis), pl. epididymides, a cordlike structure in which sperm are stored
	THORAX (tho'raks), pl. thoraces, the chest
	APPENDIX (a-pen'diks), pl. appendices, an appendage, the appendix
	POLLEX (pol-eks), pl. pollices, the thumb
	MENINX (me'ninks), pl. meninges, a membrane, the meninges—the coverings of the brain or spinal cord
	CARIES (ca'rez), pl. caries, decay

*Also pronounced sal-ping-o-ouf'or-o-seel.

Plural ending	*Words that form their plural in this way*
-ta	DERMA (der'ma), pl. dermata, the skin
	SARCOMA (sar-ko'ma), pl. sarcomata,* cancer developing from underlying tissue
	STOMA (sto'ma), pl. stomata,* mouth
-a	FLAGELLUM (fla-jel'um), pl. flagella, a whiplike structure by which bacteria and protozoa move themselves
	LABIUM (la'bi-um), pl. labia, lip
	PROTOZOON (pro-to-zo'on), pl. protozoa, simplest animal forms

EXERCISES

I. Pronounce each term. Mark the position of the primary accent and write out the sound of the underlined letter(s). *Example:*

HEMORRHAGIC ....J........

1. EXODONTIA ....

2. AUTOGENESIS ....

3. MYOTIC ....

4. ROENTGENOGRAPHY ....

5. PHALANGES ....

6. DYSPEPSIA ....

7. GUSTATORY ....

8. XIPHOID ....

9. EUPNEA ....

10. PHLEBOLOGY ....

11. JEJUNITIS ....

12. FUNGI ....

13. APOPLEXY ....

14. GLYCEMIC ....

15. CHONDRIC ....

16. PNEUMATIC ....

17. PSEUDOPARALYSIS ....

18. SEISMOTHERAPY ....

19. EUTHANASIA ....

20. OOPHORITIS ....

21. PHLEBOSTASIA ....

22. THROMBOCYTOPOIESIS ....

23. GASTROMYXORRHEA ....

24. APPENDICOLITHIASIS ....

25. CORTEX ....

Can you give the meanings of any of these words? Their meanings are given with the answers to the exercise.

*More frequently, sarcomas, stomas.

II. Divide the following words into syllables and mark the primary stress. *Example:*

HEMATOLOGY .... hem-a-tol'-o-gy ....

1. HEPATOTOMY ....

2. GASTROPATHY ....

3. PANCREATOLYSIS ....

4. NEPHRECTOMY ....

5. LARYNGOSCOPY ....

6. ERYTHREMIA ....

7. ANTIPATHY ....

8. GLOSSOTOMY ....

9. EUPNEA ....

10. NEURALGIC ....

III. Underline any silent letters.

1. DYSPEPSIA
2. PSEUDOPOD
3. DIAGNOSIS
4. PROPTOSIS
5. CHEILOPLASTY
6. GNATHALGIA
7. RHACHIOCENTESIS
8. PTOMAINE
9. APNEA
10. THROMBOSIS
11. PNEUMATOSCOPE

IV. Provide the full form for each of the following words. *Example:*

HYPALGIA for .... hypoalgia ....

1. MEGALGIA for ....

2. ERYTHROPENIA for ....

3. THORACENTESIS for ....

4. UROSTEALITH for ....

5. PARETHESIA for ....

6. APIECTOMY for ....

V. Make combining forms from the following words. Give an example. *Example:*

Word	Combining form	Example
FEMUR	FEMOR/	FEMORAL

1. CORTEX ....

2. LARYNX ....

3. ONYX ....

4. CERVIX ....

5. APEX ....

VI. Divide the following words into prefixes and bases.

1. APPERCEPTION ....

2. COMPLEXUS ....

3. SYMPARALYSIS ....

4. ARRECTOR ....

5. IMMUNOGENIC ....

VII. Make plural forms for the following words.

1. APEX ....

2. ALVEOLUS ....

3. NEUROSIS ....

4. DENDRON ....

5. LYMPHOMA ....

6. VALVA ....

7. SPECIES ....

8. RADIX ....

9. SOMA ....

10. CORPUS ....

11. RHABDOS ....

12. RIMA ....

13. AXIS ....

14. ARTHRON ....

15. VARIX ....

ANSWERS TO EXERCISES

I.

1. eks-o-don'she-a, extraction of a tooth
2. o-to-jen'e-sis, self-production
3. my-ot'ik, pertaining to that which contracts the pupil of the eye
4. rent-gen-og'ra-fe, the process of making an x ray
5. fa-lan'jeez, bones of a finger or toe
6. dis-pep'se-a, poor or painful digestion, indigestion
7. gus'ta-to-re, pertaining to taste
8. zif'oyd, sword-shaped
9. youp-nee'a, normal breathing
10. fleb-ol'o-je, study of the veins and their diseases
11. je-jou-ny'tis, inflammation of jejunum
12. fun'ji, plural form of fungus
13. ap'o-plek-se, loss of consciousness followed by paralysis
14. gly-see'me-a, sugar in the blood
15. kon'drik, pertaining to cartilage
16. new-mat'ik, pertaining to air
17. sou-do-pa-ral'i-sis, paralysis not due to any neurological damage
18. siz-mo-ther'a-pe, treatment by means of vibratory massage
19. you-tha-nay'ze-a, dying well, with dignity
20. o-of-o-ry'tis, inflammation of the ovary
21. fleb-o-stay'ze-a, compression of the veins resulting in the trapping of an amount of blood from the general circulation

22. throm-bo-sy-to-<u>poy</u>-e′sis, formation of blood clots
23. gas-tro-miks-o-<u>re</u>′a, excessive secretion of gastric mucus
24. a-pen-di-ko-li-<u>thy</u>′a-sis, formation of stones in the appendix
25. k<u>or</u>′teks, the outer layer of an organ or structure

II.

1. hep-a-tot′o-me;   2. gas-trop′-a-the;   3. pan-kre-a-tol′-i-sis;
4. ne-frek′toe-me;   5. lar-in-gos′ko-pe;   6. er-i-three′me-a;   7. an-tip′a-thee;
8. glo-sot′o-me;   9. youp-nee′a;   10. new-ral′jik.

III.

1. dyspepsia none;   2. pseudopod;   3. diagnosis none;   4. proptosis none;
5. cheiloplasty;   6. gnathalgia;   7. rhachiocentesis;   8. ptomaine;
9. apnea none;   10. thrombosis none;   11. pneumatoscope.

IV.

1. mega-algia;   2. erythrocytopenia;   3. thoracocentesis;   4. urosteatolith;
5. para-esthesia;   6. apicectomy.

V.

1. cortic/o, cortical, pertaining to the outer layer of an organ
2. laryng/o, laryngologist
3. onych/o nail, onychitis, inflammation of a nail bed
4. cervic/o neck, or an organ resembling the neck: uterus, cervical
5. apic/o top or tip of anything, apical

VI.

1. ad-perception;   2. con-plexus;   3. syn-paralysis;   4. ad-rector;
5. in-munogenic.

VII.

1. apices (ap′i-seez);   2. alveoli (al-vey′o-lie);   3. neuroses (nēw-roe′seez);
4. dendra (den′dra);   5. lymphomata (lim-fŏ′ma-ta);   6. valvae (val′vie);
7. species (spee′sheez);   8. radices (ra′di-seez);   9. somata (so′ma-ta);
10. corpora (kor′po-ra);   11. rhabdi (rab′die);   12. rimae (rē′my);
13. axes (ak′seez);   14. arthra (ar′thra);   15. varices (var′i-seez).

5 Anatomy of the Cell; Common Medical Expressions

ANATOMY OF THE CELL

The *cell* (Figure 5-1) is the basic structure of all living things. All body parts are made up of thousands of cells that group together to perform specific functions.

The *nucleus* (Figure 5-2) is the control center of the cell. It contains the genes that are the repositories of hereditary traits. All the cell's chemical activity is controlled by the nucleus, where two substances, DNA (deoxyribonucleic acid) and RNA (ribonucleic acid), control cellular reproduction and transmit instructions to the rest of the cell. The nucleus is surrounded by a thick liquid called *protoplasm* (PROT/O first, PLASM/O formation, growth). *Cytoplasm* (CYT/O, cell) the protoplasm within a cell, contains two types of structures: *inclusions* and *organelles*. The inclusions are nonliving particles; the organelles are living structures.

Here are some of the important structures found in cytoplasm.

Mitochondria (mit-o-kon′dre-a, MIT/O thread).   In these thread- or rod-shaped structures energy is produced by the oxidation of proteins, carbohydrates, and fats.

Golgi (gol′jee) *apparatus.*   This is a group of vessels that probably transports substances to the nucleus. The Golgi apparatus may participate in cellular metabolism and may release enzymes.

Fibrils.   These are threadlike strands that form the contractile tissue of muscles.

Varioles.   These are the storage receptacles of the cell.

Tubules.   These are tubes for transporting cellular substances.

Cell membrane.   This is a porous membrane surrounding the cell and continuing within the cell as a series of folds called *endoplasmic reticulum* (network). Attached to the endoplasmic reticulum are small granular substances called *ribosomes* (ry′bosooms). The ribosomes contain RNA and are the centers in which proteins are synthesized (called *anabolism*, BOL/O cast, throw).

Substances enter and leave the cells by *osmosis*. Osmosis is a simple method of diffusion: solutions of a greater concentration (*hypertonic*) diffuse into a solution of a lesser concentration. This is how substances are exchanged between the capillaries and surrounding cells. Substances can also enter a cell by becoming attached to a *carrier*

48

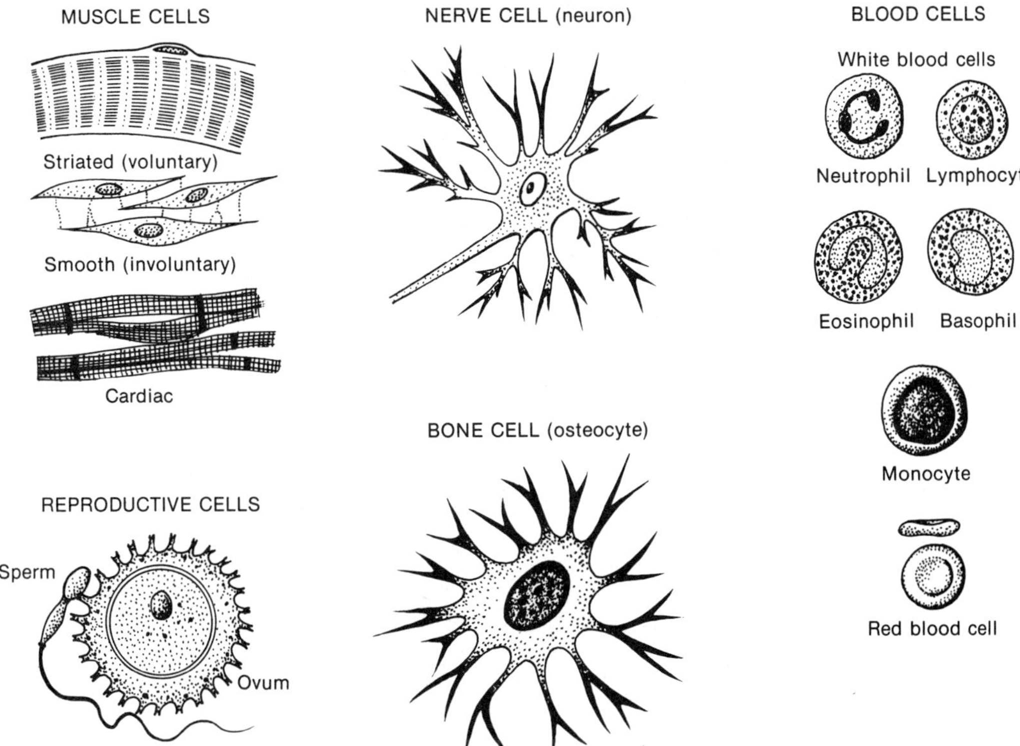

Figure 5-1 Various types of cells.

substance, such as an enzyme. Some cells can engulf entire particles in a process called *phagocytosis* (fag-o-sy-toe'sis). A cell can also draw in water by the process known as *pinocytosis* (pee-no-sy-toe'sis).

Cell division begins in the nucleus, which divides by a process called *mitosis* (my-toe'sis, MIT/O thread). Next, the cytoplasm divides (called *cytokinesis*, sy-to-kin-ee'sis). In mitosis or *karyokinesis*, as it is sometimes called, the genetic material is formed into 23 pairs of rodlike structures called *chromosomes*. Before cell division is completed, the chromosomes are duplicated and a groove called a *cleavage furrow* develops. This cleavage furrow eventually passes through the entire cell, resulting in two separate cells.

Cells having a similar structure and function group together to form *tissues*. *Histology* (HIST/O tissue) is the study of tissue, both normal and diseased. There are four classes of tissues: epithelial, connective, muscle, and nervous. *Epithelial tissue* covers the entire exterior of the body and lines all body cavities and vessels. There are several varieties of epithelial tissue: simple epithelial squamous, cuboidal, columnar, and combinations of them. *Connective tissue* is of two types: solid and fluid. Fibrous tissue, bones, cartilage, ligaments, and tendons are solid connective tissue. Blood and

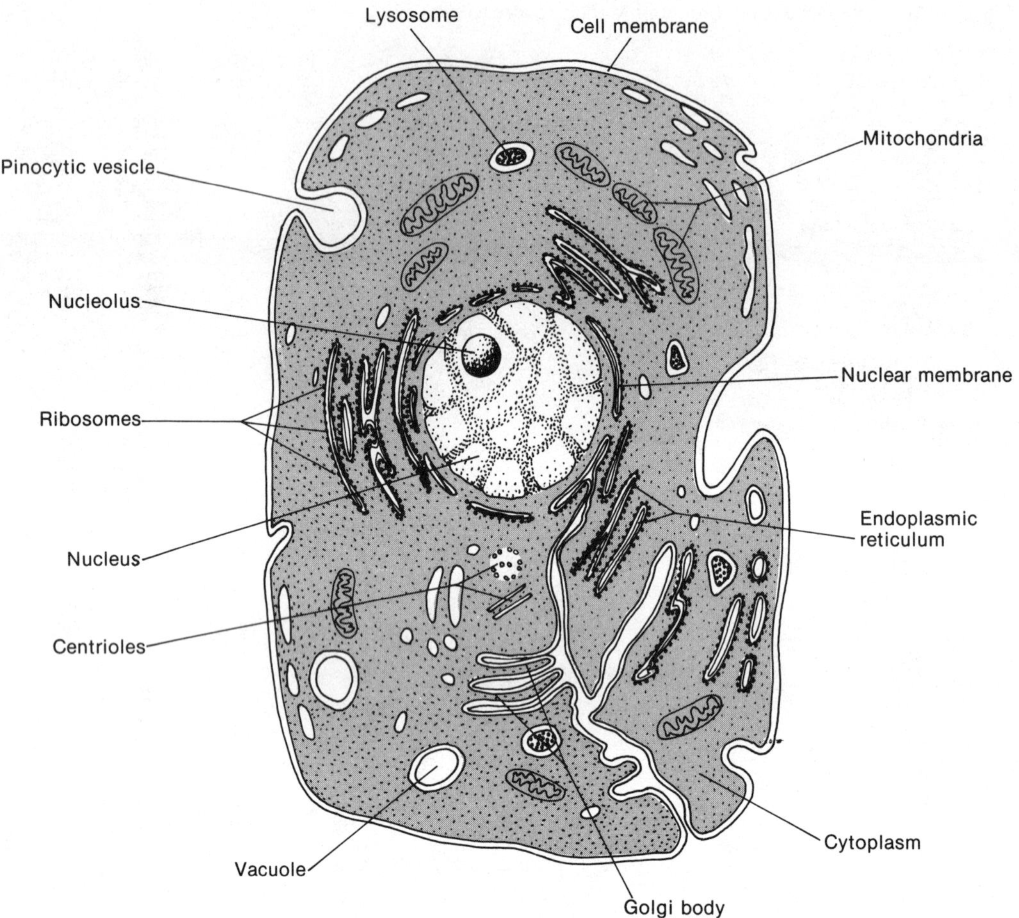

Figure 5-2   Major parts of a cell: (above) electron-microscopic structure; (facing page) three-dimensional structure. Both are diagrammatic.

plasma are fluid connective tissue. *Muscle tissue* is capable of contraction that results in movement. Skeletal, smooth, and cardiac are the three types of muscle tissue. *Nervous tissue* is specialized tissue that can respond to stimuli and conduct impulses.

Two or more tissues combine to form *organs*. Organs are structures that have a specific function. The heart, the stomach, and the brain are all organs. The organs, in turn, group together to form systems that perform specific functions. In anatomy several body systems are recognized. The number of these systems is not fixed, however, because any grouping of tissues or organs to perform a specific function can be viewed as a system. For example, we can refer to the *hematopoietic system*, the groups of tissues and structures that produce new blood cells and break down worn-out blood cells. Our treatment of medical terminology will center around the systems shown in the table.

50

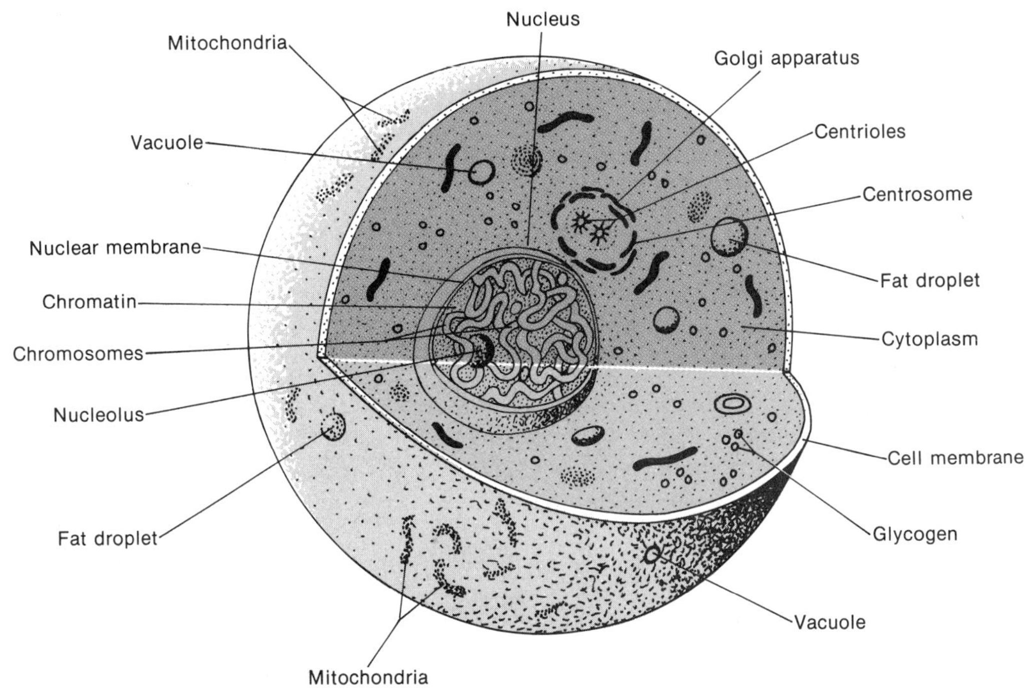

System	*Organs*
The skin or integumentary system	skin, hair, and nails
The musculoskeletal system	bones, cartilage, joints, ligaments, tendons, muscles
The nervous system	brain, spinal cord, nerves, (the various receptor organs)
The cardiovascular system	heart, blood vessels, blood, lymph and lymph vessels and nodes, spleen
The respiratory system	nose, pharynx, larynx, trachea, bronchial tubes, lungs, and diaphragm
The digestive system	tongue, teeth, esophagus, stomach, intestines, liver, gallbladder, pancreas
The urinary system	kidneys, ureters, bladder, urethra
The reproductive system	male: testes, epididymis, urethra, prostate, penis female: ovaries, fallopian tubes, uterus, vagina, mammary glands
The endocrine system	hormone-producing glands: pituitary, thyroid, parathyroid, and adrenal glands; also, the secretions of the pancreas, ovaries, testes, and several other organs

COMMON MEDICAL EXPRESSIONS

Because the following terms are used so frequently in medicine, they are presented to you now, at the outset of your study of medical terminology, so that you can become familiar with them.

A *disease* is a disorder of the body (or mind) in which body structures and functions are affected. An *organic* disease is an illness arising from a body structure, such as a tissue or organ.

Clinical is a term used to describe what is observable, capable of being examined, and treatable. *Pathology* is the study of diseases. The causes of diseases, their effects on the body, and their diagnosis form the basis of pathology. *Physiology* is the study of the normal functioning of cells, tissues, organs, and systems.

Etiology (ee-tee-ol'o-je) is the examination of the causes of a disease. *Symptoms* are the signs of a disease that are discovered upon observation, examination, and interrogation of a patient. A *syndrome* is a group of signs and symptoms that occur in a specific pattern and indicate a particular disease. An *asymptomatic* disease occurs without any observable signs. *Atypical* refers to a condition that is unusual, irregular, or abnormal.

A *diagnosis* is the determination of disease or disorder based on an examination of a patient, the patient's history and complaints, and any laboratory tests. A *prognosis* is the determination of the course and outcome of a disease and the patient's chance for recovery. *Treatment* is the application of some form of therapy either to cure the disease or to relieve its symptoms.

A *complication* is a secondary disease or disorder following the first condition. The second condition occurs as a result of the first condition or because of the body's weakened state from the first condition.

Vital signs are the indications of those processes necessary to sustain the life of an organism. They are blood pressure, body temperature, respiration, and heart rate.

Congenital refers to a condition present at birth. A *congenital anomaly* (a-nom'a-le) is a birth defect. *Genetic* refers to any condition developing from or caused by normal or abnormal genes. For example, a genetic disease is an abnormality developing from an abnormal gene. *Neonatal* (nee-o-nay'tal) refers to the newborn child or the first four weeks after birth. *Acquired* refers to a condition that has occurred after the birth of an individual.

Infection is the invasion of the body or part of the body by disease-causing microorganisms.

Inflammation is the reaction of body tissues to injury. The symptoms of inflammation are heat, redness, swelling, pain, and disrupted function. *Purulent* (pour'ou-lent) and *suppurative* (sup'per-a-tiv) are two commonly used words to indicate pus-producing.

Degeneration refers to the deterioration of cells or tissues, possibly leading to their destruction. Degeneration is reversible either by *regeneration*, the repair of the original cells or tissue, or by *replacement*, the growth of new cells or tissues.

Acute refers to a disease or illness that has a short duration but whose symptoms appear quickly and are severe. *Chronic* refers to a disease or illness that has a long duration with milder symptoms.

Atrophy is the decrease in tissue size resulting from the reduction in the number or the size of cells, or both. *Hypertrophy* is an increase of cell size. *Hyperplasia* is an increase in the number of cells.

An *enlargement* is the abnormal increase in the size of an organ. *Edema* (e-dee'ma) is the swelling of body tissue caused by an accumulation of fluid.

Dilatation or *distension* is the stretching of an organ.

A *prolapse* is the falling or slipping downward of an organ from its normal place. *Displacement* is the movement of a structure to a place or position different from its original place or position.

An *occlusion* is the blocking of a passageway. To *occlude* means to block.

A *trauma* is a wound to tissue caused by an external agent.

EXERCISES

I.   Match the following phrases with their medical words.

1. control center of the cell	a.	cytoplasm
2. necessary for protein synthesis	b.	endoplasmic reticulum
3. genetic substance	c.	karyokinesis
4. thick cellular liquid	d.	varioles
5. nonliving structures in cytoplasm	e.	RNA
6. living structures in cytoplasm	f.	organ
7. energy is produced here	g.	ribosomes
8. storage receptacles	h.	tubules

9.   transporters of cellular matter ....   i.   hypertonic

10. encloses the cell ....   j.   nucleus

11. membranous folds within the cell ....   k.   tissue

12. proteins are synthesized here ....   l.   osmosis

13. process by which substances enter and leave cell ....   m.   mitochondria

14. highly concentrated solution ....   n.   inclusions

15. nuclear division ....   o.   mitosis

16. another name for nuclear division ....   p.   DNA

17. division of the cellular protoplasm ....   q.   cytokinesis

18. carry genetic traits during nuclear division ....   r.   cell membrane

19. similar cells coming together for a specific function .... s.   chromosomes

20. two or more tissues coming together for a specific   t.   organelles
     function ....

   II.   List the type of tissue being described.

1.   .... capable of contraction

2.   .... joins parts of the body—e.g., ligament

3.   .... capable of conducting impulses

4.   .... lines body cavities

   III.   Identify the system to which the following organs belong.

1. thyroid gland ....   a.   skin

2. heart ....   b.   musculoskeletal system

3. bladder ....   c.   nervous system

4. lungs ....   d.   cardiovascular system

5. ovaries ....   e. respiratory system

6. spleen ....   f. digestive system

7. prostate ....   g. urinary system

8. kidney ....   h. reproductive system

9. nails ....   i. endocrine system

10. blood vessels ....

11. brain ....

12. trachea ....

13. intestines ....

14. hair ....

15. adrenal glands ....

16. mammary glands ....

17. tendons ....

18. fallopian tubes ....

19. spinal cord ....

20. bones ....

IV. Match the following descriptions with their medical words.

1. describes a disease that has a short duration ....   a. pathology

2. a secondary disorder following a previous disorder ....   b. purulent

3. capable of being examined and treated ....   c. edema

4. referring to a condition produced by the genes ....   d. treatment

5. a group of signs and symptoms occurring in a   e. congenital

    pattern ....   f. symptoms

6. invasion of the body by disease-causing

microorganisms ....

7. blocking of a passageway ....

8. the repair of damaged cells or tissue ....

9. the study of the cause of a disease ....

10. the study of the normal function of cells, tissues, and

organs ....

11. the growth of new cells or tissue to replace cells or tissue that

have been destroyed ....

12. an abnormal increase in the size of an organ ....

13. pertaining to a condition present at birth ....

14. a disorder of the body affecting body structures and

functions ....

15. a degenerative decrease in the size of a tissue or

organ ....

16. pus producing ....

17. the study of the causes, effects, and diagnoses of

diseases ....

18. describes a disease that has a long duration ....

19. an increase in the number of cells ....

20. referring to a situation or condition that is unusual or

abnormal ....

21. the signs of a disease ....

22. the swelling of body tissue caused by excess fluid ....

23. the determination of the outcome of a disease ....

24. the slipping downward of an organ ....

g. acute

h. chronic

i. dilatation

j. trauma

k. clinical

l. prognosis

m. diagnosis

n. etiology

o. syndrome

p. disease

q. occlusion

r. asymptomatic

s. inflammation

t. infection

u. enlargement

v. neonatal

w. vital signs

x. complication

y. prolapse

z. atrophy

aa. hypertrophy

bb. genetic

25. developing from or originating in a body structure, such as an organ or tissue	cc. hyperplasia
	dd. physiology
26. the progressive deterioration of cells or tissue	ee. atypical
27. the stretching of a body structure	ff. replacement
28. referring to a disease occurring without signs	gg. organic
29. the determination of a disease or disorder	hh. degeneration
30. indications of life-sustaining processes	ii. regeneration
31. the reaction of body tissue to injury	
32. pertaining to the newborn	
33. the application of therapy	
34. injury to tissue caused by an external agent	
35. an increase in cell size	

ANSWERS TO EXERCISES

I.

1. j; **2.** e; **3.** p; **4.** a; **5.** n; **6.** t; **7.** m; **8.** d; **9.** h;
10. r; **11.** b; **12.** g; **13.** l; **14.** i; **15.** o; **16.** c; **17.** q;
18. s; **19.** k; **20.** f.

II.

1. muscular tissue;
2. connective tissue;
3. nervous tissue;
4. epithelial tissue.

III.

1. i; **2.** d; **3.** g; **4.** e; **5.** h/i; **6.** d; **7.** h; **8.** g;
9. a; **10.** d; **11.** c; **12.** e; **13.** f; **14.** a; **15.** i; **16.** h;
17. b; **18.** h; **19.** c; **20.** b.

IV.

1. g; **2.** x; **3.** k; **4.** bb; **5.** o; **6.** t; **7.** q; **8.** ii; **9.** n
10. dd; **11.** ff; **12.** u; **13.** e; **14.** p; **15.** z; **16.** b; **17.** a;
18. h; **19.** cc; **20.** ee; **21.** f; **22.** c; **23.** l; **24.** y; **25.** gg;
26. hh; **27.** i; **28.** r; **29.** m; **30.** w; **31.** s; **32.** v; **33.** d;
34. j; **35.** aa.

6 Body Regions, Directions, Numbers, and Colors

MAJOR BODY REGIONS

In *gross anatomy* (examination of structures with the naked eye) the body can be divided visually into three major parts: the head and neck, the trunk, and the extremities (limbs).

Major Division	*Subdivision*	
Head and neck	Cranium Face Neck	
Trunk	*Front*	*Back*
	Thorax (chest)	Upper back (between and below shoulder blades)
	Abdomen	Lower back (lumbar region)
	Pubic region (groin)	Gluteal region (buttocks)
	Perineum (region between the legs; contains the external sex organs and anal opening)	
Extremities	*Upper*	*Lower*
	Shoulder	Thigh
	Upper arm	Leg
	Forearm	
	Hand	Foot

Study the major body regions in Figure 6.1 and become familiar with the scientific names. Here is a list of these terms. In most cases, you can form the base by removing the adjective suffix (ar, ary, ic).

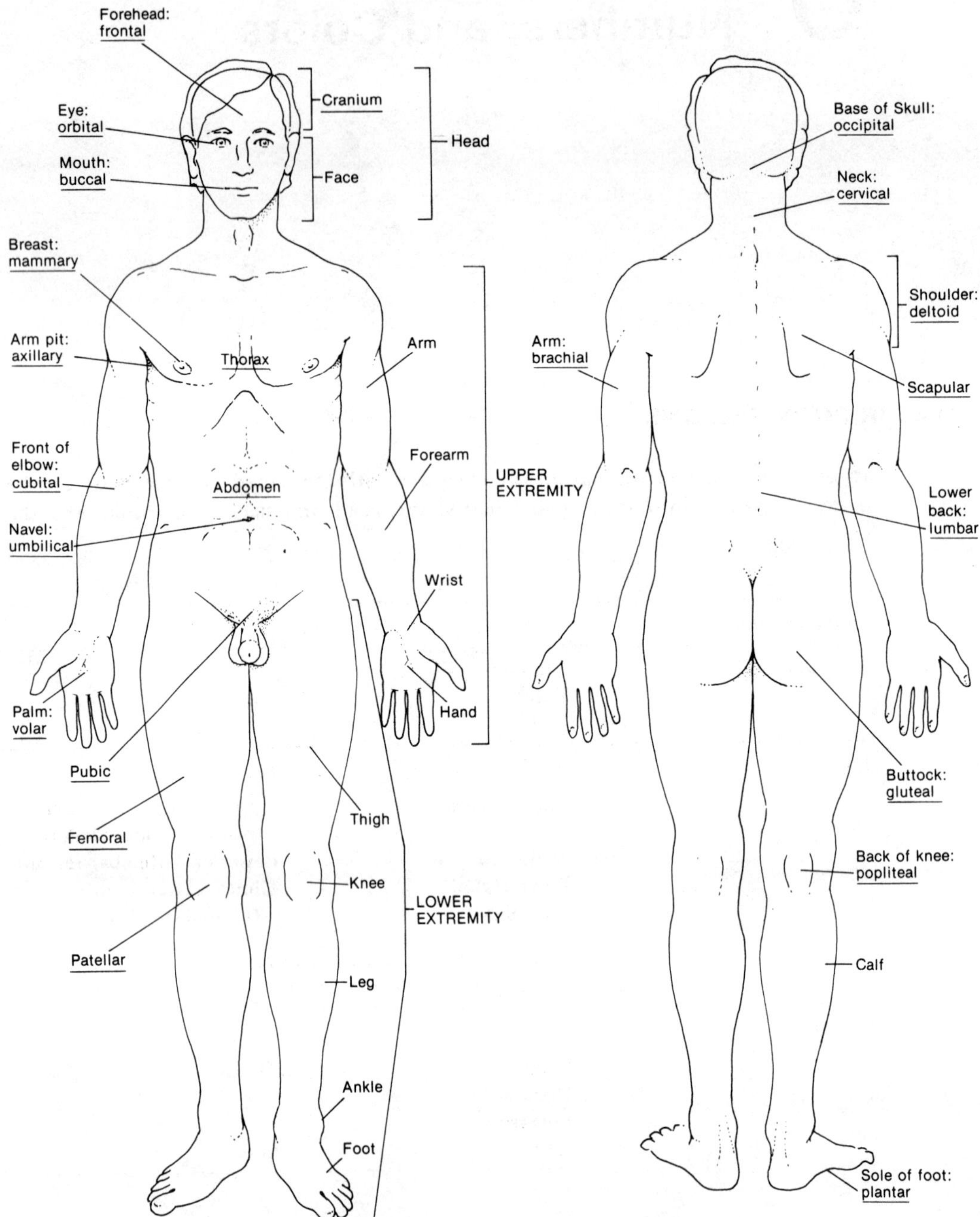

Figure 6-1 Major body regions. Some are labeled with common and scientific terms, with the latter indicated by underscores. The subject is standing in the anatomical position.

Term	Region
frontal (front'al)	forehead
orbital (or'bit-al)	eye
buccal (buk'al)	cheek, mouth
cervical (ser'vik-al)	neck
thoracic (tho-ra'sik)	chest
mammary (mam'ari)	breast
abdominal (ab-dom'in-al)	abdomen
umbilical (om-bil'ik-al)	navel
pubic (pu'bik)	groin
perineal (per-i-nee'al)	base or floor of the trunk
occipital (ok-sip'i-tal)	base of the skull
deltoid (del'toyd)	shoulder
scapular (skap'u-lar)	shoulderblade
lumbar (lum'bar)	lower back
gluteal (glue-tee'al)	buttocks
brachial (bray'key-al)	arm
cubital (ku'bi-tal)	front of elbow
carpal (kar'pal)	wrist
volar (vol'ar)	palm
femoral (fem'or-al)	thigh
patellar (pa-tel'ar)	knee
popliteal (pop-lit-tee'al)	back of the knee
plantar (plan'tar)	sole of the foot

BODY CAVITIES

The body cavities (Figure 6-2) are hollows or spaces in the body that house body organs and structures. The body cavities are divided into two groups according to their location in the body. Posterior cavities are located in the back of the body whereas the anterior cavities are located in the front.

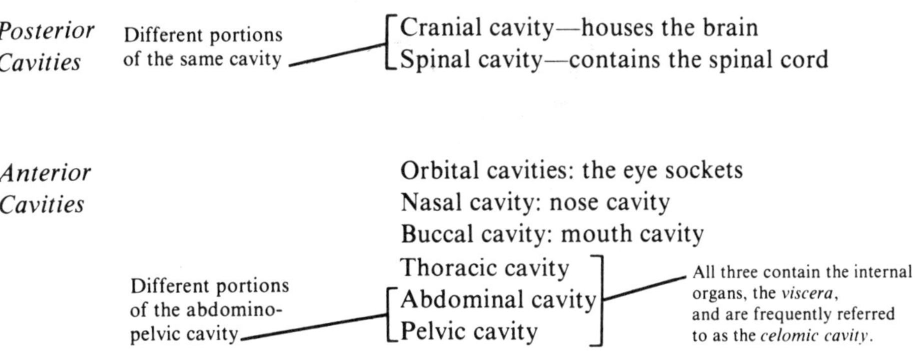

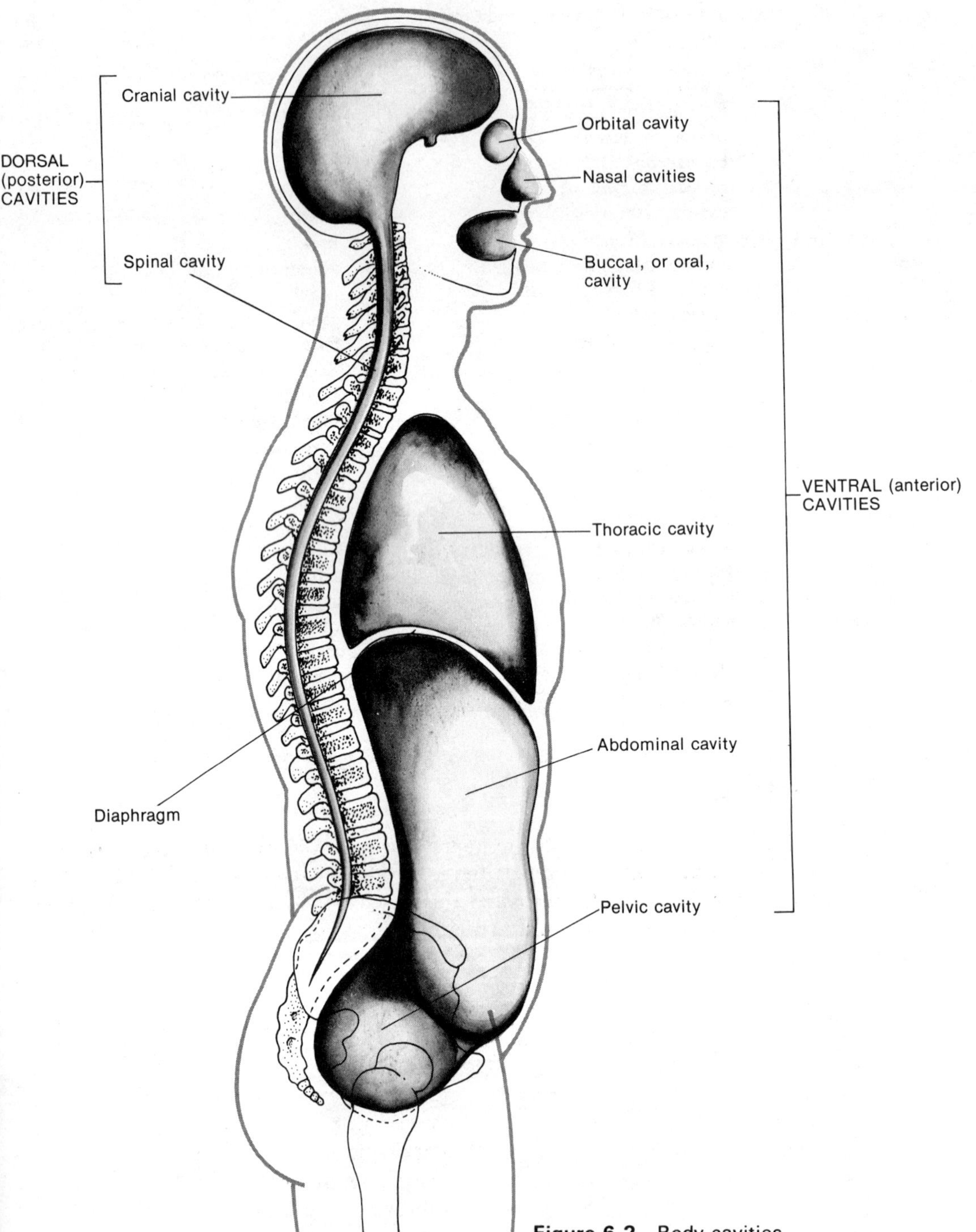

Figure 6-2 Body cavities.

The *alimentary canal* (digestive tract) is also a cavity that passes through the celomic (se-loo'mik) cavity but doesn't open to it. Instead it opens by means of the mouth and anus to the outside of the body.

DIRECTIONAL TERMS

Directional terms are used to indicate the position of one structure in relation to another structure. For example, the nose is *inferior* (located below) to the eyes but *superior* (located above) to the mouth. Directional terms indicate the position of body structures when the body is in the *anatomical position*—that is, a standing position, head and palms facing forward, and the feet spread slightly apart (see Figure 6-1).

Directional term	*Meaning*
anterior (synonym: ventral)	*toward the front* of the body or structure
posterior (synonym: dorsal)	*toward the back* of the body or structure
superior	*situated higher or above* another structure
inferior	*situated lower or below* another structure
medial	*near the middle*—refers to a structure located near the middle of the body or to a part of a structure located near the middle of the structure itself
lateral	*on the side*, away from the middle of the body or body structure
proximal ⎤ Describe the positions of extremities	*located near the trunk* of the body
distal ⎦	*located away from the trunk* of the body
superficial	*located near the surface* of the body or structure
deep	*located away from the surface* of the body or structure

TERMS FOR BODY MOVEMENTS

Flexion. By a bending action, two portions of an extremity are brought closer together. For example, the hand is moved toward the shoulder.

Extension. Two ends of an extremity are separated, as in moving the hand away from the shoulder.

Rotation. Here a structure turns on its long axis, as in the rotation of the head. The rotation of the palm of the hand into the anatomical position (facing forward) is called *supination;* the rotation of the palm in the backward position is called *pronation.*

Inversion and *Eversion.*   Both terms refer to the movements of the feet. In inversion the feet are turned inward with the soles facing one another whereas in eversion the soles face outward.

Abduction.   The movement of an extremity *away from* the median plane of the body is known as abduction. For instance, in abduction the hand and arm move away from the trunk of the body.

Adduction.   Adduction is the movement of an extremity *toward* the median plane of the body, as in the movement of the hand and arm toward the trunk of the body.

Circumduction.   Circumduction refers to a cone-shaped movement of an extremity, such as in the circular rotation of the arm.

Protraction and *retraction.*   Protraction indicates the *forward movement* or *protrusion* of a body part, such as the protrusion of the lower jaw. In retraction a body part is drawn *backward.* The lower jaw is retracted when the mouth is open.

Elevation and *depression.*   Elevation refers to the *raising* of a body part. The lower jaw is elevated when the mouth is closed. Depression indicates the *lowering* of a body part. For example, the lower jaw is depressed when the mouth is open.

BODY PLANES

The body planes (Figure 6-3) are artificial sections of the entire body or body structure, such as an organ, that are used as points of reference to indicate the position of a body structure in relation to the body as a whole or the position of a part of the same structure in relation to the structure itself. Remember that the body is in the anatomical position.

Median or *midsagittal plane.*   The body (or body structure) is cut from front to back (anterior to posterior) to form two equal right and left halves.

Transverse plane.   The body (or body structure) is cut horizontally.

Coronal plane.   The body (or body structure) is divided into front and rear sections that are not necessarily equal.

SURFACE ANATOMY

Frequently the position of body structures can be determined by surface examination through *palpation* (feeling) or the use of *imaginary lines* drawn over the body.

The following structures can be located by palpation.

1. The *point of the shoulder* is formed by the acromion process.
2. The *suprasternal notch* is located at the front end of the sternum.
3. Below the suprasternal notch is the *sternal angle*, which slightly projects anteriorly.

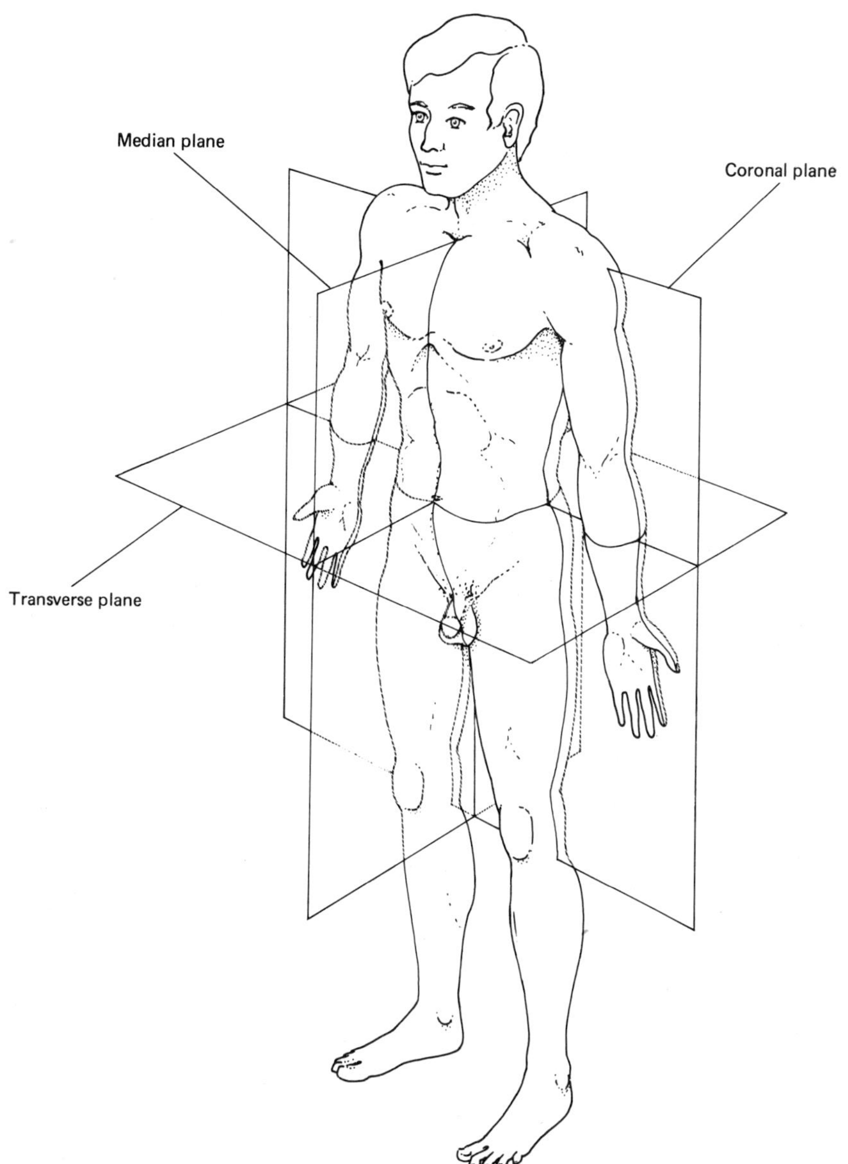

Figure 6-3 The body planes.

4. The *xiphisternal junction* (zif'i-stern-al) is the cartilaginous portion of the sternum; it locates the pit of the stomach.
5. The *iliac crests* are located on either side of the lower trunk. They are formed by the upper portion of the ilium.
6. The *lateral malleolus* (end portion of the fibula bone) is the bony projection located on the side of the ankle whereas the *medial malleolus* (end portion of the tibia bone) lies on the medial surface of the ankle.

The nine regions of the abdomen can be sectioned off by the use of imaginary lines running transversely and vertically across the abdominal region (Figure 6-4).

1. The upper third of the abdomen is divided into the *right and left hypochondriac areas* on either side and the *epigastric region* medially.
2. The middle third of the abdomen is divided into the *right and left lumbar areas* and the *umbilical region* medially.

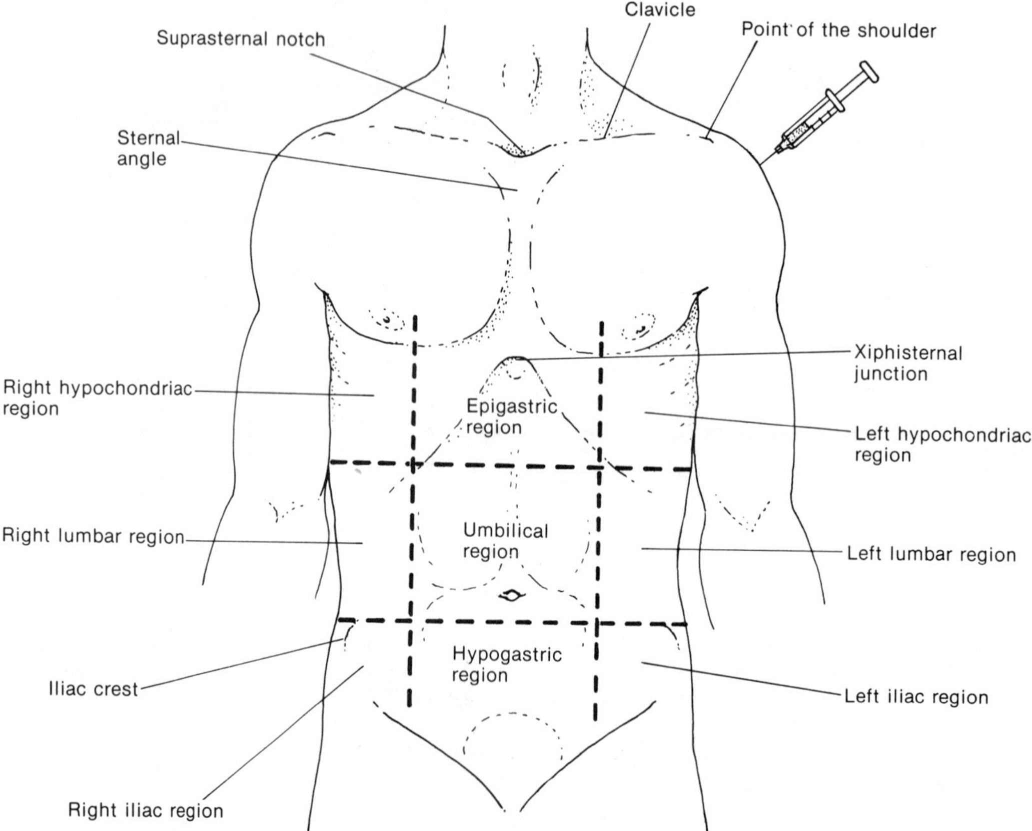

Figure 6-4 Surface anatomy.

3. The lower third of the abdomen is divided into the *right and left iliac regions* on either side and the *hypogastric region* medially.

NUMBERS AND COLORS

mono- uni- haplo-	one, single
di- diplo- bi	two, double
tri- triplo-	three, triple
tetra- quadri- quarto-	four, fourfold
hecto	one hundred
centi	one-hundredth
kilo-	one thousand
milli-	one-thousandth
poly- multi-	many

Combining Forms for Colors

leuk/o, leuc/o alb/o	white
melan/o nigr/o	black
erythr/o rub/o	red
chlor/o	green
cyan/o	blue
xanth/o	yellow
glauc/o	gray, greenish gray
poli/o	gray, whitish gray

Only those numbers and colors that are used with some frequency are listed here. Numbers are frequently prefixed to words indicating chemical compounds:

pentose (pent/o, five): a sugar containing five atoms of carbon

triglyceride: a combination of fatty acids and glycerol, characteristic of most animal and vegetable fats

diethylstilbestrol: a synthetic estrogen compound

EXERCISES

I. List each body region under the major body regions.

1. pubic region	**2.** shoulder	**3.** foot	**4.** cranium
5. thorax	**6.** gluteal region	**7.** forearm	**8.** upper back
9. lower back	**10.** leg	**11.** upper arm	**12.** thigh
13. neck	**14.** hand	**15.** abdomen	**16.** face

Head and Neck	*Trunk*	*Extremities*
. . . .	. . . .	. . . .
. . . .	. . . .	. . . .
. . . .	. . . .	. . . .
	. . . .	. . . .
	. . . .	. . . .
	. . . .	. . . .

II. Match the medical terms for the body regions with their common names.

1. frontal . . . .   a. abdomen

2. orbital . . . .   b. shoulder

3. buccal . . . .   c. back of knee

4. cervical . . . .   d. buttocks

5. thoracic . . . .   e. base/floor of the trunk

6. mammary . . . .   f. knee

7. abdominal ....   g. eye

8. umbilical ....   h. palm

9. pubic ....   i. neck

10. perineal ....   j. front of elbow

11. occipital ....   k. wrist

12. deltoid ....   l. mouth/cheek

13. scapular ....   m. groin

14. lumbar ....   n. lower back

15. gluteal ....   o. thigh

16. brachial ....   p. breast

17. cubital ....   q. forehead

18. carpal ....   r. arm

19. volar ....   s. sole of the foot

20. femoral ....   t. navel

21. patellar ....   u. shoulder blade

22. popliteal ....   v. chest

23. plantar ....   w. base of the skull

III. Make five pairs of antonyms from the following directional terms.

1. inferior   1. ....
2. distal
3. medial   2. ....
4. anterior
5. superficial   3. ....
6. posterior
7. superior   4. ....
8. deep
9. proximal   5. ....
10. lateral

IV. Multiple choice: Choose the term that most closely identifies the movement of the body part.

1. Movement of the legs away from the median plane of the body
   (a) eversion
   (b) adduction
   (c) abduction
   (d) inversion

2. The raising of the lower jaw to close the mouth
   (a) extension
   (b) elevation
   (c) depression
   (d) protraction

3. The forward movement of the lower jaw
   (a) protraction
   (b) adduction
   (c) extension
   (d) none of the above

4. Movement in which the soles of the feet face one another
   (a) elevation
   (b) extension
   (c) eversion
   (d) inversion

5. The lowering of the shoulders from a raised or shrugged position
   (a) depression
   (b) retraction
   (c) extension
   (d) abduction

6. Movement in which the soles of the feet face outward
   (a) adduction
   (b) inversion
   (c) eversion
   (d) extension

7. Movement of the tongue back into the mouth
   (a) abduction
   (b) retraction
   (c) protraction
   (d) circumduction

8. Movement of the heel toward the back of the knee
   (a) flexion
   (b) extension
   (c) inversion
   (d) retraction

9. A series of movements involving flexion, extension, and rotation
   (a) adduction
   (b) elevation
   (c) circumduction
   (d) eversion

10. A straightening movement bringing the hand away from the shoulder
    (a) flexion
    (b) extension
    (c) retraction
    (d) protraction

11. Movement of the arm toward the trunk of the body
    (a) extension
    (b) retraction
    (c) adduction
    (d) abduction

12. A twisting movement of the body or body part, such as the twisting of the neck
    (a) rotation
    (b) circumduction
    (c) adduction
    (d) protraction

V. True or false: Circle T or F for each of the following statements. If the statement is false, provide the correct answer.

1. Another name for the median body plane is the midsagittal plane.

   T / F ....

2. The median plane cuts the body horizontally.

   T / F ....

3. The transverse plane divides the body into front and rear sections.

   T / F ....

4. The plane that divides the body into front and rear sections is called the coronal plane.

   T / F ....

5. Palpation involves the use of certain imaginary lines to locate key body areas.

   T / F ....

VI. Indicate in the boxes below the nine abdominal regions.

1	2	3
4	5	6
7	8	9

VII. Give the meaning for each of the following medical words.* Divide each word into bases, prefix, and suffix; underline the letter or letters that have the primary stress. *Example:*

UNINUCLEAR   having only one nucleus   uni/<u>nucle</u>/ar

1. DIMORPHOUS   ....

2. QUADRILATERAL   ....

3. KILOGRAM   ....

4. LEUKODERMA   ....

5. CHLOROMA   ....

6. ERYTHROBLASTOSIS   ....

7. POLIOENCEPHALITIS   ....

8. CYANODERMA   ....

9. BICEPS   ....

*You may use a dictionary for any unfamiliar forms.

10. **POLYARTHRITIS** ....

11. **MELANOCYTE** ....

12. **RUBEFACIENT** ....

13. **XANTHOSIS** ....

14. **ALBUMIN** ....

15. **CENTIGRADE** ....

VIII. Make medical words from the following phrases. Indicate the primary stress by underlining the stressed letter(s). *Example:*

formation of red blood cells

erythropoi<u>e</u>sis
....

1. a tooth having two points or protrusions

....

2. having many nuclei

....

3. blood containing dark pigment

....

4. abnormal bluish color (of the skin)

....

5. single/simple inflammation of the skin

....

6. abnormal increase in the number of white blood cells

....

7. inflammation of the gray matter of the spinal cord

....

8. yellowish, having a yellow color

....

9. disease/diseased condition that affects only one area of the body

....

10. a red blood cell

....

ANSWERS TO EXERCISES

I.

Head and neck: 4, 16, 13
Trunk: 5, 15, 1, 8, 9, 6
Extremities: 2, 11, 7, 14, 12, 10, 3

II.

1. q; **2.** g; **3.** l; **4.** i; **5.** v; **6.** p; **7.** a; **8.** t; **9.** m;
10. e; **11.** w; **12.** b; **13.** u; **14.** n; **15.** d; **16.** r; **17.** j;
18. k; **19.** h; **20.** o; **21.** f; **22.** c; **23.** s.

III. 4 and 6; 7 and 1; 3 and 10; 9 and 2; 5 and 8.

IV.

1. (c); **2.** (b); **3.** (a); **4.** (d); **5.** (a); **6.** (c); **7.** (b); **8.** (a);
9. (c); **10.** (b); **11.** (c); **12.** (a).

V.

1. T
2. F, cuts the body from front to back (anterior to posterior)
3. F, cuts the body horizontally
4. T
5. F, location of body structures through feeling or touching

VI.

1. right hypochondriac region; **2.** epigastric region; **3.** left hypochondriac region;
4. right lumbar region; **5.** umbilical region; **6.** left lumbar region;
7. right iliac region; **8.** hypogastric region; **9.** left iliac region.

VII.

1. having two forms or shapes, di/morph/ous
2. four-sided, quadri/later/al
3. one-thousand grams, kilo/gram

4. patches on the skin that lack pigmentation, vitiligo, leuk/o/<u>derm</u>a
5. greenish fleshy tumor (of the cranial bones), chlor/oma
6. abnormal presence of erythroblasts in the blood: erythroblastosis fetalis—the breakdown of blood in a newborn child characterized by anemia, jaundice, enlargement of the spleen and liver, and generalized edema (swelling), erythr/o/blast/osis
7. inflammation of the gray matter of the brain, poli/o/encephal/<u>it</u>is
8. blue discoloring of the skin, cyan/o/<u>derm</u>a
9. a muscle with two heads, <u>bi</u>/ceps
10. inflammation of several joints, poly/arthr/<u>it</u>is
11. dark pigment cell, <u>mela</u>n/o/cyte
12. any agent that causes the skin to become red, rube/<u>fa</u>cient
13. condition characterized by a yellowing of the skin, <u>xanth</u>/osis
14. protein found in the blood, al<u>bu</u>min
15. divided into a hundred, <u>cen</u>ti/grade

VIII.

1. bi<u>cu</u>spid;   2. multi<u>nu</u>clear;   3. melan<u>e</u>mia;   4. cyan<u>o</u>sis;
5. haplodermat<u>it</u>is;   6. leukocy<u>to</u>sis;   7. poliomyel<u>it</u>is;   8. <u>xan</u>thous;
9. mon<u>o</u>pathy;   10. e<u>ry</u>throcyte.

7 The Skin

COMBINING FORMS

	Meaning	Example
CUT/I (ku'ti)	skin	SUBCUTANEOUS (sub-ku-tay'ne-us), under the skin
DERM/O (der/mo)	skin	EPIDERMIS (ep-e-der'mis), outer layer of skin
DERMAT/O (der'ma-to)	skin	DERMATOSIS (der-ma-toe'sis), any disease of the skin
KERAT/O (ker'a-to)	horny, hard	KERATONOSIS (ker-a-to-no'sis, NOS/O, disease), any disease of the outer layer of the skin
ACANTH/O (a-kan'tho)	thorn, spine	ACANTHOMA (ak-an-tho'ma), benign skin tumor
TRICH/O (tri'ko)	hair	TRICHOSIS (tri-ko'sis), any abnormal condition of the hair
PIL/O (py'lo)	hair	PILOUS (py'lus), hairy
FOLLICUL/O (fo-lik'you-lo)	small cavity or sac, a follicule	FOLLICULITIS (fo-lik-you-ly'tis), inflammation of a follicule
SEB/O (see'bo)	sebum, fatty secretion	SEBACEOUS (see-bay'shus), containing or excreting sebum
SUDOR/O (su'dor-o)	sweat	SUDORIFIC (su-dor-if'ik), sweat-producing
DIAPHOR/O (di-af'o-ro)	sweat	DIAPHORESIS (di-a-fo-re'sis), profuse sweating

76

	Meaning	*Example*
HIDR/O (hi'dro)	sweat	HIDROPOIESIS (hi-dro-poy-e'sis), formation of sweat
HOL/O (hol'o)	whole, entire	HOLOCRINE (hol'o-krin), pertaining to a gland that consumes its cells in producing a secretion
MER/O (mer'o)	part	MEROCRINE (mer'o-krin) pertaining to a gland that produces its secretion without destroying its cells
UNGU/O (un-gwo)	nail	UNGUAL (un'gwal), pertaining to the nail
ONYCH/O (on'i-ko)	nail, nailbed	ONYCHOLYSIS (on-i-kol'i-sis), the separation of a nail from its nail bed
ADIP/O (ad'i-po)	fat	ADIPOSE (ad'i-poz), pertaining to fat
-CRINE (krin')	to secrete	ENDOCRINE (en'do-krin), pertaining to a gland that secretes directly into the bloodstream

The skin covers the external surface of the body and constitutes what is called the *integumentary* (in-teg-you-men'te-re) *system*. Two qualities of skin are *elasticity* and *resiliency*, which means that it can be stretched and will return to its former shape. In addition to covering and, in a sense, shaping the body, the skin performs four essential functions: protection, sensation, regulation of body heat, and the synthesis of certain substances.

The skin protects the body in two ways. Sebaceous and sweat glands provide a secretion that properly moistens the skin and protects it from harmful bacteria and fungi. Secondly, the horny layer of skin composed of *keratinized cells* presents a physical barrier to substances attempting to enter the body. Although gases and fatty substances called *lipids* penetrate rather easily, the skin remains impermeable to water and *electrolytes* (acids, bases, and salts).

The skin is sensitive to four types of sensations: touch, cold, warmth, and pain. Each sensation has its own receptor, and these receptors or *sensory spots* occur throughout the entire area of the skin. A light touch activates *Meissner's corpuscles* (kor'pus-el, little body), whereas a heavy touch stimulates the *Pacinian corpuscles*, which are located deep within the dermis. Warmth is sensed by the *Ruffini corpuscles*, cold by the *Krause corpuscles*. The skin senses pain as either sharp and localized or burning and generalized.

The skin has two other important functions. It draws unnecessary heat from the body by acting as a *radiant surface* and through evaporation and sweating. This important function of the skin is known as *thermoregulation*. In addition to producing substances such as keratin for its own use, the skin also produces vitamin D.

ANATOMY OF THE SKIN

Although the skin contains many layers, there are two major divisions: the outermost layer called the *epidermis*, and the innermost layer called the *dermis* (Figure 7-1). The *epidermis* consists of four layers of *stratified* (layered) *squamous* (skwa'mus, squam/o, scaly) epithelium: the *stratum corneum* (stra'tum kor'ne-um), the *stratum lucidum* (lu'si-dum), the *stratum granulosum* (gran-you-lo'sum), and the *stratum germinativum* (jer-min-a-tie'vum). The corneum (CORNE/O horny) is composed of scaly cells without nuclei and containing *keratin*, a horny protein. The lucidum is a thinner, less-structured layer and contains a keratinous substance called *eleidin* (e-lay'i-din). The granulosum is composed of layers of cells containing granules of *keratohyalin*, which begins the keratinization process as the cells move toward the corneum. In the several layers of the germinativum cells multiply and begin to surface toward the corneum. Melanocytes, cells responsible for the skin's pigment, are located in the germinativum.

The *dermis*, also called the *corium* (ko're-um, KORI/O skin) or true skin, is dense connective tissue that gives the entire skin its elasticity. Two layers make up the dermis: the outer *papillary layer*, a vascular layer that nourishes both the dermis and germinativum, and the deep *reticular layer*. Blood vessels, sweat and oil glands, hair follicles, and sensory receptors all lie in the reticular layer. The *subcutaneous layer*, which is not a layer of skin, is below the dermis and is composed of loose connective tissue and numerous fatty deposits (*adipose* tissue).

APPENDAGES OF THE SKIN

The hair, nails, and glands are structures of the skin and are closely associated with it. Hair develops from a folding inward (*invagination*) of the epidermis to form a *follicle*. Most of the body with some notable exceptions (e.g., the palms and soles of the feet) has some hair. Infants are covered with fine hair called *lanugo* (la-nou'go); a protective coating, called *vernix caseosa* (ver'niks ka-se-o'sa, cheeselike coating), of peelings of skin, lanugo, and sebum produced by the glands of the skin covers the fetus at birth. The growth of hair in the axillary and pubic regions accompanies puberty.

A hair has two parts—the *root* and the *shaft*. Hair cells are formed in the *bulb* portion of the root where they become cornified before appearing on the surface of the skin as the hair shaft. The hair shaft is lubricated with *sebum*, which is produced by the *sebaceous glands*. The scalp itself consists of five layers of tissue: *s*kin, *c*onnective tissue, *a*poneurosis (fibrous connective tissue), *l*oose connective tissue, and *perio*steum connecting it to the cranium.

The nails (Figure 7-2) are hard, cornified layers of the epidermis of the fingers.

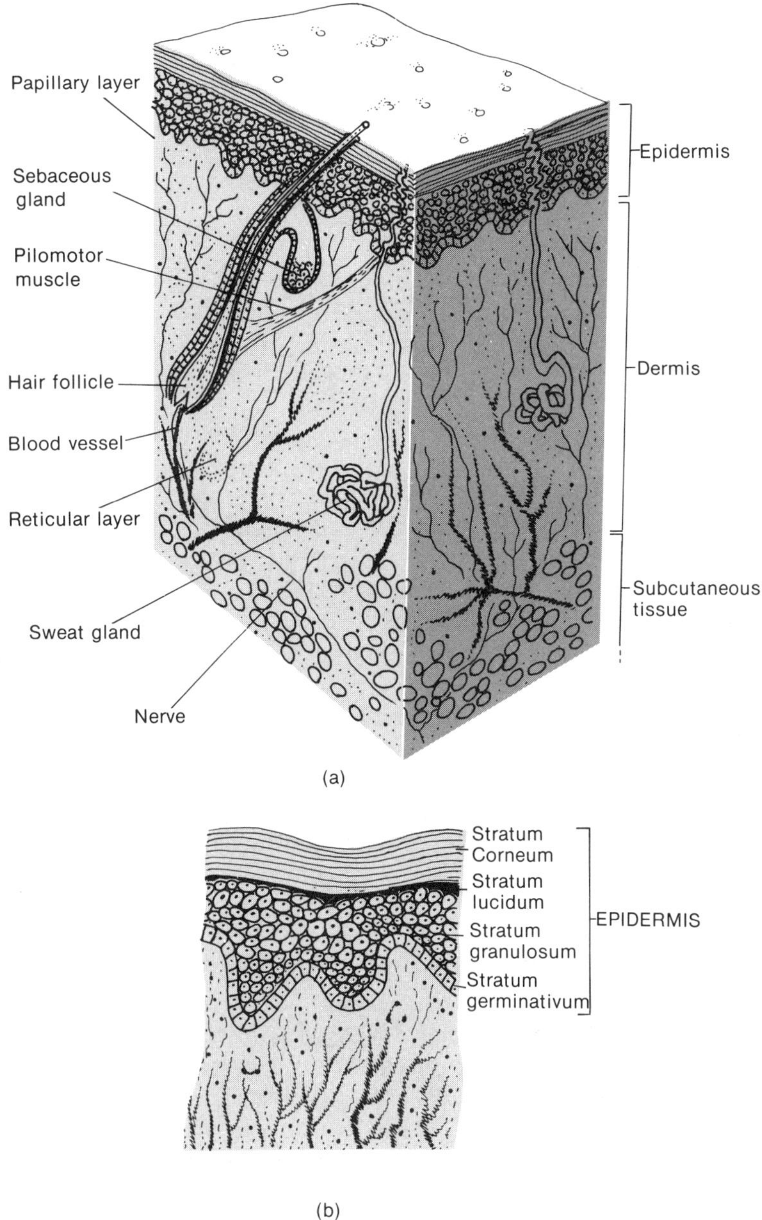

Figure 7-1 (a) Three-dimensional view of the skin. (b) Layers of the epidermis.

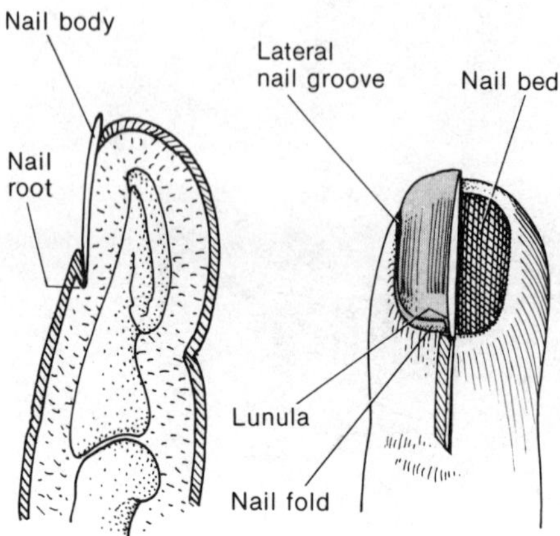

Figure 7-2 Construction of the nails.

Like the hair, each nail consists of a *root* and a *body* resting on the *nail bed*. The light portion near the *nail fold* is the *lunula* (lou'nou-la, LUN/O moon). New nail growth takes place in the lunula.

Two types of glands are located in the skin: *sebaceous* or sebum-producing glands and *sudoriferous* or sweat-producing glands. The sebaceous glands produce and secrete *sebum*, an oily substance that lubricates the hair shafts. These glands are classified as *holocrine glands*, which means that the secretory cells themselves break down and become the secretion. There are two types of sweat glands: *merocrine* and *apocrine*. Merocrine glands produce a secretion without destroying the secreting cells whereas apocrine glands lose part of their cytoplasm in the secretion. Apocrine glands tend to be larger than merocrine glands; they are located in the axillary region, nipples, anus, and groin. Much of the odor characteristic of sweat is produced by apocrine glands.

EFFECTS OF AGING ON THE SKIN

Many of the skin changes associated with aging are the result of years of exposure to sunlight. The collagen of the dermis gradually degenerates while the epithelium thins out and the subcutaneous deposits of fat decrease. The result is a loss of elasticity so that the skin begins to wrinkle. Several lesions (localized areas of damaged skin) may develop as a result of this degeneration. *Telangiectasia* (tel-an-je-ek-tay'ze-a) is the appearance of blood vessels close to the body surface. Patches of pigment (*lentigo*, len-tie'go) or areas where pigmentation is lacking (*vitiligo*, vit-il-eye'go) may also occur. Scaly lesions called *actinic keratoses* may also develop and, in some instances, are precancerous lesions. The decrease (atrophy) in the number of sweat glands produces a decrease in the amount of sweating, thus reducing the skin's role as a thermoregulator.

CLINICAL AND PATHOLOGICAL CONDITIONS

Lesions

Lesions (lee'shuns) are damaged portions of the skin resulting from disease or injury. A lesion goes through various stages and may begin or stop at any stage; also, lesions are commonly divided into two groups: primary and secondary lesions.

Examples of lesions:

macule (mak'yul, MACUL/O spot): colored patches on the skin.

papule (pap'yul, PAPUL/O pimple): a raised area of the skin that is solid and may become suppurative.

wheal (wheel): a raised area of the skin having a white center surrounded by a red outer area—for instance, an insect bite.

vesicle (ve'sik-ul): a raised area of the skin filled with fluid.

pustule (pus'tul): a pus-filled vesicle.

blister or *bulla* (bul'la): a large vesicle.

abrasion or *excoriation:* a wearing away or scraping of the skin as a result of injury or burns.

crusts: a scab or covering of the skin either dry or exuding fluid, pus, or both.

scar: connective tissue covering a wound or sore.

keloid (key'loyd): an elevated, red scar.

Acne

Acne is an inflammation of the sebaceous glands and hair follicles caused by androgenic (ANDR/O male) hormones. Dried sebum or keratin plugs a sebaceous gland, forming a *comedo* (kom'ee-do) or blackhead. Bacteria act on the sebum, which spills over into the surrounding tissue, irritating it. As a result, a pustule is formed. In more serious forms of acne tissue is destroyed and scars occur; in some instances, scars extend to other areas of the body, such as the neck and arms.

Alopecia (al-o-pee'she-a)

Alopecia, the loss of hair, may result from aging, illness, disease, or drugs.

Ecchymosis (ek-i-mo'sis)

Ecchymosis refers to "black and blue" marks caused by hemorrhaging into the skin. *Petechiae* (pee-tee'ke-eye) are small hemorrhagic marks on the skin. *Purpura* (pur'pu-ra) or purple patches occur from hemorrhaging into the skin, mucous membranes, and other tissue.

Eczema (ek′ze-ma)

Eczema is a severe inflammation of the skin characterized by both primary and secondary lesions. Its cause is unknown; it is more common, however, among those with dry skin.

Impetigo (im-pe-tee′go)

Impetigo is an inflammatory skin disease caused by bacteria. Pustules at various stages develop. The disease appears chiefly around the mouth and nostrils.

Keratosis

A thick horny growth develops out of the epidermis. *Seborrheic keratosis* is a benign skin tumor that occurs frequently in old age. Keratosis may result from dry skin and overexposure to sunlight.

Leukoplakia (lu-ko-play′ke-a)

White patches form on the mucous membranes of the tongue, gums, and cheeks. The affected areas become dry and irritated; the lesions may become malignant. Smokers are particularly susceptible to leukoplakia.

Lupus (lou′pus, LUP/O wolf)

Lupus is an *autoimmune* (the body forms an antibody against one of its own antigens) disease characterized by a rash that appears on the face, especially the nose (called a butterfly rash). There are two types of lupus: *systemic lupus erythematosis* (erythema, er-i-thee′ma, red spots) and *discoid* (dis′koyd, dislike) *lupus erythematosis*. Systemic lupus is often a fatal form of lupus in which the vascular system and body organs, especially the kidneys, are affected. In systemic lupus the face has a rash whereas in discoid lupus scaly patches are produced.

Pemphigus (pem′fe-gus)

This is a skin disease in which groups of blisters appear and suddenly disappear, leaving pigmented spots.

Pruritus (prou-ry′tus)

Pruritus is abnormal and severe itching. It frequently accompanies other skin diseases and allergies.

Psoriasis (so-ry′a-sis)

This is a type of dermatitis in which the affected area is covered with red patches marked by a grayish scaling. The scalp, elbow, and knee are the most common areas affected.

Tinea (tin′ee-a, TINE/O worm)

Tinea is a general term for any fungus disease of the skin. Itching, red patches, and scaling are characteristic of tinea. Common forms of tinea are athlete's foot, ringworm, and jock itch.

Urticaria (ur-te-ka're-a)
Urticaria or hives are white eruptions of the skin accompanied by itching. Contact with an allergic substance is the usual cause of urticaria.

Burns
A burn is an injury to tissue as a result of overexposure to fire, heat, electricity, caustics (CAUST/O, burning), and radiation. The extent of the damage caused by burns is reported in two ways: the depth of the burn and the amount of body surface affected.

In the first method, the depth of the burn, there are three degrees.

First-degree burn. The burn is superficial and only the epidermis is injured. The skin is red and tender.

Second-degree burn. Here there is considerable destruction of the epidermis and the dermis is also affected. Blisters appear and the area is extremely painful.

Third-degree burn. Both epidermal and dermal layers are penetrated; underlying tissues, muscles, and bones may be affected. Nerves are destroyed and, as the affected area heals, *eschars* (es'karz, ESCHAR/O dead tissue mass) may form.

In the second method the amount of surface area burned is used to describe the extent of the burn. The greater the body area exposed to burns, the greater the loss of essential body fluids, accompanied by an increased chance of infection. In describing the burn in this way, each area of the body is given a certain percentage. This is known as the "rule of nines."

Head	9%
Chest	18% (front and back)
Arms	18%
Abdomen	18% (front and back)
Legs	36%
Perineum	1%
Total	100%

Skin cancers
Skin cancer is a common form of cancer, usually caused by overexposure to sunlight. The three main forms of skin cancer are *basal cell carcinoma, squamous cell carcinoma,* and *malignant melanoma.* Basal cell carcinoma is a malignant tumor developing from the epidermis. It is generally found on the face and trunk of older adults. It does not metastasize and can be easily treated. Squamous cell carcinoma originates in the keratinocytes of the epidermis. Lesions in the form of nodules and ulcers develop. The great danger is that it can metastasize to other tissue and the lymph channels. Squamous cell carcinoma is caused by an overexposure to sunlight and occurs most frequently among the elderly. Melanocytes in the epidermis are the source

of *malignant melanoma*, which most often develops from benign moles (*nevi*, ne-vie, NEV/O, mole). Melanomas are highly malignant and metastasize quickly. Nearly half of those affected die within four to six years.

EXERCISES

I. Give the meaning for each of the following medical words. Divide each word into base(s), prefix, and suffix; underline the letter(s) that has the primary stress. *Example:*

DERMATITIS   inflammation of the skin   dermat/itis

1. TRICHORRHEXIS ....

2. SUDORIFEROUS ....

3. DERMATOHETEROPLASTY (HETER/O other)

   ....

4. ACANTHOSIS ....

5. ADIPOGENOUS ....

6. HOLOTRICHOUS ....

7. PILOSIS ....

8. PACHYDERMIA (PACHY/ thick)

   ....

9. MEROGENESIS ....

10. KERATOSIS ....

11. ONYCHOPHAGY ....

12. DIAPHORETIC ....

13. TRICHOTROPHY ....

14. EPIDERMITIS ....

15. DERMATOPHYTOSIS (PHYT/O plant)

   ....

16. HOLISTIC ....

17. ONYCHITIS ....

18. ADIAPHORESIS ....

19. DERMATOMYOSITIS ....

20. PILOSEBACEOUS ....

II. Make medical words from the following phrases. Indicate the primary stress by underlining the stressed letter(s). *Example:*

under the skin

subcutaneous or hypodermic
....

1. infection of the skin caused by a fungus

....

2. pertaining to a follicle

....

3. abnormal discharge of sebum

....

4. an instrument for measuring the skin to determine the degree of subcutaneous fat

....

5. cut into parts or segments

....

6. a suppurative skin disease

....

7. resembling a thorn

....

 8. the study of the hair, its diseases, and their treatment

. . . .

 9. abnormal softening of the nails

. . . .

10. producing sweat

. . . .

11. pertaining to the skin

. . . .

12. pertaining to sweat

. . . .

13. hair-shaped

. . . .

14. abnormal accumulation of fat

. . . .

15. inflammation of the sweat glands

. . . .

III.   Match the following descriptions with their medical names.

1. the outermost layer of skin . . . .   a. melanocytes

2. the innermost layer of skin . . . .   b. holocrine gland

3. cells multiply in this layer of skin   c. apocrine gland

      . . . .   d. stratum germinativum

4. pigmented cells . . . .   e. lanugo

5. another name for the dermis . . . .   f. merocrine gland

6. the area where adipose tissue is found   g.   epidermis

....   h.   dermis

7. fine hair covering infants ....   i.   corium

8. the place where new nail growth occurs   j.   subcutaneous layer

....   k.   lunula

9. a type of gland that breaks down its

own cells to make the secretion

....

10. a sweat gland that does not destroy its

own cells to produce a secretion

....

11. the sweat gland responsible for the

offensive odor of sweat ....

      IV.   Put the layers of epidermis in their correct order. Begin with the outermost layer.

1. stratum germinativum ....

2. stratum lucidum ....

3. stratum granulosum ....

4. stratum corneum ....

      V.   Fill in the blank(s) for each of the following statements.

1. Two qualities of skin are .... and ....

2. The ability of the skin to control heat loss is called ....

3. The receptors on the skin are called ....

4. The sense of touch stimulates .... (light touch) and the

   .... (heavy touch).

5. Warmth is sensed by ...., cold by

   ....

6. The four layers of the epidermis are .... which means scaly.

7. The two layers of the skin that constitute the dermis are the .... and

   .... layers.

8. A hair can be divided into two parts: the .... and the ....

9. The fatty substance that lubricates the hair shaft is called ....

10. A damaged portion of the skin is called a ....

   VI. List the five layers of tissue that comprise the scalp.

1. S...

2. C...

3. A...

4. L...

5. P...

   VII. Multiple choice: Underline the correct letter.

1. An inflammatory skin disease of bacterial origin and chiefly affecting the mouth and
   nostrils
   (a) ecchymosis
   (b) petechia
   (c) urticaria
   (d) impetigo

2. A fluid-filled lesion
   (a) vesicle
   (b) papule
   (c) wheal
   (d) macule

3. A general term denoting a fungus disease of the skin
    (a) urticaria
    (b) pemphigus
    (c) lupus
    (d) tinea

4. A burn in which the epidermis is considerably destroyed and the dermis is also damaged
    (a) first-degree burn
    (b) second-degree burn
    (c) third-degree burn

5. White erruptions of the skin as a result of contact with an allergic substance
    (a) pruritus
    (b) tinea
    (c) urticaria
    (d) eczema

6. A solid, raised type of lesion
    (a) macule
    (b) papule
    (c) excoriation
    (d) crusts

7. "Black and blue" marks
    (a) impetigo
    (b) leukoplakia
    (c) ecchymosis
    (d) keratosis

8. A form of dermatitis characterized by red patches covered with grayish scales
    (a) pruritis
    (b) psoriasis
    (c) tinea
    (d) ecchymosis

9. The "rule of nines" refers to
    (a) the degree of subcutaneous tissue burned
    (b) the amount of surface area burned
    (c) the depth of a burn
    (d) the quality of the burn

10. A disease common among smokers and characterized by white patches on the tongue, gums, and cheeks
    (a) keratosis
    (b) leukoplakia
    (c) petechia
    (d) pemphigus

11. Abnormal, persistent itching
     (a) petechia
     (b) pruritus
     (c) alopecia
     (d) tinea

12. A burn in which eschars may form
     (a) first degree
     (b) second degree
     (c) third degree

13. A skin inflammation characterized by both primary and secondary lesions
     (a) eczema
     (b) pruritis
     (c) psoriasis
     (d) alopecia

14. A tumor developing from the scaly epidermal cells
     (a) basal cell carcinoma
     (b) squamous cell carcinoma
     (c) malignant melanoma
     (d) melanoma

15. An insect bite is a lesion called
     (a) pustule
     (b) blister
     (c) papule
     (d) wheal

16. Basal cell carcinoma is a malignant tumor of the
     (a) epidermis
     (b) dermis
     (c) subcutaneous tissue
     (d) corium

17. A progressive disease characterized by a butterfly rash on the face and renal failure
     (a) systemic lupus erythematosis
     (b) discoid lupus erythematosis
     (c) erythema
     (d) leukoplakia

18. A thick, horny growth developing from the epidermis
     (a) leukoplakia
     (b) tinea
     (c) keratosis
     (d) urticaria

19. A scab
     (a) scar
     (b) crust
     (c) excoriation
     (d) wheal

20. A superficial burn
    (a) first-degree burn
    (b) second-degree burn
    (c) third-degree burn
    (d) none of the above

21. A condition in which blisters appear and disappear, leaving spots
    (a) impetigo
    (b) lupus
    (c) leukoplakia
    (d) pemphigus

22. Patches of purple as a result of hemorrhaging into the skin
    (a) pruritis
    (b) tinea
    (c) purpura
    (d) urticaria

23. A tumor developing from the pigment-producing cells
    (a) epidermoid carcinoma
    (b) malignant melanoma
    (c) squamous cell carcinoma
    (d) basal cell carcinoma

24. The medical word for baldness
    (a) urticaria
    (b) ecchymosis
    (c) alopecia
    (d) psoriasis

ANSWERS TO EXERCISES

I.

1. splitting of the hair, trich/o/rrhexis
2. sweat producing, sudor/i/ferous
3. skin grafting using grafts from another person's skin, dermat/o/heter/o/plasty
4. abnormal thickening of the outer layer of skin, acanth/osis
5. causing the production of fat, adip/o/gen/ous
6. covered with hair (cilia), hol/o/trich/ous
7. excessive amount of hair, hirsute, pil/osis
8. abnormal thickening of the skin, pachy/derm/ia
9. reproduction by parts, segmentation, mer/o/gen/e/sis
10. any abnormal horny growth of the skin, kerat/osis
11. nail biting, onych/o/phag/y
12. producing sweat, diaphor/e/tic
13. nourishment of the hair, trich/o/trophy
14. inflammation of the outer layer of the skin, epi/derm/itis
15. fungus disease of the skin, especially athlete's foot, dermat/o/phyt/o/sis

16. pertaining to the whole, hol/istic
17. inflammation of the nail bed, onych/itis
18. absence of sweat, a/diaphor/esis
19. inflammation of connective (muscle) tissue (skin), dermat/o/myos/itis
20. pertaining to the hair and sebaceous oil glands, pil/o/seb/aceous

II.

1. dermatomycosis;　　2. follicular;　　3. seborrhea;　　4. adipometer;
5. merotomy;　　6. pyodermia;　　7. acanthoid;　　8. trichology;
9. onychomalacia;　　10. hidrotic;　　11. cutaneous;　　12. sudoral;
13. piliform;　　14. adiposis;　　15. hidroadenitis.

III.

1. g;　　2. h;　　3. d;　　4. a;　　5. i;　　6. j;　　7. e;　　8. k;　　9. b;
10. f;　　11. c.

IV.

4;　　2;　　3;　　1.

V.

1. elasticity, resiliency;　　2. thermoregulation;　　3. sensory spots;
4. Meissner's corpuscles, Pacinian corpuscles;　　5. Ruffini corpuscles, Krause corpuscles;
6. squamous;　　7. papillary, reticular;　　8. root, shaft;　　9. sebum;
10. lesion.

VI.

1. skin;　　2. connective tissue;　　3. aponeurosis;　　4. loose connective tissue;
5. periosteum.

VII.

1. (d);　　2. (a);　　3. (d);　　4. (b);　　5. (c);　　6. (b);　　7. (c);　　8. (b);
9. (b);　　10. (b);　　11. (b);　　12. (c);　　13. (a);　　14. (b);　　15. (d);
16. (a);　　17. (a);　　18. (c);　　19. (b);　　20. (a);　　21. (d);　　22. (c);
23. (b);　　24. (c).

8 The Musculoskeletal System

COMBINING FORMS

	Meaning	*Example*
THE SKELETON		
OSTE/O (os'tee-o)	bone	OSTEOBLAST (os'tee-o-blast), a bone-forming cell
CHONDR/O (kon'dro)	cartilage	CHONDRAL (kon'dral), pertaining to cartilage
MAXILL/O (maks-il'o)	the maxilla, the jawbone	MAXILLARY (maks'il-ary), pertaining to the jawbone
MANDIBUL/O (man-dib'you-lo) SUBMAXILL/O (sub-maks-il'o)	the mandible, the lower jawbone	MANDIBULAR (man-dib'you-lar), pertaining to the mandible
PALAT/O (pal'a-to)	the palate, roof of the mouth	PALATAL (pal'a-tal), pertaining to the palate
CRANI/O (kray'ne-o)	the cranium, the skull bones that enclose the brain	CRANIOTOME (kray'ne-o-tome), instrument to cut through the skull
CERVIC/O (ser'vi-ko)	the cervix, the neck	CERVICAL (ser'vi-kal), pertaining to the neck
THORAC/O (tho'ra-ko)	the thorax, the chest	THORACIC (tho-ras'ik), pertaining to the chest
LUMB/O (lum'bo)	the loins, the lower back	LUMBAR (lum'bar), pertaining to the loins or lower back
SPONDYL/O (spon'di-lo)	a vertebra	SPONDYLOSYNDESIS (spon-di-lo-sin'de-sis), surgical fixation of a joint between two vertebrae

	Meaning	*Example*
VERTEBR/O (ver'te-bro)	a vertebra	INTERVERTEBRAL (in-ter-ver'te-bral), between vertebrae
RACHI/O (ray-ke-o)	the spinal column	RACHIOTOMY (ray-ke-ot'o-me), incision of the vertebral column
LAMIN/O (lam'in-o)	a lamina, the flat bone of the neural arch of a vertebra	LAMINECTOMY (lam-in-ek'to-me), surgical removal of a lamina
MYEL/O (my'el-o)	the spinal cord, bone marrow	MYELITIS (my-e-lie'tis), inflammation of the spinal cord or bone marrow
KYPH/O (ky'fo)	humped	KYPHOSIS (ky-fo'sis), abnormal posterior curvature of the spine
SCOLI/O (sko'le-o)	curved	SCOLIOSIS (sko-le-o'sis), abnormal lateral spinal curvature
LORD/O (lor'do)	bent	LORDOSIS (lor-do'sis), abnormal anterior bending of the spine
SACR/O (sa'kro)	the sacrum, located between the fifth lumbar vertebra and coccyx	SACROILIAC (sa-kro-il'e-ak), pertaining to the sacrum and the ilium
COCCYG/O (kok'sig-o)	the coccyx, tailbone	COCCYGEAL (kok-sig'e-al), pertaining to the coccyx
COST/O (kos'to)	rib	INTERCOSTAL (in-ter-kos'tal), located between the ribs
STERN/O (ster'no)	the sternum, the breastbone	STERNOCLAVICULAR (ster-no-kla-vik'you-lar), pertaining to the sternum and the clavicle
CLAVICUL/O (kla-vik'you-lo)	the clavicle, the collarbone	CLAVICULAR (kla-vik'you-lar), pertaining to the clavicle
SCAPUL/O (skap'you-lo)	the scapula, the shoulder bone	SCAPULAR (skap'you-lar), pertaining to the scapula
ACROMI/O (a-kro'me-o)	the acromion, the portion of the scapula that articulates with the clavicle	ACROMIOCLAVICULAR (a-kro-me-o-kla-vik'you-lar), pertaining to the acromion and clavicle
HUMER/O (hu'mer-o)	the humerus, the upper arm	HUMERAL (hu'mer-al), pertaining to the humerus

	Meaning	*Example*
RADI/O (ray'de-o)	the radius, the outer bone of the forearm	RADIAL (ray'de-al), pertaining to the radius
ULN/O (ul'no)	the ulna, the inner bone of the forearm	ULNAR (ul'nar), pertaining to the ulna
OLECRAN/O (o-lek'ran-o)	the olecranon, the elbow	OLECRANAL (o-lek'ran-al), pertaining to the olecranon
CARPO (kar'po)	the carpus, the wrist	CARPAL (kar'pal), pertaining to the carpus
METACARP/O (meta-kar'po)	the metacarpals, the bones of the hand	METACARPAL (meta-kar'pal), pertaining to the metacarpals
PHALANG/O (fay-lang'o)	the phalanges, the finger or toe bones	PHALANGEAL (fa-lan'je-al), pertaining to the phalanges
PELV/O (pel'vo)	the pelvis	PELVIC (pel'vik), pertaining to the pelvis
ILI/O (il'e-o)	the ilium, the superior part of the hipbone	ILIAC (il'e-al), pertaining to the ilium
ISCHI/O (is'ke-o)	the ischium, the lower portion of the hipbone	ISCHIAL (is'ke-al), pertaining to the ischium
PUB/O or PUBI/O (pū'bō, pu'be-o)	the pubis, the pubic bone	PUBIOTOMY (pu-be-ot'o-me), incision of the pubic bone
ACETABUL/O (a-se-tab'you-lo)	the acetabulum, the saucerlike cavity of the hipbone that articulates with the head of the femur	ACETABULAR (a-se-tab'you-lar), pertaining to the acetabulum
FEMOR/O (fem'or-o)	the femur, the thighbone	FEMORAL (fem'or-al), pertaining to the femur
PATELL/O (pa-tel'o)	the patella, the kneecap	PATELLAR (pa-tel'ar), pertaining to the kneecap
TIBI/O (tib'e-o)	the tibia, the shinbone	TIBIOFEMORAL (tib-e-o-fem'or-al), pertaining to the tibia and the femur
FIBUL/O (fib'you-lo)	the fibula, the calf bone, also called the PERONEAL (per-o-ne'al) bone	FIBULAR (fib'you-lar), pertaining to the fibula
TARS/O (tar'so)	the tarsus, the ankle	TARSAL (tar'sal), pertaining to the tarsus
TAL/O (ta'lo)	the talus, the anklebone	TALAR (ta'lar), pertaining to the talus

	Meaning	*Example*
CALCANE/O (kal-kay'nee-o)	the calcaneus, the heel bone	CALCANEAL (kal-kay'nee-al), pertaining to the calcaneus
METATARS/O (me-ta-tar'so)	the metatarsals, the bones of the foot	METATARSAL (me-ta-tar'sal), pertaining to the metatarsals

THE JOINTS

	Meaning	*Example*
ARTHR/O (ar'thro)	joint	ARTHRITIS (ar-thry'tis), inflammation of a joint
ARTICUL/O (ar-tik'you-lo)	joint	ARTICULATION (ar-tik-you-lay'shun), the junction of two bones to form a joint
SYNOVI/O (sin-o've-o)	synovia, the lubricating fluid of joints	SYNOVIAL (sin-o've-al), pertaining to synovia
BURS/O (bur'so)	bursa, the sac containing synovial fluid	BURSAL (bur'sal), pertaining to a bursa
FIBR/O (fy'bro)	fiber or fibrous tissue	FIBROBLAST (fy'bro-blast), a cell that develops into fibrous tissue
TEN/O (ten'o)	tendon	TENOMYOPLASTY (ten-o-my'o-plas-te), surgical repair of a tendon and a muscle
TEND/O (ten'do)	tendon	TENDOTOME (ten'do-tome), instrument for cutting a tendon
TENDIN/O (ten'di-no)	tendon	TENDINITIS (ten-di-ny'tis), inflammation of a tendon
SYNDESM/O (sin-dez'mo)	ligament	SYNDESMOSIS (sin-dez-mo'sis), a joint where the bones are brought together by ligaments

THE MUSCLES

	Meaning	*Example*
MY/O (my'o) MYOS/O (my'o-so)	muscle	myitis (my-eye'tis) or myositis (my-o-sy'tis), inflammation of a muscle
MUSCUL/O (mus'ku-lo)	muscle	MUSCULAR (mus'ku-lar), pertaining to or having muscles
SARC/O (sar'ko)	flesh	SARCOLEMMA (sar-ko-lem'a), the thin membrane that covers a striated muscle fiber

	Meaning	*Example*
FASCI/O (fash′e-o)	fascia, a fibrous membrane that covers and separates muscles	FASCIAL (fash′e-al), pertaining to a fascia
FASCICUL/O (fa′sik′you-lo)	fasciculus, a bundle of muscle (or nerve) fibers	FASCICULAR (fa-sik′you-lar), pertaining to a fasciculus
amphi- (am′fi)	both, both sides	AMPHIARTHROSIS (am″fi-ar-thro′sis), a joint that permits slight movement in all directions
apo- (ap′o)	away, from	APONEUROSIS (ap-o-nu-ro′sis), flat connective tissue that attaches a muscle to a bone at its insertion or origin

ANATOMY OF THE SKELETON

The skeletal system (Figure 8-1) performs several important functions.

1. It gives support and shape to the body.
2. With the muscles it allows the body to move.
3. It houses and protects many of the body organs.
4. It stores minerals, such as calcium and phosphorus.
5. It helps to filter poisonous substances from the blood.

Characteristics of a Bone

A typical long bone (Figure 8-2) has two wide ends called *epiphyses* (e-pif′i-sez, -PHYSIS, growth) and a shaft termed the *diaphysis* (di-af′i-sis). The epiphyses are composed primarily of porous, or *cancellous* (kan′sel-us, CANCELL/O, lattice, reticular), bone and an outside layer of *compact bone*. The shaft, however, contains a thick layer of compact bone. The *medullary* (med′you-lar-e, MEDULL/O, marrow, inner portion) *canal* runs the length of the shaft. The canal is lined with a membrane, the *endosteum* (en-dos′te-um) and contains the substance that forms bone marrow. The *periosteal* (per-e-os′te-al) membrane covers the outer surface of the bone; it contains the bone-forming cells called *osteoblasts* (os′te-o-blasts) that enable bones to grow and repair themselves. Tendons and ligaments bind the muscles to bones or bones to bones by embedding themselves in the periosteum. The bone marrow, which is composed of netlike cells, called *reticular* (re-tik′you-lar, RETICUL/O, net) cells, produces red blood cells in the red marrow. This process is known as *hemopoiesis* (he-mo-poy-e′sis). In addition to red blood cells, the hemopoietic tissue of the bone marrow produces platelets (thrombocytes) and white blood cells (leukocytes).

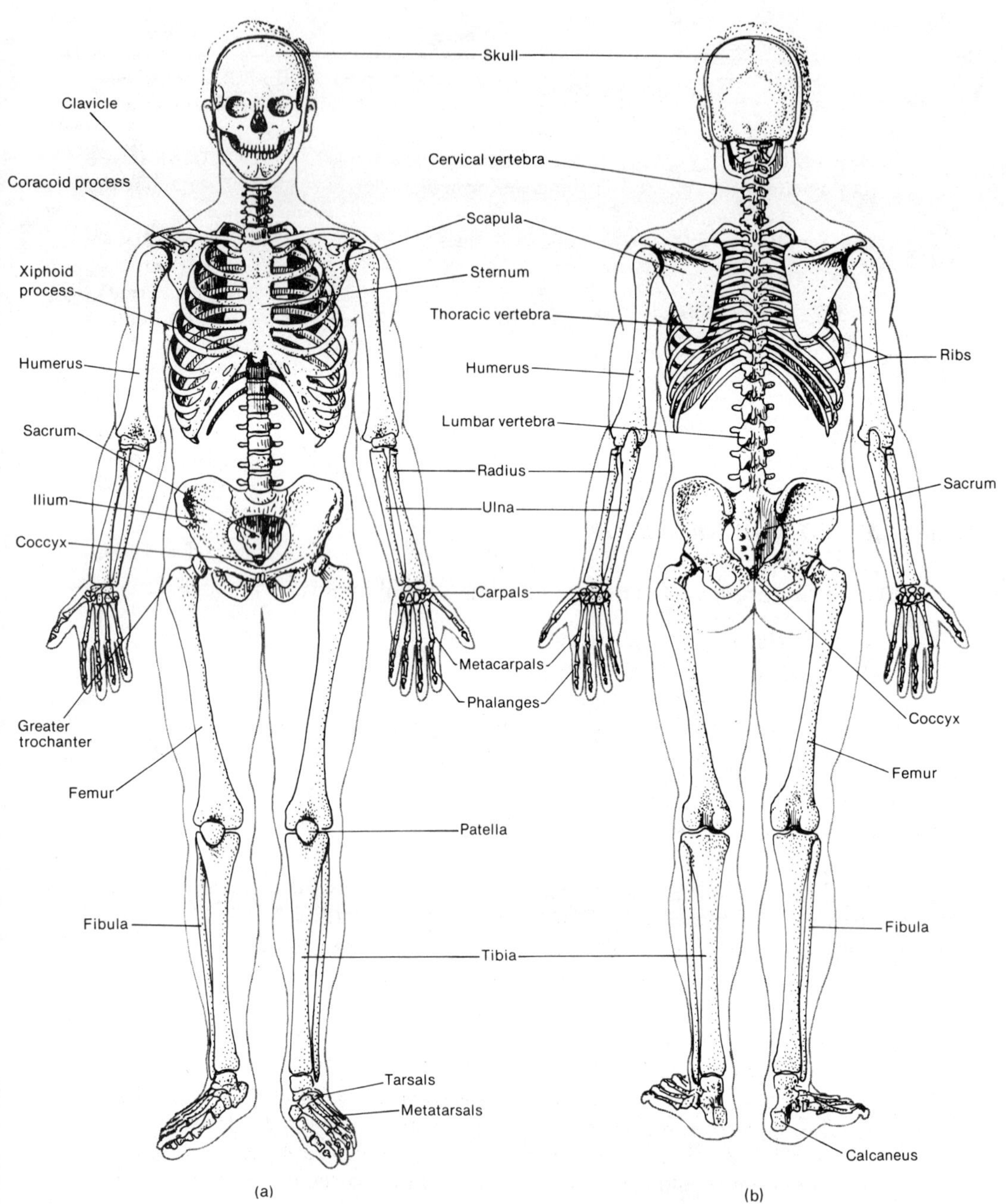

Figure 8-1 The skeleton: (a) anterior view, (b) posterior view.

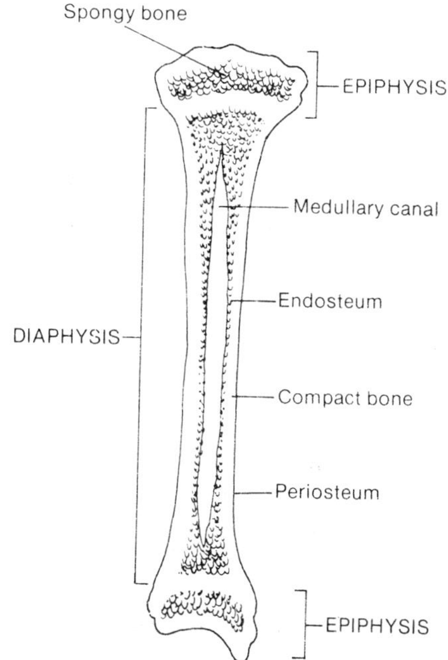

Figure 8-2 The structure of a long bone (tibia).

Besides the typical long bone, several other bone shapes exist. Like the long bone, they are composed of cancellous bone covered with a layer of compact bone; they do not, however, have a shaft. The three other bone shapes are (a) *short*, such as the wrist and anklebones, (b) *flat*, such as the rib bones, and (c) *sesamoid* (sesame seed shaped), such as the kneecap. Bones that cannot be classified as long, short, flat, or sesamoid are called *irregular* (the vertebrae).

Bones possess several types of markings, holes, and projections where they join with one another or with muscles or where blood vessels and nerves pass. You should be familiar with the following terms.

A *process* is the projecting portion of a bone.

A *fossa* (fos′a) is a shallow depression in a bone.

A *foramen* (for-a′men) is a hole in a bone through which blood vessels and nerves pass.

A *condyle* (kon′dial, CONDYL/O, knuckle) is a large process located where two bones articulate (join with one another).

An *epicondyle* (ep-e-kon′dial, EPICONDYL/O) is a process on a condyle.

A *crest* is a ridge of a bone, such as the iliac crest.

A *spine* is the pointed projection of a bone.

A *trochlea* (trok′le-a) is the smooth surface of a bone upon which another bone can smoothly move.

A *tubercle* (tou′ber-kul) is a small, round bone process.

A *trochanter* (tro-kan′ter) is either one of the two bony processes of the femur.

A *sinus* is a hollow or cavity within a bone, such as the sinuses of the skull.

A *sulcus* (sul′kus) is a groove in the bone surface.

Development of Bones

Bone tissue is made up of countless units called *Haversian* systems. Each system consists of layers of inorganic substances, such as minerals, arranged in a circle with blood, lymph, and nerve vessels passing through the middle of the circle. Mature bone cells are located in small depressions along this passage (the Haversian canal). These depressions are connected to one another by a network of canals containing cytoplasm. Compact bone consists mainly of Haversian systems whereas cancellous bone contains many spaces that contain bone-forming material.

Bones originate from the embryonic mesoderm and are initially cartilaginous or membranous. By the end of pregnancy much of this cartilage and membrane *ossifies*. Bones usually mature by age 21; growth stops around age 25. Throughout life, however, osteoblasts produce new bone and old bone is broken down and absorbed by osteoclasts (-clast, break).

Cartilage

Cartilage is a gristlelike substance found on bones at the places where they articulate. Cartilage, which is rather flexible because of its gel-type matrix (may′triks, the substance from which something is made), reduces both friction and shock. Its cells, *chondrocytes*, receive nutrients and oxygen by the diffusion of these substances from the capillaries of the *perichondrium*, the fibrous covering of cartilage. The most common form of cartilage is *hyaline* (hi′a-lin, HYAL/O, glass) cartilage; elastic and fibrous cartilage are less common.

The Axial Skeleton

The axial skeleton consists of bones of the skull, the vertebral column, bones of the thorax, and the hyoid bone.

The Skull Bones: Facial

Nasal bones.   These two thin bones form the upper portion of the bridge of the nose. (See Figure 8-3.)

Maxillae.   These two bones form the upper jaw and most of the palate.

Zygomatic bones.   The two cheekbones.

Mandible.   The lower jawbone.

Palatine bones.   With the maxillae they form the palate.

Vomer.   This small, plough-shaped (vomer) bone forms the posterior portion of the partition (called a *septum*, sep'tum) between the two nasal cavities.

Lacrimal (lak're-mal) *bones.*   These bones help form the lateral wall of each nasal cavity and the middle wall of the eye socket.

Conchae (kon'kae, concha, shell).   Shell-like bones that project from the sides of the nasal cavity.

The Skull Bones: Cranial

Occipital bone.   Forms the base and underside of the skull. Through a large opening, the *foramen magnum*, the spinal cord enters the skull. (See Figures 8-4 and 8-5).

Parietal bones.   These bones form the upper sides and roof of the skull.

Frontal bone.   The bone of the forehead. It forms the top portion of each eye socket and separates the skull interior from the nasal cavities.

Temporal bones.   Form the lower sides and base of the cranium. Each temporal bone houses the middle and internal portion of the ear.

Ethmoid bone.   An irregularly shaped bone located deep within the skull. It supports the nasal cavity, and through its process, the *cribriform* (sieve-shaped) *plate*, branches of the olfactory nerve pass.

Sphenoid (wedge-shaped) *bone.*   The "butterfly"-shaped bone in the base of the skull. It helps to support the brain, and through one of its openings, the *optic foramen*, the optic nerve passes.

The cranial bones are joined at points called *sutures* (seams) that look like jagged lines on the surface of the skull. There are four of these immovable joints: the *coronal* (crown shaped), the *sagittal* (arrow shaped), the *squamous* (scalelike), and the *lambdoidal* (resembling the Greek letter lambda: Λ). A fifth, the *metopic suture*, occurs when the frontal bones do not completely fuse.

At birth there are six areas of the cranium where bone formation is incomplete. These *fontanels* (fon-ta-nel'z), which are nothing more than membrane covered by the scalp, allow for bone movement and brain growth. By age 2 all fontanels are replaced by bone. (See Figure 8-6).

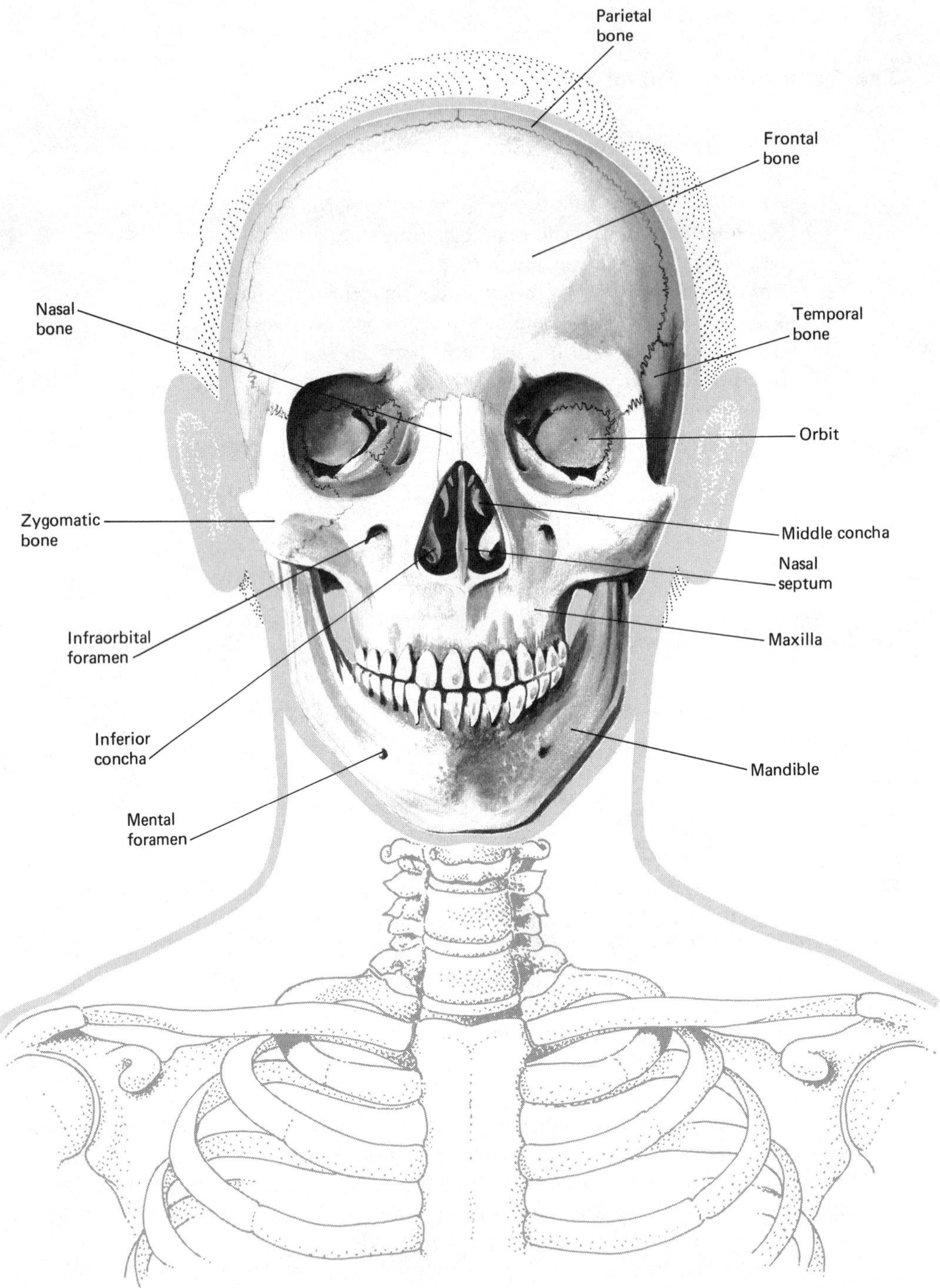

Figure 8-3 The skull, front view.

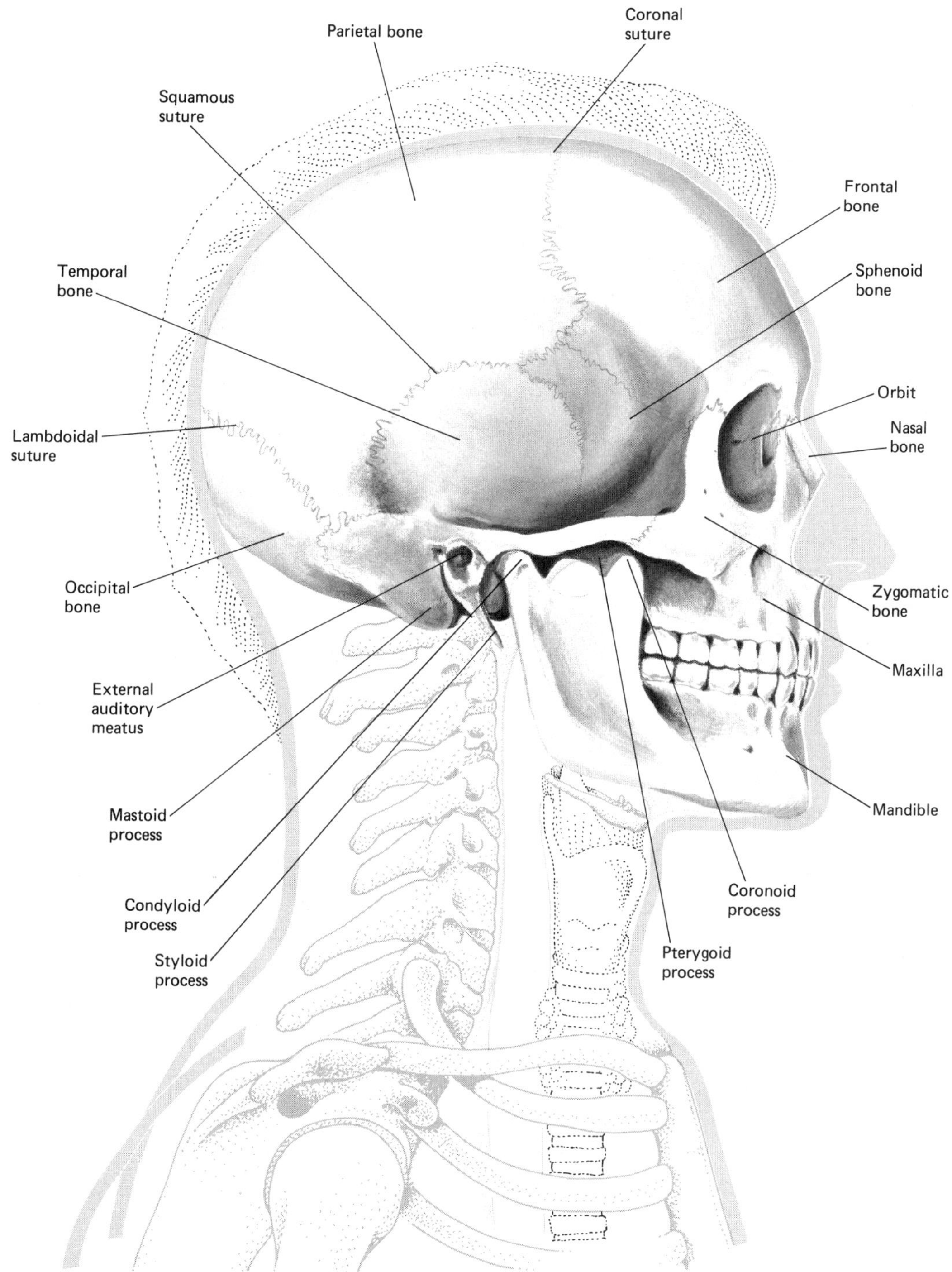

Figure 8-4 The skull, lateral view.

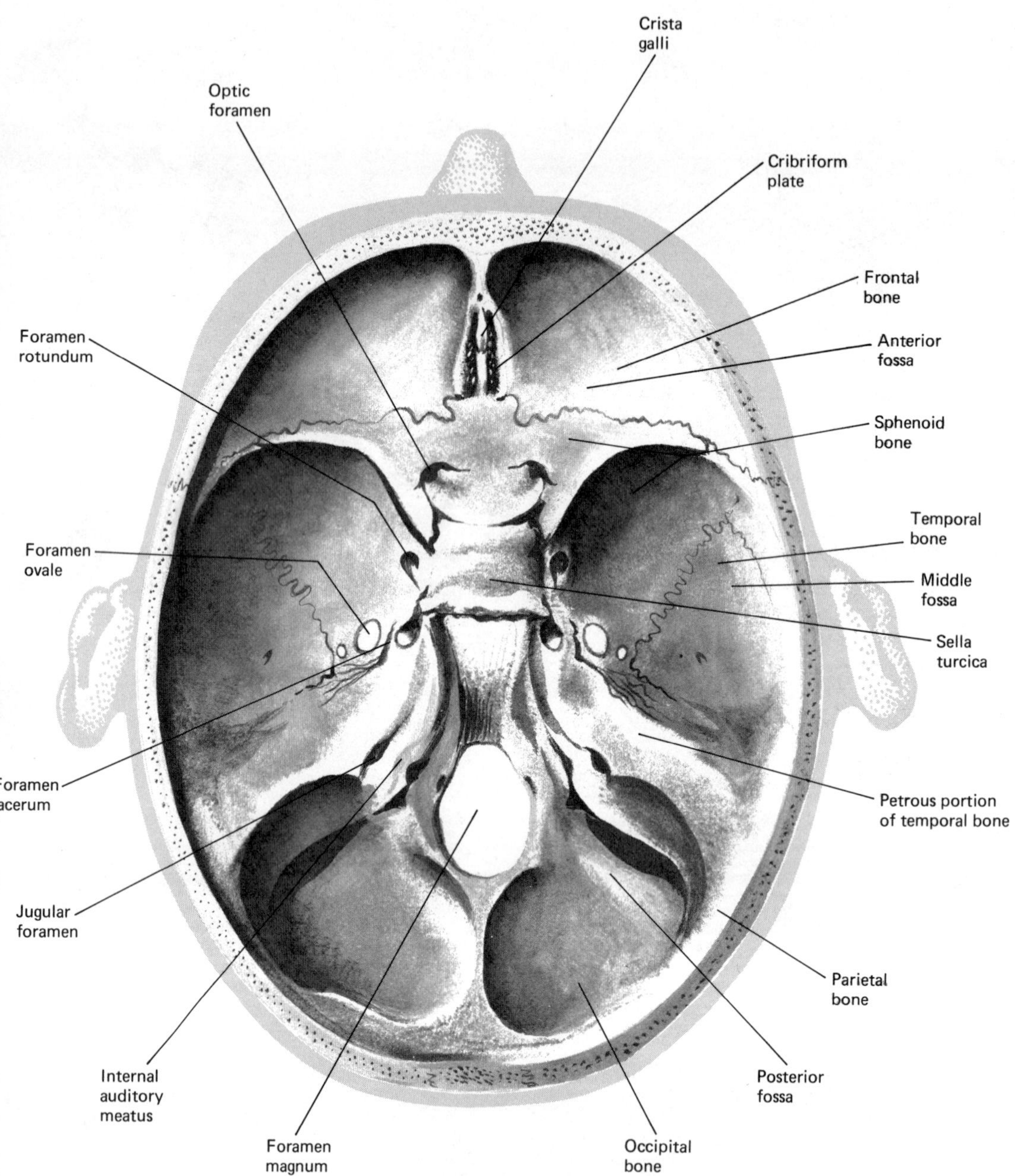

Figure 8-5   The floor of the cranium.

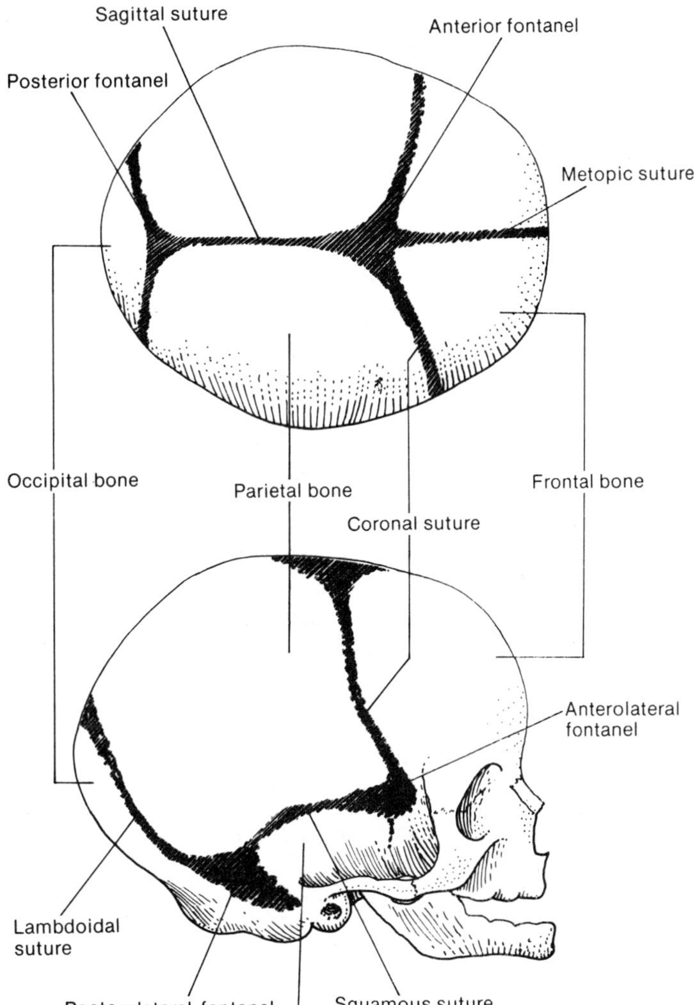

Figure 8-6
The sutures
and fontanels.

The Vertebral Column

The vertebral column (Figure 8-7) is a set of bones arranged one on the other that extend from the base of the skull to the pelvic region. The vertebra column is divided into five sets.

1. The *cervical* portion
2. The *thoracic* portion (The ribs are attached to this portion.)
3. The *lumbar* portion
4. The *sacral* portion (In the adult this is fused into one triangular-shaped bone.)
5. The *coccygeal* portion (fused into what we call the tailbone)

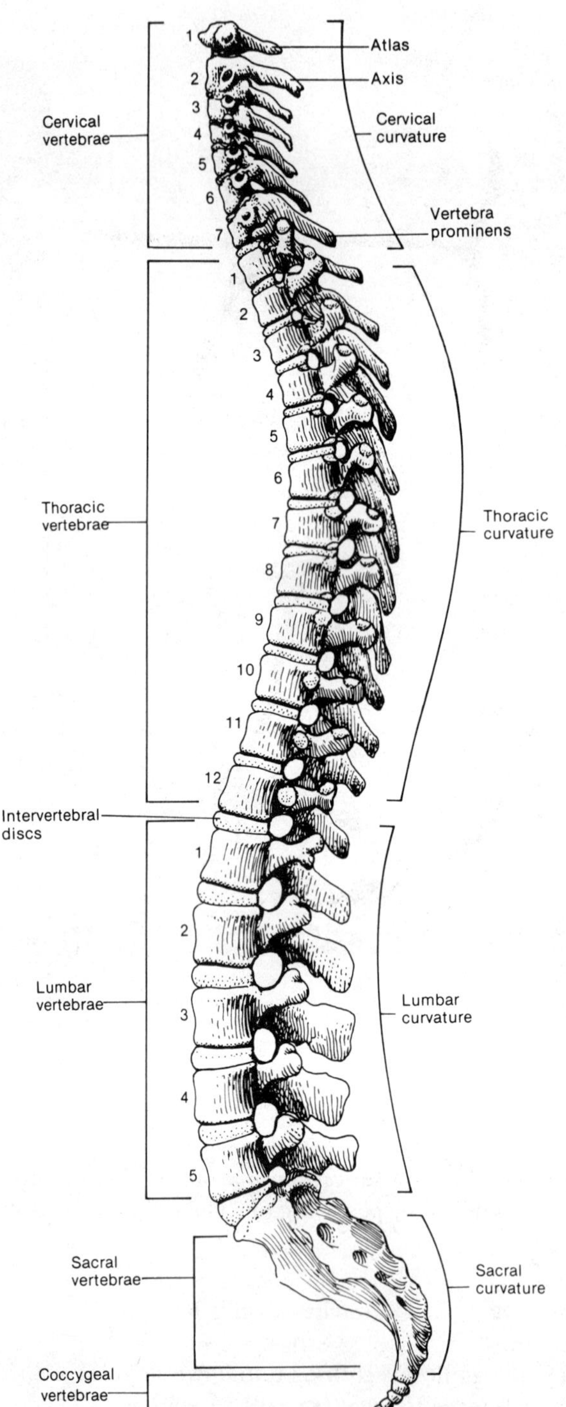

Figure 8-7 The vertebral column, showing the different types of vertebrae and curvatures.

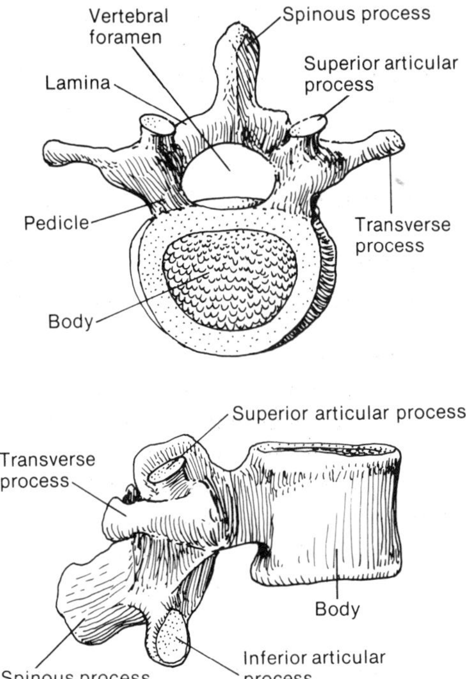

Figure 8-8   A vertebra

A typical vertebra (Figure 8-8) has a body called a *centrum* and an arched portion, called the *neural arch*, that encloses the spinal cord. The neural arch is formed by several processes joined by flat bones called *laminae*.

Bones of the Thorax

Ribs

There are 12 (sometimes 11 or 13) pairs of ribs. All the ribs are attached posteriorly to the vertebral column. The first ten pairs are joined anteriorly to the sternum. The last two pairs are called *floating ribs* because they are not attached to the sternum. (See Figure 8-1.)

Sternum

The sternum, or breastbone, provides a place for both the ribs and the clavicles to articulate. The sternum has three parts: the upper bone, called the *manubrium* (ma-nu'bri-um, handle shaped), the *body*, and the *xiphoid* (zif'oyd, sword-shaped) process.

Hyoid Bone

The *hyoid* (hi'oyd, U-shaped) bone is located in the throat region where it is attached to some of muscles of the tongue and floor of the mouth; it is not joined to any other bone.

The Appendicular Skeleton

The appendicular skeleton consists of bones of the shoulder girdle and upper extremity and bones of the pelvic girdle and lower extremity. (See Figure 8-1).

Bones of the Shoulder Girdle and Upper Extremity

These bones are attached to the rest of the skeletal system by means of the *clavicles* (the collarbones) and the large, triangular breastbones, the *scapulae*. The sternoclavicular articulation is the only point at which the upper extremity is connected to the rest of the skeletal system.

Humerus.   The upper arm bone.

Radius and ulna.   Bones of the forearm. The radius is the shorter of the two bones and revolves partially around the ulna.

Carpus.   The carpus or wrist bone is actually two sets of four bones. The carpal bones not only join the hand and forearm but also allow a variety of wrist movements.

Metacarpals.   The bones of the hand.

Phalanges.   The 14 finger bones.

Bones of the Pelvic Girdle and Lower Extremity

Os coxae (os kok' si, hipbone).   A fusion of three bones: the *ilium*, which is the largest of the pelvic bones; the *ischium*, the lower portion of the hipbone; and the *pubis*, the pubic bone. The *rami* (ra'my, RAM/O, branch), branches or extensions of both the pubis and ischium, form a good portion of the *obturator* (ob'tou-ray-tor, obstructor) *foramen*, the largest hole in the skeleton. (See Figure 8-1.)

Femur.   The thighbone. It extends from the hip to the knee and is the largest and strongest bone in the skeleton.

Patella.   The kneecap, a flat, sesmoidal bone located in front of the knee in the tendon of the quadriceps femoris muscle.

Tibia.   The shinbone.

Fibula.   The calf bone. It is not part of the knee joint but articulates with the tibia at its proximal end and with the tibia and talus at its distal end.

Bones of the Ankle and Foot

Tarsals.   The seven bones of the ankle: *talus, calcaneus, navicular* (na-vik'you-lar), *cuboid* (ku'boid), and three *cuneiform* (ku-nee'i-form).

Metatarsals.   The five foot bones between the ankle and toe bones.

Phalanges.   The 14 toe bones. (See Figure 8-9.)

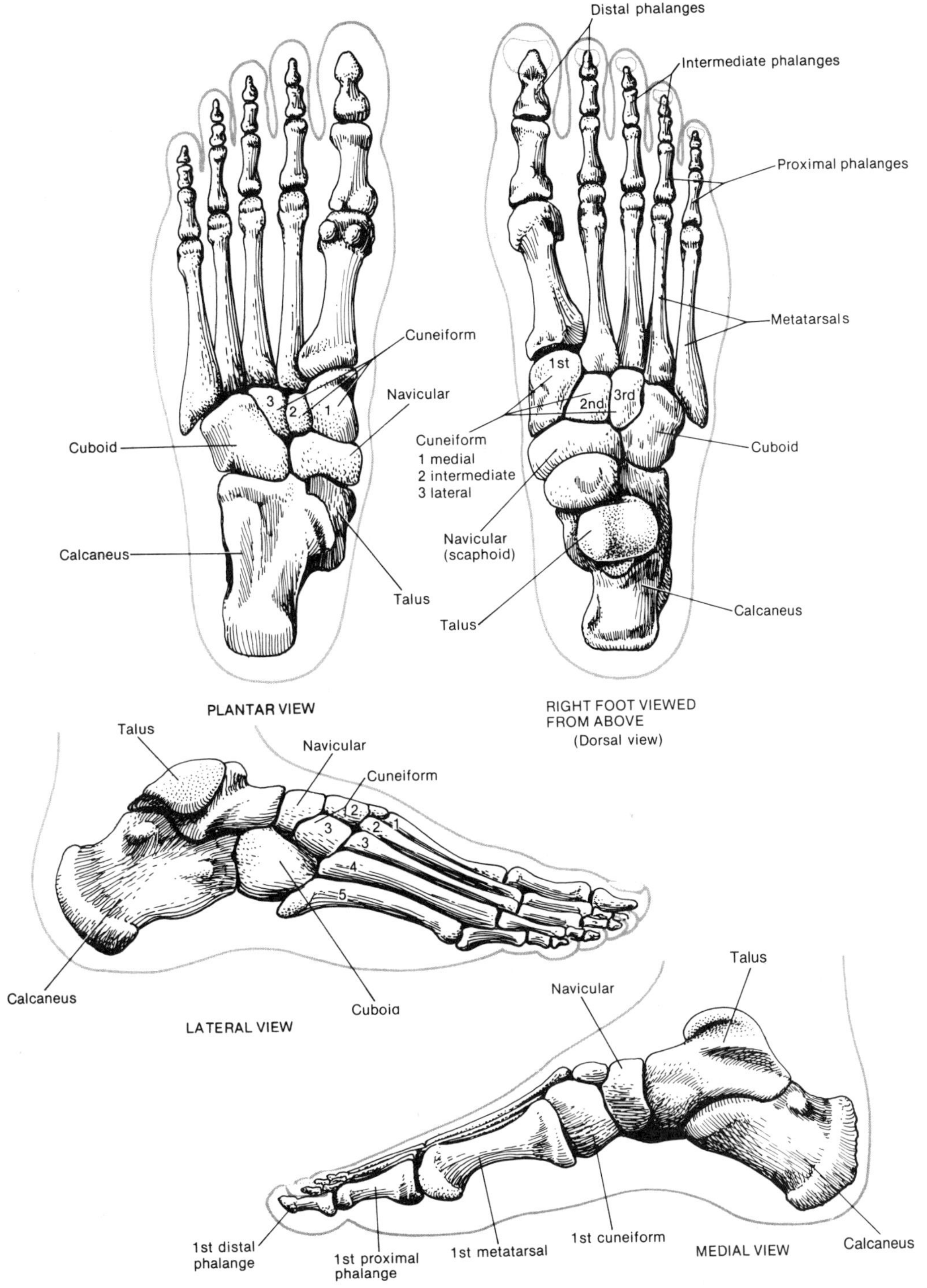

Figure 8-9 Bones of the right ankle and foot

THE JOINTS

Joints or *articulations* are the sites at which bones come together. Movable bones have joints that are held together by *ligaments* (connect bones to bones), *fibrous joint capsules*, and *muscles* (held to bones by *tendons*). Capsulated joints have joint cavities that are covered with a membrane called the *synovial membrane*, which secretes *synovial fluid*, a clear lubricating fluid. Near many joints are little sacs, *bursae*, which also secrete synovial fluid. Some joints have cartilaginous discs (such as the intervertebral disc) that help to reduce friction.

Types of Joints

Synarthrodial (sin-arth-ro'de-al)
No joint cavity, no movement. There are three forms of synarthrodial joints.
    Suture.   Found in the bones of the skull.
    Synchondrosis (sin-kon-dro'sis).   Maturing bone composed of hyaline cartilage.
    Syndesmosis (sin-des-mo'sis).   A joint held together by ligaments.

Amphiarthrodial (am-fe-ar-thro'de-al)
Only slight movement is permitted, as in the joints of the vertebrae.

Diarthrodial (dy-ar-thro'de-al)
These joints permit a maximum amount of movement. Diarthrodial joints are divided into the following categories.
    Gliding or arthrodial.   As in the joints between the carpals.
    Pivot or trochoid (tro'koid).   As in the articulation of the radius and the humerus.
    Hinge or ginglymus (jing'le-mus).   As in the kneecap.
    Saddle or biaxial.   As in the radiocarpal articulation.
    Ball-and-socket.   As in the shoulder joints.

THE MUSCLES

Muscles are responsible for our body movements. *Contractility* is the quality that enables them to cause movement.

Classification of Muscles

Smooth (LEIOMY/O, ly-o-my'o)
Also called *involuntary* because we have no control over them. The cells are spindle

shaped and arranged in layers. Smooth muscles are found mainly in the internal organs.

Cardiac (CARDIOMY/O)

Involuntary muscles of the heart, an intermediate type between the smooth and the skeletal muscles. The muscle fibers (the name given to muscle cells) are striated (marked with stripes) and are formed into a network where the cell nuclei form a *syncytium* (sin-sit'e-um), a multinucleate mass of protoplasm.

Skeletal (RHABDOMY/O, rab-do-my'o)

Voluntary muscle attached to the skeleton. The muscle fibers are grouped in bundles called *fasciculi* (fa-sik'you-lie)—hence the origin of the name (RHABD/O, rod). Each muscle fiber is surrounded by a thin membrane, the *sarcolemma* (sar-ko-lem'a).

Muscle Attachments

Skeletal muscles are attached to a fixed bone on one end, called the *origin*, and to a movable bone, called the *insertion*, on the other. A muscle may be directly attached to the periosteum of the bone or may be attached indirectly by cords of connective tissue called *tendons* or by flat sheets of connective tissue called *aponeuroses* (a-po-new-row'sez).

CLINICAL AND PATHOLOGICAL CONDITIONS

The Bones

Fractures

Broken bones are called fractures. Fractures occur as the result of too much stress being placed on a bone. *Simple fractures* involve only a broken bone. In a *compound fracture* the bone protrudes through the skin. Fractures heal in the following manner.

1. A blood clot forms at the site of the fracture.
2. Fibroblasts and osteoblasts produce collagen.
3. A *callus* develops and connective tissue forms.
4. The connective tissue ossifies.

Osteomyelitis

The bone and bone marrow become inflamed as a result of a bacterial infection. The inflammation becomes *abscessed* (pus deposits form) and the portion of bone affected dies. A bone that has undergone *necrosis* or death is called a *sequestrum* because it becomes detached from surrounding tissue. Treatment is with antibiotics and the removal of dead tissue.

Metabolic bone disorders (osteodystrophy, os-te-o-dis'tro-fe)

Osteitis deformans (also called Paget's disease).   This bone disease occurs in older people and is caused by the excessive reabsorption and repair of bones. The long bones thicken and the flat bones lose their shape. Body height diminishes and the skull becomes enlarged, making the face look small and irregular.

Osteitis fibrosa cystica.   The overactivity of the parathyroid glands causes the bones to decalcify so that they become soft (osteomalacia) and porous (osteoporosis).

Rickets (rachitis).   This is an inflammation of the spine. Occurring in children, rickets is a softening of the bones as a result of a vitamin D deficiency that inhibits the body's ability to absorb calcium and phosphorus, both essential for normal bone formation. In adults rickets is called *osteomalacia.*

Bone tumors

Osteoma.   An osteoma is a benign bone tumor that frequently arises in the skull.

Osteoid osteoma.   This benign bone tumor is accompanied by severe pain.

Osteogenic sarcoma.   This is a malignant tumor developing from bone tissue. It spreads rapidly to other parts of the body, especially the lungs. The prognosis is usually poor.

Multiple myeloma.   This is a malignant tumor originating in the bone marrow.

Cartilaginous tumors

Osteochondromas (classified as an *exostosis*, a bony protrusion).   These are benign tumors that develop at the metaphysis of a bone. They are composed of both bone and cartilage.

Enchondromas.   These are benign cartilaginous tumors forming inside bone cavities.

Chondrosarcomas.   These are malignant tumors developing from cartilage.

The Joints

Dislocation

A dislocation is the separation of a bone from its position in a joint. Dislocations occur as a result of pulling or stretching movements that put severe strain on the joints. For example, falling with one's arm in an extended position can cause the scapulo-humeral joint to become dislocated.

Sprain

A sprain is a traumatic joint injury involving the tearing of ligaments and muscles. It causes both pain and swelling.

Arthritis

Arthritis is an inflammation of the joints and is the most commonly occurring disease of the joints. There are several forms of arthritis; the most common are listed below.

Rheumatoid arthritis (rou'ma-toid, RHEUMAT/O discharge).   This is a chronic form of arthritis that results in severe deformities. It usually begins in the joints of the hand, which become stiff in the morning. The synovial membrane of the hand joints becomes swollen and the synovial fluid becomes thick. Eventually granulated tissue forms between the synovium and the cartilage and spreads to the bone itself.

Gouty arthritis.   This form of arthritis is usually associated with arthritis of the knee or foot but can affect any joint. It is caused by an excess of uric acid in the blood (*hyperuricemia*, hi-per-your-i-see'me-a).

The Muscles

Muscular dystrophy

This is a progressive destruction of the muscle fibers. At first muscles appear to be developing normally but are, in fact, being replaced by fat tissue (the process is called *pseudohypertrophy*, PSEUD/O false), which leads to a general atrophy of muscle tissue.

Neurogenic muscular disease

The blocking of nerve impulses to the muscles causes them to atrophy (become reduced in size). The muscle decreases in size and is weakened but is capable of sensory stimulation. Polio and *myasthenia gravis* (my-as-then'e-a gra'vis) are examples of neurogenic muscular diseases.

Muscle tumors

A *rhabdomyoma* is a benign tumor originating in skeletal muscle. A *rhabdomyosarcoma* is a malignant tumor of the skeletal muscle. Rhabdomyosarcomas spread rapidly and have an unfavorable prognosis.

EXERCISES

I.   Give the meaning for each of the following medical words. Divide each word into bases, prefix and suffix; underline the letter or letters that have the primary stress. *Example:*

OSTEITIS   inflammation of a bone   oste/<u>i</u>tis

1. CHONDROLYSIS   ....

2. ILIOFEMORAL   ....

  3. KYPHOTIC ....

  4. MAXILLITIS ....

  5. ARTHRORRHAGIA ....

  6. SYNOVIOMA ....

  7. THORACOCENTESIS ....

  8. OSTEOCLAST ....

  9. CRANIOMALACIA ....

10. TENODESIS ....

11. SARCOGENIC ....

12. PHALANGECTOMY ....

13. SPONDYLALGIA ....

14. STERNOCOSTAL ....

15. SYNDESMOPEXY ....

16. MYITIS or MYOSITIS ....

     ....

17. MYELITIS ....

18. SCOLIOSOMETRY ....

19. VERTEBRECTOMY ....

20. RACHITIS ....

21. ACROMIAL ....

22. ARTHROTOME ....

23. TENDINOPLASTY ....

24. PUBIC ....

25. SYNOVITIS ....

> **II.** Make medical words from the following phrases. Indicate the primary stress by underlining the stressed letter(s). *Example:*
>
> pertaining to the cartilage of the rib
>
> chondro<u>cos</u>tal

....

1. pertaining to the thoracic and lumbar regions

....

2. excision of the coccyx

....

3. pertaining to the scapula and clavicle

....

4. to form a joint

....

5. inflammation of the synovial membrane of a joint

....

6. inflammation of the sac containing synovial fluid

....

7. fleshy (cancerous) tumor

....

8. surgical reshaping of the palate

....

9. formation or production of cartilage

....

10. (congenital) split of the vertebral column

....

11. pertaining to the sacrum and coccyx bones

....

12. formation of bone marrow

....

13. inflammation of the synovial membrane of a tendon

....

14. tumor composed of muscle tissue

....

15. inflammation of cartilage

....

16. breaking down of a vertebra

....

17. anterior and lateral curvature of the spine

....

18. excision of a rib

....

19. swelling of a joint (-edema, swelling)

....

20. elbow shaped

....

21. softening of muscle tissue

....

22. pertaining to the loins and ribs

....

23. pertaining to the lower jaw

....

24. surgical fastening of a joint

....

25. suture of a ligament

....

III.   Match the following bones with their medical names.

1. tailbone ....   a.   maxilla

2. elbow ....   b.   mandible

3. ankle ....   c.   palate

4. collarbone ....   d.   cranium

5. upper jawbone ....   e.   coccyx

6. kneecap ....   f.   sternum

7. upper arm bone ....   g.   clavicle

8. roof of the mouth ....   h.   scapula

9. hand bones ....   i.   humerus

10. heel bone ....   j.   ulna

11. lower jawbone ....   k.   olecranon

12.	calf bone	l.	carpus
13.	thighbone	m.	metacarpals
14.	shinbone	n.	phalanges
15.	the bones of the head	o.	femur
16.	a bone of the forearm	p.	patella
17.	breastbone	q.	tibia
18.	wrist	r.	fibula
19.	shoulder bone	s.	tarsus
20.	foot bones	t.	talus
21.	finger or toe bones	u.	calcaneus
22.	anklebones	v.	metatarsals

IV. Give the meaning for the following medical words; indicate the primary stress by underlining the stressed letter(s).

1. epiphyses ....

2. diaphysis ....

3. cancellous ....

4. compact bone ....

5. medullary canal ....

6. periosteum ....

7. osteoblast ....

8. hemopoiesis ....

V. Multiple choice: Choose only one answer.

1. A projecting portion of a bone is known as a
   (a) fossa
   (b) process
   (c) sulcus
   (d) sinus

2. A *foramen* is a
   (a) groove in a bone
   (b) ridge of a bone
   (c) small, round bone process
   (d) hole in a bone

3. A large bone process located where two bones articulate is called a
   (a) condyle
   (b) sinus
   (c) sulcus
   (d) crest

4. A groove in the surface of a bone is known as a
   (a) epicondyle
   (b) sulcus
   (c) spine
   (d) trochlea

5. A *fossa* is a
   (a) small, rounded bone process
   (b) hole in a bone
   (c) ridge of a bone
   (d) shallow depression in a bone

6. A hollow or cavity within a bone is called a
   (a) sinus
   (b) trochanter
   (c) process
   (d) foramen

VI. From the following list make two groups of bones: bones of the face and bones
of the skull.

	Bones of the Face	*Bones of the Skull*
1. palatine bones	....	....
2. conchae	....	....
3. frontal bone	....	....
4. mandible	....	....
5. occipital bone	....	....
6. parietal bone	....	....
7. sphenoid bone	....	....

	Bones of the Face	*Bones of the Skull*
8. maxillae	....	....
9. zygomatic bones	....	....
10. temporal bones	....	....
11. vomer	....	....
12. ethmoid bone	....	....
13. lacrimal bones	....	....

VII. Put the five portions of the vertebral column in order.

1. lumbar ....

2. coccygeal ....

3. thoracic ....

4. cervical ....

5. sacral ....

VIII. Match the following.

1. "soft" spots on a baby's head ....   a. bursae

2. the type of joint found on the skull ....   b. synarthrodial

3. a joint that permits no movement ....   c. tendons

4. a joint that permits slight movement ....   d. aponeurosis

5. a joint that permits maximum movement ....   e. smooth

6. a clear fluid that lubricates joints ....   f. suture

7. sacs that contain the fluid that lubricates   g. cardiac

joints ....   h. fasciculi

8. involuntary muscles found chiefly in the internal

   organs ....

9. involuntary muscles of the heart ....

10. striated, voluntary muscles ....

11. bundles of muscle fibers ....

12. connect bones to bones ....

13. hold muscles to bones ....

14. immovable bone to which a muscle is attached ....

15. movable bone to which a muscle is attached ....

16. flat sheet of connective tissue that attaches a muscle to

    a bone ....

i. ligaments

j. synovial

k. amphiarthrodial

l. fontanels

m. skeletal

n. origin

o. diarthrodial

p. insertion

    IX. Match the following descriptions with their medical names.

1. a break in a bone ....

2. inflammation of both the bone and bone

   marrow ....

3. pus deposits ....

4. a general term for metabolic bone disorders ....

5. a bone disease occurring among the elderly and
   characterized by a reduction in body height and an

   enlarged skull ....

6. dead bone tissue ....

7. a bone disease occurring in children and caused by a

   vitamin D deficiency ....

a. osteitis fibrosa
   cystica

b. rheumatoid arthritis

c. muscular dystrophy

d. chondrosarcoma

e. rhabdomyosarcoma

f. sequestrum

g. osteoma

h. sprain

i. fracture

8. bone disease caused by a hypersecretion of the parathyroid glands ....

9. a malignancy of the bone marrow ....

10. benign tumors of the metaphysis of a bone ....

11. a malignancy developing from bone tissue ....

12. the separation of a bone from its position in a

    joint ....

13. chronic inflammation of the joints, usually beginning in

    the joints of the hand ....

14. a progressive destruction of muscular fibers that causes

    the muscles to atrophy ....

15. an example of a neurogenic muscular disease ....

16. a malignant muscle tumor ....

17. injury to a joint involving the tearing of ligaments and

    muscles ....

18. arthritis resulting from an excess of uric acid in the

    blood ....

19. a benign bone tumor ....

20. a malignant tumor developing from cartilage ....

j. osteochondromas

k. osteogenic sarcoma

l. osteitis deformans

m. abscesses

n. gout

o. osteomyelitis

p. rickets

q. multiple myoma

r. myasthenia gravis

s. dislocation

t. osteodystrophy

ANSWERS TO EXERCISES

I.

1. breaking down of cartilage, chondr/o/lysis
2. pertaining to the ilium and femur, ili/o/femor/al
3. pertaining to kyphosis, kyph/o/tic
4. inflammation of the upper jawbone, maxill/itis
5. hemorrhaging into a joint, arthr/o/rrhagia
6. a tumor developing from a synovial membrane, synovi/oma
7. surgical puncture of the thoracic cavity to remove fluid, thorac/o/centesis

8. cell that breaks up and absorbs bone matter, oste/o/clast
9. softening of the skull bones, crani/o/malacia
10. surgical fastening of a tendon, ten/o/desis
11. pertaining to that which produces flesh or muscle, sarc/o/gen/ic
12. excision of one or more of the phalanges, phalang/ectomy
13. pain in a vertebra, spondyl/algia
14. pertaining to the sternum and ribs, stern/o/cost/al
15. surgical fastening of a ligament, syndesm/o/pexy
16. inflammation of a muscle, my/itis, myos/itis
17. inflammation of the spinal cord or bone marrow, myel/itis
18. measurement of the degree of spinal curvature, scolios/o/metry
19. excision of a vertebra, vertebr/ectomy
20. inflammation of the spine, rickets, rach/itis
21. pertaining to the acromion process, acromi/al
22. instrument for cutting a joint, arthr/o/tome
23. surgical repair of tendon, tendin/o/plasty
24. pertaining to the pubis, pub/ic
25. inflammation of a synovial membrane, synov/itis

II.

1. thoracolumbar;   2. coccygectomy;   3. scapuloclavicular;   4. articulate;
5. arthrosynovitis;   6. bursitis;   7. sarcoma;   8. palatoplasty;
9. chondrogenesis;   10. rachischisis;   11. sacrococcygeal;   12. myelopoiesis;
13. tenosynovitis;   14. myoma;   15. chondritis;   16. spondylosis;
17. lordoscoliosis;   18. costectomy;   19. arthredema;   20. olecranoid;
21. myomalacia;   22. lumbocostal;   23. mandibular, or submaxillary;
24. arthrodosis;   25. syndesmorrhaphy.

III.

1. e;   2. k;   3. s;   4. g;   5. a;   6. p;   7. i;   8. c;   9. m;
10. u;   11. b;   12. r;   13. o;   14. q;   15. d;   16. j;   17. f;
18. l;   19. h;   20. v;   21. n;   22. t.

IV.

1. epiphyses, the wide ends of long bones
2. diaphysis, the shaft of a long bone
3. cancellous, porous bone
4. compact bone, hard bone
5. medullary canal, a bone's inner portion that runs through the shaft
6. periosteum, the membrane that covers the outer surface of a bone
7. osteoblast, bone-forming cell
8. hemopoiesis, the production of blood cells in the red bone marrow

V.

1. (b);   2. (d);   3. (a);   4. (b);   5. (d);   6. (a).

VI.

Bones of the Face	Bones of the Skull
8	5
9	6
4	3
1	10
11	12
13	7
2	

VII.

1. 4;   **2.** 3;   **3.** 1;   **4.** 5;   **5.** 2.

VIII.

1. l;   **2.** f;   **3.** b;   **4.** k;   **5.** o;   **6.** j;   **7.** a;   **8.** e;   **9.** g;
10. m;   **11.** h;   **12.** i;   **13.** c;   **14.** n;   **15.** p;   **16.** d.

IX.

1. i;   **2.** o;   **3.** m;   **4.** t;   **5.** l;   **6.** f;   **7.** p;   **8.** a;   **9.** q;
10. j;   **11.** k;   **12.** s;   **13.** b;   **14.** c;   **15.** r;   **16.** e;   **17.** h;
18. n;   **19.** g;   **20.** d.

9 The Nervous System

COMBINING FORMS

	Meaning	*Example*
NEUR/O (new'ro)	nerve	NEUROBLAST (new'ro-blast), nerve-forming cell
MYELIN/O (my-el-in'-o)	myelin, fatty substance covering nerve fibers	MYELINIC (my-el-in'ic), composed of or containing myelin
MYEL/O (my-el'o)	spinal cord	MYELOCELE (my-el'o-seel), herniation of the spine, spina bifida with sac
GLI/O (gle'o)	glue, adhesive	NEUROGLIA (new-rog'lee-a), nontransmitting, supportive nervous tissue
ASTR/O (as'tro)	star shaped	ASTROGLIA (as-trog'-lee-a), a type of neuroglia
OLIG/O (o-le'go)	few, deficient in	OLIGODENDROGLIA (o-lee-go-den-drog'lee-a), another type of neuroglia
MICR/O (my-kro)	small	MICROGLIA (my-krog'lee-a), a neuroglia that acts as a phagocyte
GANGLI/O (gang'le-o) GANGLION/O (gang'le-on-o)	a ganglion, a collection of nerve cell bodies outside the central nervous system	GANGLIONIC (gang'le-on-ic), pertaining to a ganglion GANGLIAL (gang'le-al), pertaining to a ganglion

	Meaning	*Example*
CEREBR/O (ser'e-bro)	the cerebrum	CEREBRAL (ser'e-bral), pertaining to the cerebrum
CEREBELL/O (ser-e-bel'lo)	the cerebellum	CEREBELLAR (ser-e-bel'lar), pertaining to the cerebellum
ENCEPHAL/O (en-sef'a-lo)	brain	ENCEPHALOMENINGO-CELE (en-sef-a-lo-mening'go-seal) saclike protrusion of the brain and protective membranes through the cranium
VENTRICUL/O (ven-trik'u-lo)	a small hollow or cavity, a ventricle of the brain	VENTRICULAR (ven-trik'u-lar), pertaining to a ventricle
MES/O (mez'o)	middle	MESENCEPHALON (mez-en-sef'a-lon), midbrain
THALAM/O (thal'a-mo)	the thalamus	THALAMIC (thal-am'ik), pertaining to the thalamus
MENING/O (men-in'go) MENINGI/O (men-in'je-o)	meninges, membranes of the spinal cord and brain	MENINGITIS (men-in-jy'tis), inflammation of the coverings of the brain and spinal cord MENINGIOMA (men-in-je-o'ma) a tumor originating in the meninges
SPIN/O (spi'no)	spinal cord	SPINOCEREBELLAR (spi-no-ser-e-bel'ar), pertaining to the spine and cerebellum
RAM/O (ra'mo)	branch, offshoot	RAMOSE (ram'os), having or being full of branches
AUT/O (aw'toe)	self	AUTONOMIC (au-to-no'mik) self-controlling
SYMPATH/O (sim-path'o) SYMPATHIC/O (sim-path'i-ko) SYMPATHETIC/O (sim-pa-the'ti-ko)	sympathetic portion of the autonomic nervous system	SYMPATHOMIMETIC (sim-path-o-my-met'ik), imitating the sympathetic nervous system SYMPATHICOBLAST (sim-path'i-ko-blast), embryonic cell of the sympathetic nervous system

	Meaning	*Example*
		SYMPATHETIC (sim-pa-the′tik), pertaining to the sympathetic nervous system
PARASYMPATH/O (para-sim-path′o) PARASYMPATHIC/O (para-sim-path′i-ko) PARASYMPATHETIC/O (para-sim-pa-the′ti-ko)	parasympathetic portion of the autonomic nervous system	PARASYMPATHOMIMETIC (para-sim-path-o-my-met′ik), imitating the parasympathetic nervous system PARASYMPATHICOTONIA para-sim-path-i-ko-ton′ia, TONIA, tension), abnormal condition in the autonomic nervous system in which the parasympathetic nervous portion of the ANS overpowers the sympathetic portion PARASYMPATHETIC (para-sim-pa-the′tik), pertaining to the parasympathetic portion of the ANS
FER/O (fer-o)	carry, conduct	AFFERENT (af′fer-ent), conducting impulses to the central nervous system

The nervous system is responsible for regulating body functions and body movements, keeping us aware of the changes in the external and internal environments and enabling us to carry on higher mental processes, such as thinking and remembering. All these functions—from the simple to the most complex—are carried on by nervous tissue that *respond* to stimuli and *conduct* impulses from one area of the body to another.

THE NEURON AND ITS FUNCTION

The *neuron*, the nerve cell, is the basic structural unit of the nervous system. Each neuron has a *cell body* and two protoplasmic processes: *axon*(s) and *dendrite*(s) (see Figures 9-1 and 9-2). An impulse is carried to the neuron by way of the dendrites (called *afferent* processes because they conduct impulses toward the neuron) and is carried from the neuron through the axons (called *efferent* processes because they conduct impulses away from the neuron). The impulse is passed along to the next neuron by

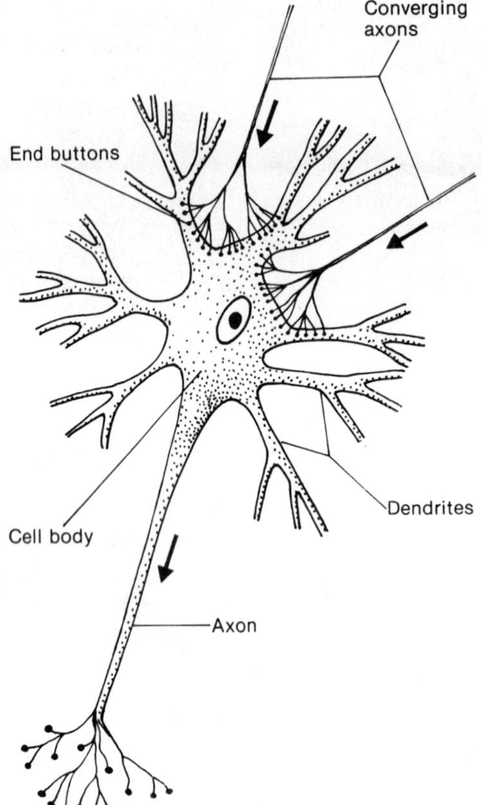

Figure 9-1 Two neurons in synapse with a third neuron.

way of a *synapse*, which is the gap between the terminal buttons of an axon and the dendrites of the next neuron receiving the impulse. The terminal buttons of the axon release a chemical, acetylcholine, which quickly breaches the synaptic gap and is then neutralized by the enzyme cholinesterase. (The central nervous system uses many chemicals to breach the synaptic gap.) Actually, acetylcholine depolarizes the receiving neuron, thus allowing the impulse to pass. The nerve impulse itself is negatively charged and continually regenerated as it moves from one neuron to the next. Since only axons can release a chemical-transmitting agent, transmission between neurons occurs only in one direction—from axons to the dendrite and cell body of the receiving neuron.

Impulses too weak to pass to another neuron can build up (a process known as *summation*) and then move to another neuron. When many nerve cells send impulses to one receiving neuron, the process is known as *convergence*. In *divergence*, however, one nerve cell sends impulses to several nerve cells at the same time. Some neurons prevent other nerve cells from discharging impulses; such neurons are called *inhibitory neurons*. This is done, for example, to coordinate body movements, such as flexing the arm.

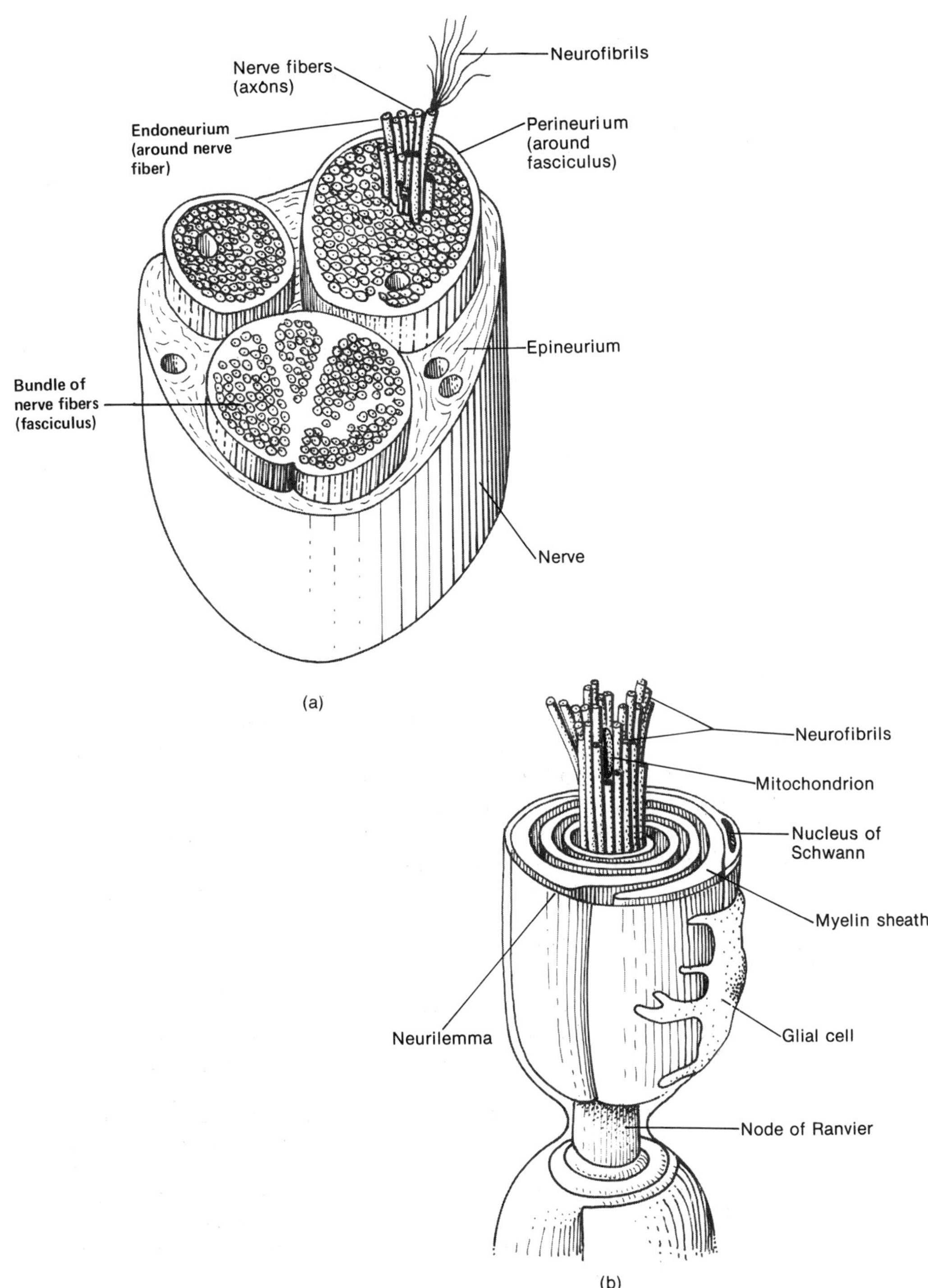

Figure 9-2 The structure of nerve cells and nerves. (a) Construction of a typical nerve. (b) The fine structure of an axon and its neurilemma sheath.

In addition to the transmitting type of neuron, the nervous system also has several types of supporting cells called *neuroglia*. The three types of neuroglia are *astrocytes, oligodendroglia,* and *microglia.* The neuroglia provide support and structure to nervous tissue; also, microglia protect nervous tissue by acting as phagocytes.

DIVISIONS OF THE NERVOUS SYSTEM

The nervous system (Table 9-1) can be divided into the following smaller systems, which are both connected and interrelated.

1.   The central nervous system (CNS), consisting of the brain and spinal cord.
2.   The peripheral nervous system (PNS), consisting of those nerves originating from the brain and spinal cord.
3.   The autonomic nervous system (ANS), consisting of those nerves and nerve cells partially coordinated by the CNS and partially by the PNS.

The Central Nervous System

The brain
The central nervous system (CNS) consists of the brain and the spinal cord (see Figure 9-3). The *brain* itself is divided into the *cerebrum,* the *cerebellum,* and the *brainstem.* The *cerebrum* is actually two halves connected deep within by a band of neural fibers called the *corpus callosum* and by three other bands of connective nerve fibers known as *commissures* (kom′i-sures). The crossing of these fibers results in the right half of the brain controlling the left side of the body and vice versa.

The surface of the cerebrum consists of numerous folds; the ridge of each fold is

Table 9-1   Divisions of the Nervous System

		Organization of the nervous system
	Central nervous system (CNS)	Brain and spinal cord
	Peripheral nervous system (PNS)	Cranial and spinal nerves (located outside the CNS)
	Autonomic nervous system (ANS)	Nerves that carry involuntary motor impulses to cardiac muscle, smooth muscle, and glands
Mainly antagonistic	Sympathetic division of the ANS	Produces change in reaction to certain stimuli
	Parasympathetic division of the ANS	Maintains normal functioning

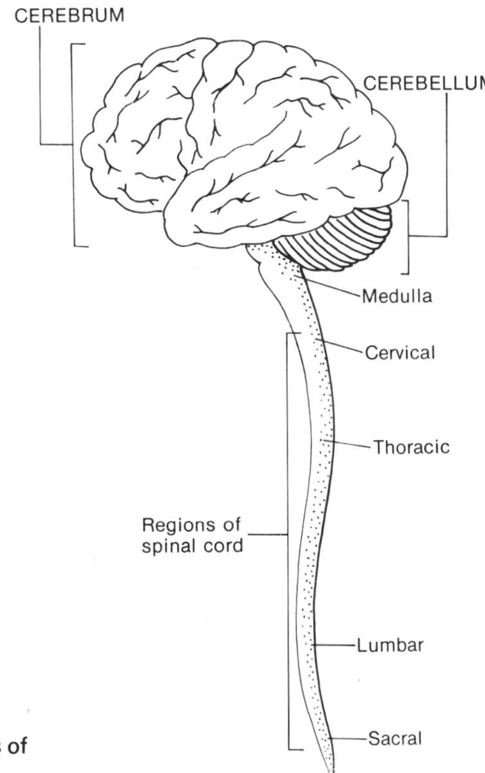

Figure 9-3 The chief organs of the central nervous system.

called a *gyrus*. The depressions or grooves on each side of a gyrus are known as *sulci*. Deep grooves are called *fissures*. A side view of the cerebrum shows the *lateral fissure* (fissure of Sylvius), which divides the cerebrum into upper and lower portions. The upper portion is separated anteriorally and posteriorally by a groove, the *central sulcus* (sulcus of Rolando). The rear of the cerebrum is marked off by the *parietooccipital* (parye-eto-ok-sip′it-al) *fissure*. By dividing each cerebral hemisphere according to sulci and fissures, we can separate the brain into four lobes: the *frontal*, the *parietal*, the *occipital*, and the *temporal*. A fifth lobe, the *insular* lobe, is located on the floor of the lateral fissure.

The functions of the cerebral lobes are as follows:

Frontal lobe: Control of voluntary muscle movements and personality, and partial control of memory and speech are centered here.

Parietal lobe: Sensations of hot and cold, pain, touch and pressure and the position of the body or body parts in space (called proprioception or stereognosis) are located here.

Occipital lobe: Vision takes place here.

Temporal lobe: Hearing (audition), smell (olfaction), and taste (gustatory sensation) are located here. Major control of speech is also found here.

The *cerebral cortex* (kor′teks, CORTIC/O, outer surface, rind), a layer of gray matter consisting of neural cell bodies, covers the surface of the cerebrum. Our ability to think and act is located in the cortical gray matter. Gray matter, called *deep gray matter,* is also located deep within the cerebrum, where it is called *basal nuclei.* (*Nucleus* here refers to a collection of nerve cell bodies within the central nervous system whereas a *ganglion* is a collection of nerve cell bodies outside the CNS.) The inside of the cerebrum consists of white matter. This white matter contains myelinated (myelin is the fatty substance that covers nerve fibers) fibers or axons. Such fibers are classified into three groups: (a) *association fibers,* which connect adjacent lobes of each cerebral hemisphere and the gyri of each lobe with one another, (b) *commissural fibers,* which join the two cerebral hemispheres with one another, and (c) *projection fibers,* which join the cerebrum to the brainstem and spinal cord.

The *cerebellum* is the part of the brain that controls and coordinates body movements. Like the cerebrum, the cerebellum is actually two lobes joined by a worm-shaped lobe called the *vermis* (VERM/I, worm). Gray matter constitutes both the outer surface, the *cerebellar cortex,* and the inner structures, the *cerebellar nuclei.* The cerebellum, too, is divided into gyri and sulci and has two types of fibers: association fibers connecting the cells of the cerebellar cortex with the cells of the nuclei situated in the white matter and projection fibers connecting the cerebellum with portions of the brainstem and the spinal cord.

The *brainstem* (Figure 9-4) is located in the midportion of the brain and consists of the *medulla oblongata* (me-dul′la ob-long-ga′ta), the *pons* (ponz′), the *mesencephalon* (mez-en-sef′a-lon), the *diencephalon* (di-en-sef′a-lon), and the *basal nuclei.* The medulla, about an inch long, is that portion of the spinal cord within the brain. In addition to manufacturing *cerebrospinal fluid,* the medulla is the source of several cranial nerves and the control center for the rate of heartbeat, the diameter of the blood vessels, breathing, coughing, swallowing, vomiting, sneezing, and hiccupping. Basically composed of white-matter nerve fibers, the medulla carries all impulses passing between the brain and the spinal cord. The *pons* (PONT/O, bridge) is also a source for several cranial nerves, and the nerve pathways for breathing, eye movements, and pupillary action pass through the pons. The *pneumotaxic center* controlling the rate of breathing is located here as well. The *mesencephalon* or midbrain is composed dorsally of four raised areas (*colliculi,* kol-lik′u-lie, hills) that control visual and auditory reflexes. The *red nucleus* of the mesencephalon acts as a communications center for the cerebrum, cerebellum, pons, and medulla. The *diencephalon* is composed of the *thalamus, epithalamus, subthalamus,* and *hypothalamus.* The subthalamus acts as a booster station, sending impulses from the mesencephalon to the cerebral cortex. The hypothalamus consists of the pituitary gland (called the *hypophysis,* hi-pof′i-sis, because it influences growth), the pituitary stalk (called the *infundibulum,* in-fun-dib′ou-lum, because it is shaped like a funnel), the base (*tuber cinerum,* too′ber sin′er-um), several pimple or breastlike bodies called *mammillary bodies,* and the *optic*

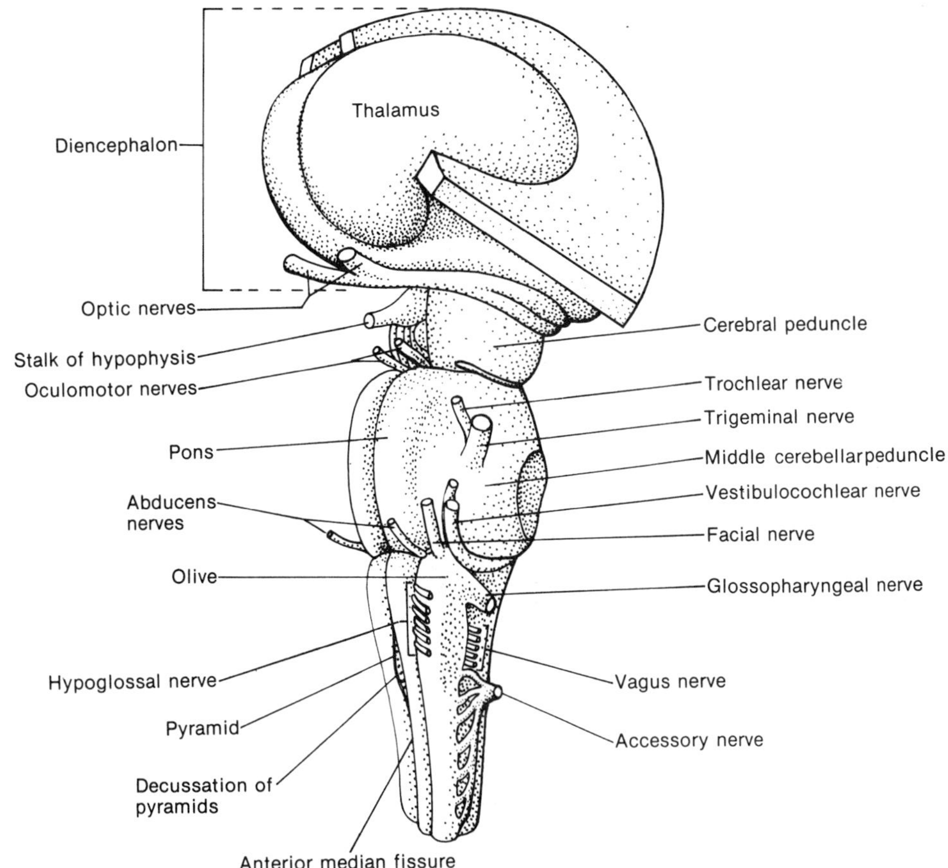

Figure 9-4 The brainstem.

chiasm, which is the gap where the optic tract becomes the optic nerve. Hormonal functions, such as growth, lactation, regulation of blood pressure, and metabolic processes, are controlled by the pituitary gland. The mammillary bodies receive impulses that will be interpreted as odors. As a whole, the hypothalamus also influences body temperature, appetite, the body's water level, hormonal secretion, sexual activity, and the coordination of the autonomic nervous system. The epithalamus, consisting of the pineal body, the habenular trigone, and a fibrous band (posterior commissure), may also influence sexual maturity and growth. The habenular trigone is a transmitter of olfactory impulses. The thalamus is actually two thalami (chambers) of gray matter, usually connected by another gray mass. The thalamus acts as a relay center, sending impulses to the appropriate parts of the cerebral cortex. The last part of the brainstem, the basal nuclei, is found in each hemisphere of the cerebrum and helps to coordinate body movements.

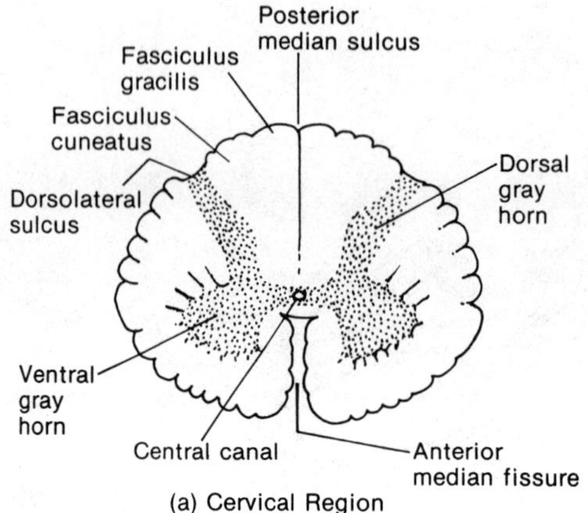

(a) Cervical Region

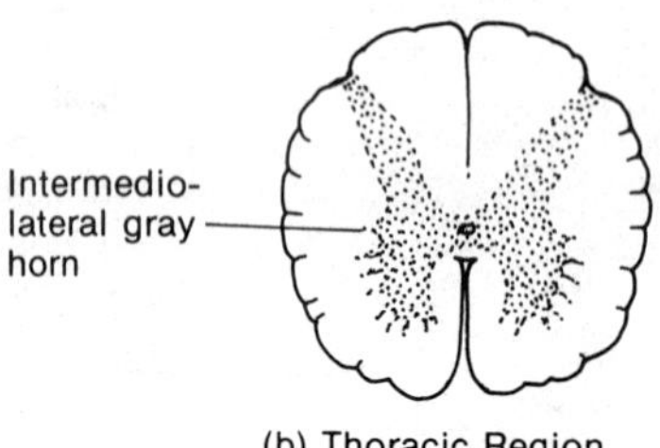

(b) Thoracic Region

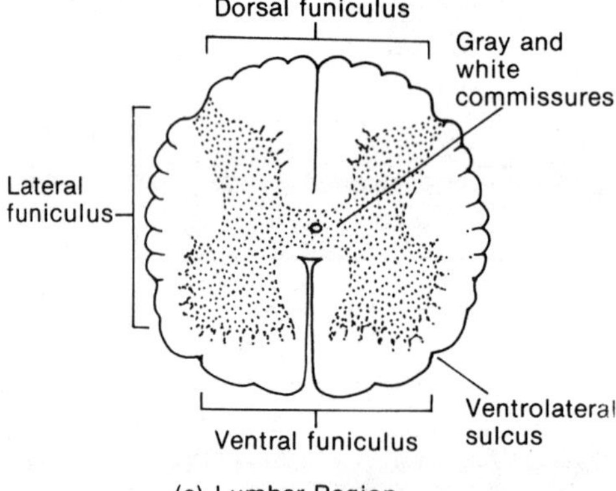

(c) Lumbar Region

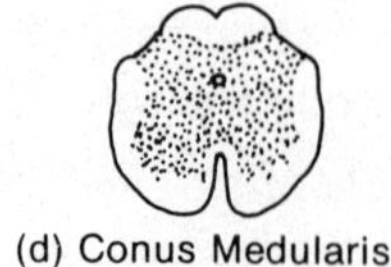
(d) Conus Medularis

Figure 9-5 Features of the spinal cord, as seen on cross-section.

The spinal cord

The spinal cord, the nerve pathway center of the body, begins at the first cervical vertebra and extends to the second lumbar vertebra. Like the cerebrum and cerebellum, the spinal cord contains both gray and white matter; here, however, the white matter is on the outside and the gray matter on the inside in an H or butterfly shape. The white matter consists of fiber tracts that act as pathways for impulses moving up or down the cord.

Without its protective covering the surface of the spinal cord (Figure 9-5) has an *anterior median fissure, posterior median sulcus*, a *dorsolateral sulcus*, and a *ventrolateral sulcus* (lumbar region only). Thirty-one pairs of spinal nerves originate from the dorsal and ventral roots along the cord itself. The dorsal roots contain a mass of nerve cell bodies, the *dorsal root ganglion* that relays impulses into the cord from nerves outside the central nervous system. The long nerve roots of the lumbar and sacral regions of the spinal cord overlap to form a horse's tail—hence their name *cauda equina* (kau'da e-queen'a). The upper and lower extremities of the body are innervated with nerves originating from the *cervical* (located between cervical vertebra 3 and thoracic vertebra 2) and lumbar (located between thoracic vertebrae 9 and 12) *enlargements.*

The Peripheral Nervous System

The peripheral nervous system (PNS) consists of cranial, spinal, and autonomic nerves. It joins the central nervous system with the rest of the body. The nerves of the peripheral nervous system are classified into three groups: *motor (efferent), sensory (afferent)*, and *mixed* (both efferent and afferent). The motor or efferent nerves carry impulses from the central nervous system to different parts of the body; sensory or afferent nerves carry impulses to the central nervous system; mixed nerves can do both. Twelve pairs of *cranial nerves* (designated by Roman numerals) form part of the peripheral nervous system (Figure 9-6). They are

    I.   Olfactory (afferent): located in the mucous membrane of the nasal cavities.

    II.   Optic (afferent): origin is in the retina of each eye.

    III.   Oculomotor (efferent): control of the skeletal muscles of the eye.

    IV.   Trochlear (mixed): control of eye movements, proprioceptive impulses.

    V.   Trigeminal (mixed): chewing, head and facial sensations.

    VI.   Abducens (efferent): control of lateral eye movement.

    VII.   Facial (mixed): facial movements, taste (front of tongue), salivation.

    VIII.   Acoustic (afferent): auditory, equilibrium.

    IX.   Glossopharyngeal (mixed): salivation, swallowing, taste (rear of tongue and the pharynx), breathing, blood pressure.

    X.   Vagus (mixed): heartbeat and movements, larynx and digestive organs.

    XI.   Accessory (efferent): head and shoulder movements, vocal movements.

    XII.   Hypoglossal (efferent): tongue movements.

There are 31 pairs of *spinal nerves* that form the spinal portion of the peripheral nervous system. Each pair is named according to the region of its orgin. For example, C2 is the second cervical nerve; T4 is the fourth thoracic nerve. A spinal nerve (Figure

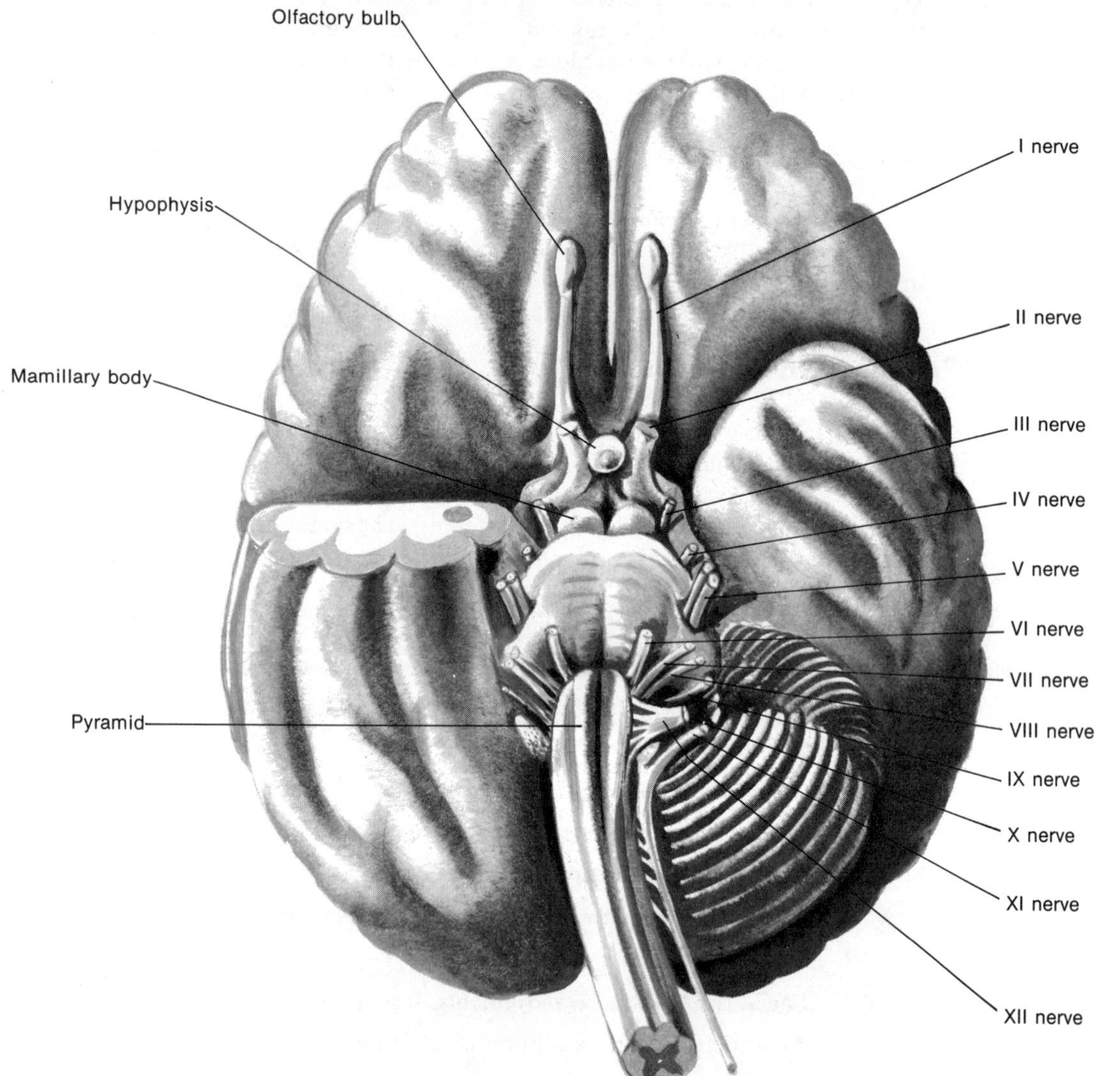

Figure 9-6 The cranial nerves.

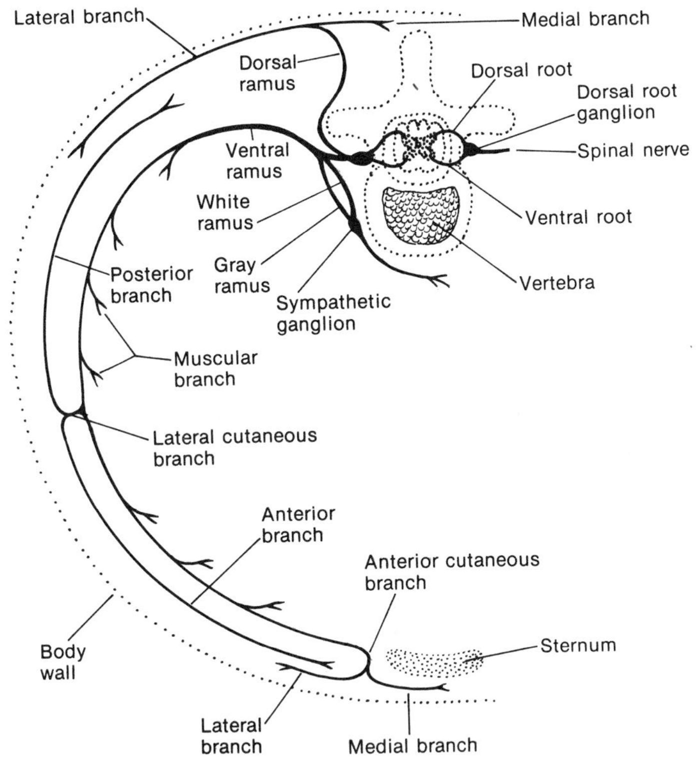

Figure 9-7   A typical spinal nerve and its branches.

9-7) is formed by the merging of a dorsal or posterior nerve root and a ventral or anterior nerve root. Immediately after a nerve is formed, it begins to branch off (forms *rami*). Spinal nerves and their branches or rami are mixed nerves—that is, they are both efferent and afferent nerves. The anterior rami (with the exception of the lower eleven thoracic spinal nerves) group together to form nerve networks called *plexuses* (pleksus′is, sing. plexus, Figure 9-8). The body nerve plexuses are the brachial plexus, the cervical plexus, the lumbosacral plexus (combination of the lumbar and sacral plexuses), and the pudental plexus (supplying nerves to the private parts). The intercostal nerves (upper eleven pairs of thoracic spinal nerves) do not form plexuses but individually innervate the area of the thorax, its walls and lining, the ribs, armpit and upper arm, and portions of the abdomen. The spinal nerves also supply the skin with sensory nerves arranged in an overlapping pattern called *dermatomes* (Figure 9-9).

Neuron pathways

Neuron pathways are chains of neurons linked together to allow impulses to travel from the brain to parts of the body or vice versa. There are two types of neuron

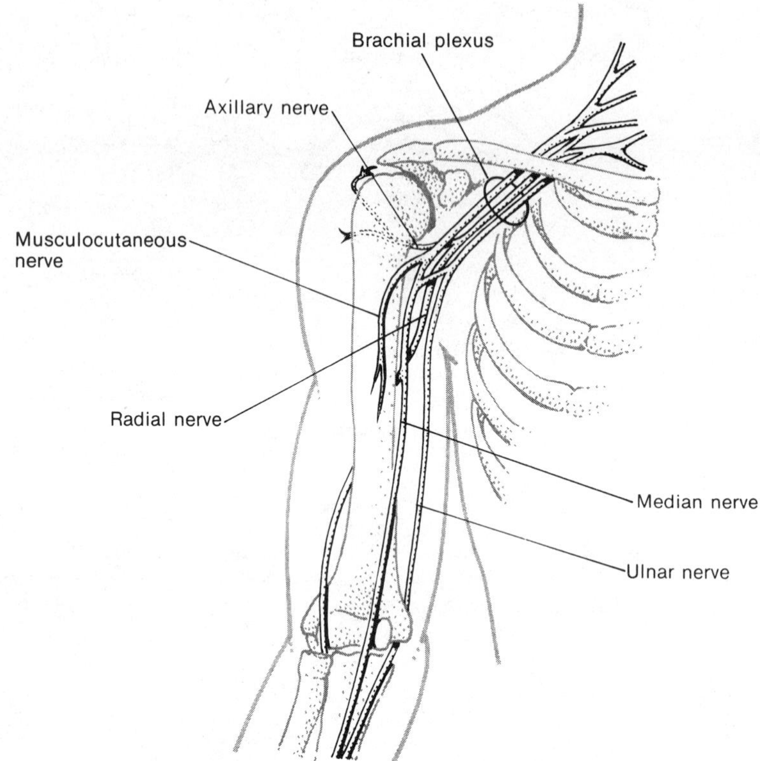

Figure 9-8 Certain spinal nerves of the upper extremity, and the position of the brachial plexus.

pathways: *sensory* or *afferent* pathways and *motor* or *efferent* pathways. In the sensory pathway a receptor is activated by an external (*exteroceptive*) or internal (*enteroceptive*) stimulus. From the receptor the impulse is carried to the spinal cord, where it is then routed to the thalamus. The thalamus next sends it to the appropriate area of the cerebral cortex. This process is known as a *three-neuron pathway* (receptor—spinal cord—thalamus). Of course, other neurons can be added to the pathway (e.g., five-neuron pathway). The spinal cord contains seven *ascending pathways* (Figure 9-10). *Motor* or *efferent pathways* are termed *descending pathways* because they carry impulses from the brain to the muscles. The three major descending pathways are the *corticospinal tract* (initiates voluntary muscle action), the *extrapyramidal system* (coordinates voluntary muscle action), and the *final common pathway* (the various routes that carry motor impulses to the muscles).

Reflexes

Reflexes are involuntary responses to stimuli that are predictable. Clinically reflexes are important because the absence of the predictable response indicates damage at

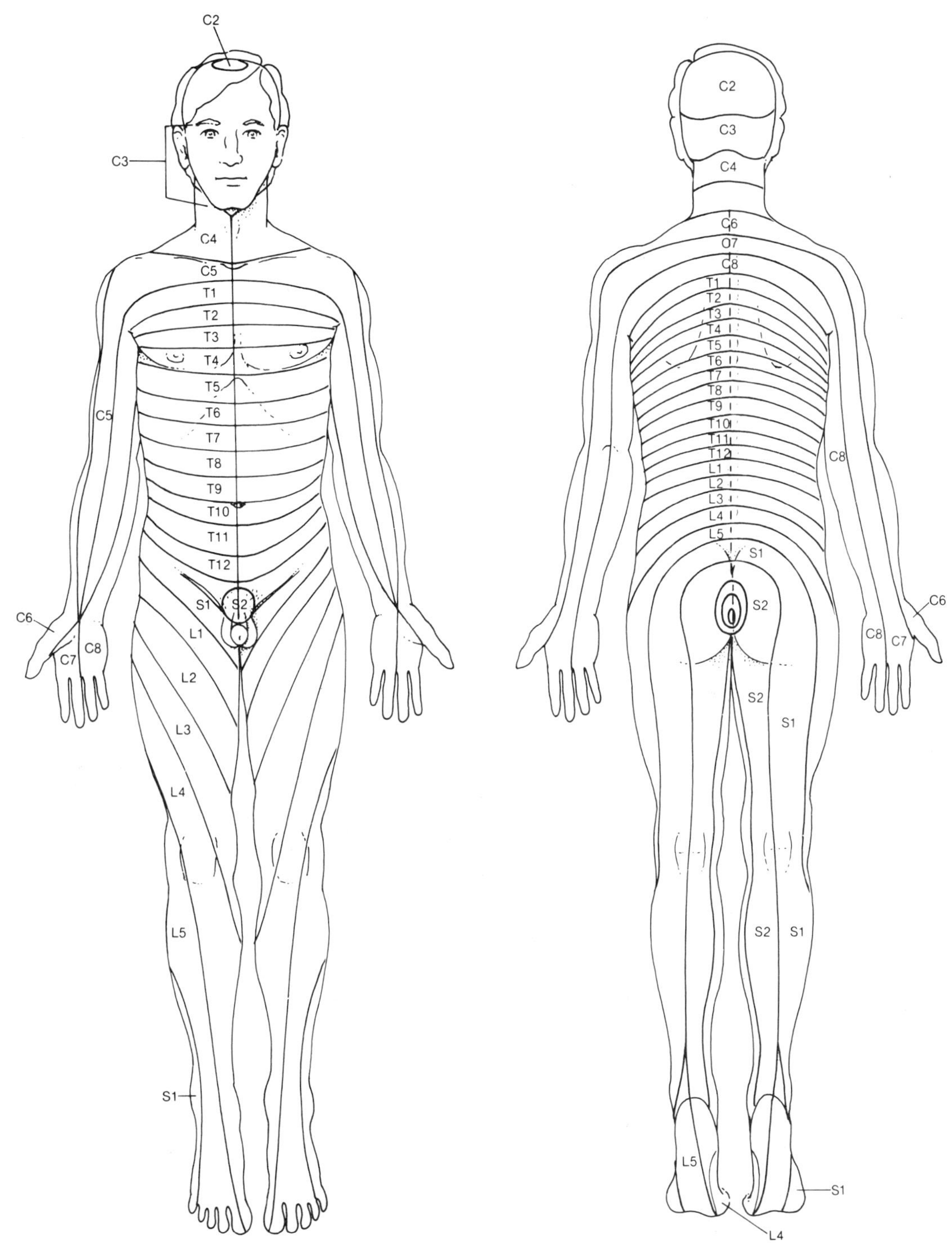

Figure 9-9. Dermatomes.

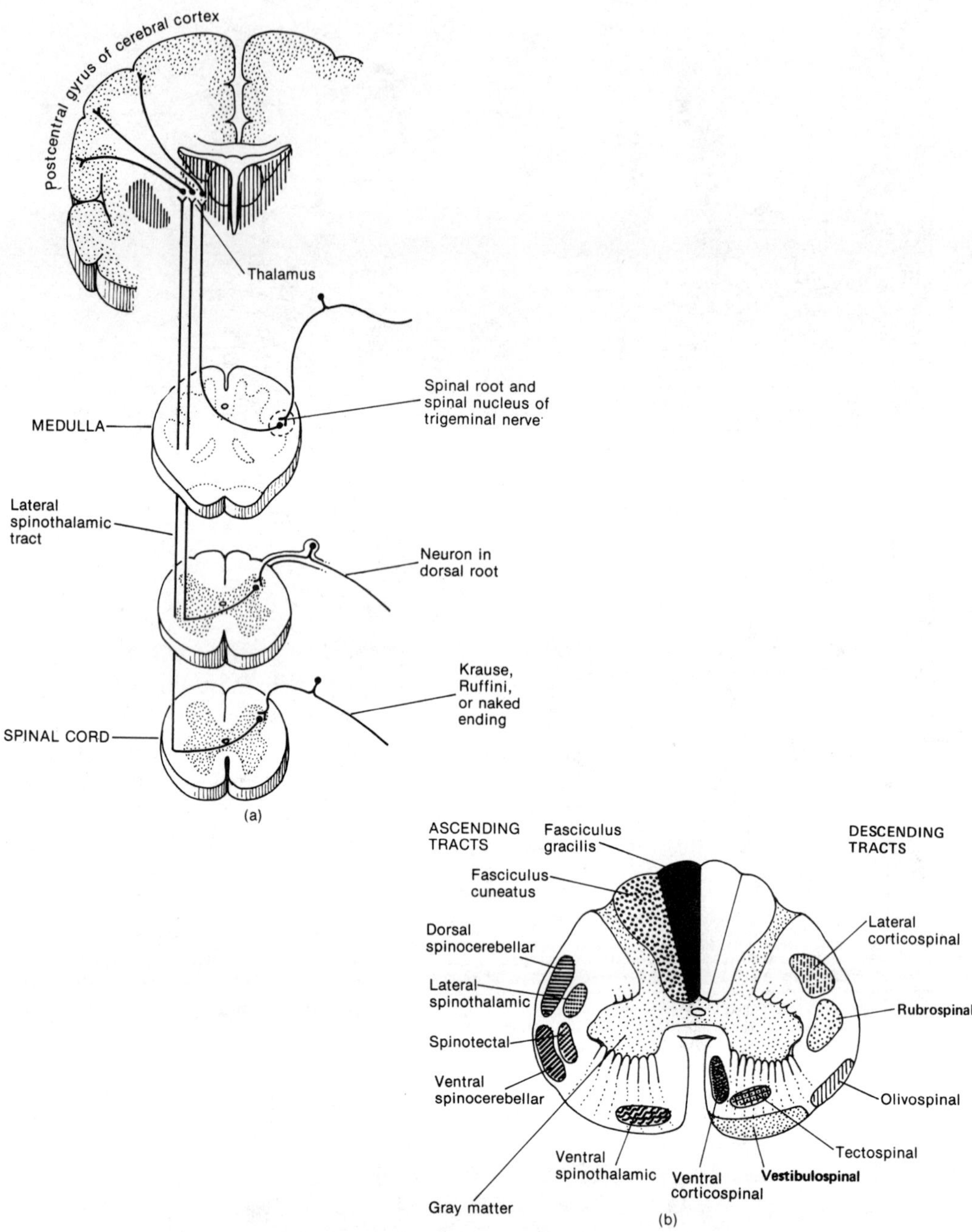

Figure 9-10 Spinal tracts or pathways. (a) A typical three-neuron pathway, the lateral spinothalamic tract, which is the pathway for pain and temperature. (b) Location of the major tracts or pathways of the spinal cord. All are bilateral but are shown on only one side of the drawing for clarity.

some point to the neural pathway (called a *reflex arc*). Most reflex arcs are five-neuron pathways: receptor—afferent neuron—connecting neuron—efferent neuron—effector. Reflexes can be classified into four groups: *superficial* (plantar reflex, abdominal wall reflex, corneal reflex), *deep* (called muscle or myotatic reflex: knee jerk or patellar reflex, Achilles reflex, biceps and triceps reflexes), *visceral* (light reflex—constriction of the iris, ciliospinal—pinching the skin causes the pupil to dilate), and *pathological* (destruction of sphincter muscles controlling defecation—individual may be unable to hold back feces).

The Autonomic Nervous System

The *autonomic nervous system* (ANS) or *visceral nervous system* carries involuntary motor impulses to the glands, cardiac muscle, and smooth (visceral) muscle. The autonomic nervous system consists of *efferent* fibers of two neuron chains: a *preganglionic neuron* having its cell body in the spinal cord or medulla and its axon connecting with a ganglion and synapsing with a *postganglionic neuron* that makes contact with the body structure. There are three types of *ganglia* (nerve cell bodies outside the brain or spinal cord) in the autonomic nervous system: *vertebral, collateral,* and *terminal.* The vertebral ganglia are two columns of ganglia parallel to the vertebral column. They are referred to as *sympathetic trunks.* The collateral ganglia (e.g., superior and inferior mesenteric ganglia) are located in the thoracic and abdomino-pelvic cavities. Terminal ganglia (e.g., ciliary, sphenopalatine ganglia) occur in the nerve plexuses of the thorax and abdomen.

The autonomic nervous system actually consists of two systems that work together: the *sympathetic* or *thoracolumbar system* and the *parasympathetic* or *craniosacral system.* Their alternate names indicate their origin in the central nervous system. In fact, many visceral organs are innervated by both systems. Both systems maintain body homeostasis by regulating body temperature, fluid balance, enzyme production, blood pressure, sugar level, heart rate and beat, hormone production, and similar factors. The process is accomplished mainly by the *antagonistic* relationship between the two systems. For instance, the sympathetic system causes coronary blood vessels to dilate whereas the parasympathetic system causes the same blood vessels to constrict.

Coverings of the Brain and Spinal Cord

The *meninges* (me-nin′jez) are the protective membranes of the brain and spinal cord and consist of three types: (a) the *dura mater* (du′ra ma′ter) is the thick, fibrous outside cover; (b) the *arachnoid mater* (a-rack′noyd) is a thin, weblike cover; and (c) the *pia mater* (pee′a) is a thin, delicate cover that is attached to the brain surface and is separated from the outer two covers by a layer of *cerebrospinal fluid.* The arachnoid mater has processes called *arachnoid villi* or *granulations* that protrude into the blood sinuses. Here cerebrospinal fluid enters the bloodstream. Cerebrospinal fluid is formed and circulated in the four spaces (*ventricles*) inside the brain. The fluid acts as a shock absorber. From the fourth ventricle it makes its way through the subarachnoid space to the spinal cord.

CLINICAL AND PATHOLOGICAL CONDITIONS

Agnosia (ag-no'she-a) refers to the inability to recognize sounds, familiar objects, and so on.

Aphasia (a-fay'ze-a) indicates the inability to understand written or spoken words or to speak meaningfully.

Apraxia (a-prak'se-a) is the inability to perform certain voluntary movements.

All three preceding conditions are associated with damage of the temporal lobe of the cerebrum.

Apoplexy (apo-plek'se) or stroke indicates damage to the brain as a result of an obstruction in one of the cerebral blood vessels [*ischemia* (ISCH/O, block), is-key'me-a, is the technical term for an obstruction of a blood vessel]. There are three reasons for such an obstruction:

1. *Hemorrhage:* hypertension, arteriosclerosis, or infections cause the cerebral arteries to weaken. The escaping blood damages cerebral tissues, causing hemiplegia, incontinence, and aphasia.
2. *Thrombosis:* a blood clot blocks arteries supplying the brain. As a result, portions of the cerebral tissue are damaged.
3. *Embolism:* a portion of a clot leaves its original site and *occludes* (blocks) a cerebral artery.

Coma is an abnormal deep sleep. Many comas result from head injuries or cerebral circulatory accidents.

Epilepsy is a fit or seizure resulting from a neurological disease. The more severe seizure, called a *grand* (grahn) *mal,* is accompanied by convulsions and unconsciousness; the less severe seizure, called a *petit mal,* is accompanied by a minor lapse in consciousness.

Hydrocephalus (hi-dro-sef'a-lus) refers to an excessive amount of cerebrospinal fluid in the ventricles of the brain as a result of overproduction, poor absorption, or a blockage. In turn, the head swells out of proportion.

Hypertension is high blood pressure as a result of increased activity of the autonomic nervous system. A *sympathectomy* in which the sympathetic ganglia (from T10 to L2) are removed can be performed to lower blood pressure.

Meningitis is the inflammation of the protective membranes of the brain and spinal cord caused by bacteria or viruses.

Multiple Sclerosis is the destruction of the myelin coverings in the brain and spinal cord and a hardening of the gray and white matter. Speech and vision are affected, and shaking is characteristic of this disorder. Both the cause and the cure are unknown.

Myasthenia Gravis (my-as-then′e-a gra′vis) is a muscular weakness and a general feeling of fatigue resulting from a lack of acetylcholine or an abundance of cholinesterase at the point where nerve axons and muscle fibers come in contact. Normal muscle contraction is prevented. Face, lip, throat, and neck muscles are usually affected.

Neuritis is a nerve inflammation characterized by a prickly, numb, or painful feeling in the affected area. Neuritis is caused by infection, poison, or trauma.

Parkinson's Disease is a disease of the brain and spinal cord, usually beginning with a tremor of the hand or foot. The tremor spreads, and the patient has a bent-forward appearance. Voluntary muscle movements become difficult and speech becomes both slow and difficult.

Poliomyelitis is a viral infection that affects the cell bodies of the neurons of the skeletal muscles and results in paralysis. Sometimes the neurons controlling the breathing reflex are affected. Immunity can be developed by vaccination.

Shingles (herpes zoster, her′pez zos′ter) is an acute viral infection that attacks sensory nerves entering the spinal cord and cause blisterlike sores on the skin.

Spina Bifida (speen′a bi′fi-da) is a congenital defect affecting the spinal column, usually in the lumbar region. The laminae of the vertebrae are imperfectly joined, and the membranes of the affected portion of the spinal cord may push through to the surface of the body to form a sac containing cerebrospinal fluid and sometimes neural tissue itself. If the vertebrae close imperfectly, but there is no saclike protrusion, the condition is called *spina bifida occulta* (o-kul′ta).

Subdural Hematoma is a blood clot beneath the dura mater as a result of a head injury.

Syncope (sin′ko-pe) refers to fainting or unconsciousness.

Thalamic Syndrome occurs when a damaged or blocked vessel of the thalamus results in a lack of awareness of a particular sensation, which finally surfaces in a painful and unbearable manner.

Tumors

Gliomas (or *gliomata*) are tumors that develop from the supporting nerve cells, the neuroglia. Generally gliomas are malignant but don't metastasize (to *metastasize* means to spread to other body parts).

Meningiomas (or *meningiomata*) are tumors, usually benign, that originate in the arachnoidal tissue.

EXERCISES

    I.   Give the meaning for each of the following medical words. Divide each word into base(s), prefix, and suffix; underline the letter(s) that has the primary stress. *Example:*

HYDROCEPHALUS   abnormal amount of cerebrospinal fluid in the ventricles of the

brain   hydro/<u>cephalus</u>

1. GANGLIONECTOMY ....

2. NEUROGLIAL ....

3. NEURORRHAPHY ....

4. MESOCEPHALIC ....

5. MENINGORRHAGIA ....

6. RAMIFICATION ....

7. EFFERENT ....

8. SYMPATHICOTONIA ....

9. AUTOGENIC ....

10. OLIGEMIA ....

11. CEREBROPATHY ....

12. ANENCEPHALUS ....

13. VENTRICULOSCOPY ....

14. MYELINOGENETIC ....

15. NEURASTHENIA ....

16. POLYNEURITIS ....

17. CEREBROMALACIA ....

18. MENINGOENCEPHALITIS ....

19. CEREBELLOSPINAL ....

20. GANGLIONITIS ....

II. Make medical words from the following phrases. Indicate the primary stress by underlining the stressed letter(s). *Example:*

inflammation of the cerebellum

    cerebell<u>i</u>tis

....

1. a star-shaped neuroglial cell

....

2. embryonic ganglion cell

....

3. incision into the cerebrum

....

4. pertaining to the cerebellum

....

5. surgically attaching one end of a severed nerve to the other end (ANASTOMOSIS means surgically joining together.)

....

6. incision of the thalamus

....

7. hernia of the spinal cord and its coverings

....

8. pertaining to the cerebral cortex and the spinal cord

....

9. excision of (a portion of) the sympathetic division of the ANS

....

10. containing myelin

....

11. tumors originating in the supporting nervous tissue

....

12. having an abnormally small head

   ....

13. pertaining to the cerebrum and spinal cord

   ....

14. x raying of the ventricles of the brain (by withdrawing cerebrospinal fluid and replacing it with air)

   ....

15. inflammation of the brain

   ....

III.   Multiple choice: Circle the correct letter.

1. The afferent processes of nerve cells are the
   (a) nerve cell bodies
   (b) dendrites
   (c) axons
   (d) synapses

2. Those processes that conduct impulses away from neurons are the
   (a) axons
   (b) dendrites
   (c) afferent processes
   (d) synapses

3. The transmission of impulses by many neurons to a single neuron is known as
   (a) summation
   (b) inhibition
   (c) divergence
   (d) convergence

4. Which of the following supportive nerve cells act as phagocytes?
   (a) oligodendroglia
   (b) astrocytes
   (c) microglia
   (d) neuroglia

5. Which of the following is NOT considered part of the central nervous system?
   (a) brain
   (b) nerves originating from the brain and spinal cord
   (c) spinal cord
   (d) all of the above

IV.   Match the following descriptions with their medical names.

1.   the band of neural fibers that connects the two halves of the

cerebrum   ....

2.   a general name for connective fibers   ....

3.   grooves in the cerebral and cerebellar surfaces   ....

4.   deep grooves in the cerebral and cerebellar

surfaces   ....

5.   the ridge of each fold of the cerebral and cerebellar

surfaces   ....

6.   the layer of gray matter covering the cerebral and cerebellar

surfaces   ....

7.   gray matter deep within the cerebrum   ....

8.   a fatty substance that coats nerve fibers   ....

9.   the worm-shaped lobe that joins the two lobes of the

cerebellum   ....

10.   nerve fibers that connect the cells of the cerebellar cortex
with the cells of the nuclei located in the white

matter   ....

11.   a term indicating that portion of the spinal cord within the
brain and forming the lower portion of the

brainstem   ....

12.   that portion of the brainstem that acts as a bridge

connecting the spinal cord to the brain proper   ....

13.   the technical term for the midbrain   ....

14.   the portion of the brain containing the thalamus   ....

15.   another name for the pituitary gland   ....

a.   gyrus

b.   association fibers

c.   hypophysis

d.   corpus callosum

e.   pons

f.   fissures

g.   myelin

h.   dorsal root
     ganglion

i.   commissure

j.   cauda equina

k.   cerebral cortex

l.   vermis

m.   sulci

n.   medulla oblongata

o.   diencephalon

p.   basal nuclei

q.   mesencephalon

16. a mass of nerve cell bodies that relays impulses to the spinal

cord from nerves outside the CNS ....

17. a term meaning horse's tail and referring to the long nerve roots

of the lumbar and sacral regions of the spinal cord ....

V. Circle true or false for each of the following statements. If the statement is false, give the correct answer in the space provided.

1. Cranial, spinal, and autonomic nerves constitute the peripheral nervous system.

T / F ....

2. Motor nerves are termed afferent nerves.

T / F ....

3. The term mixed nerves refers to sensory nerves.

T / F ....

4. Roman numerals are used to designate the 12 pairs of cranial nerves.

T / F ....

5. Olfactory nerves are the motor nerves of the sense of smell.

T / F ....

6. Tongue movements are controlled by the glossal nerves.

T / F ....

7. The term proprioceptive refers to the awareness of the position of the body or body parts in space.

T / F ....

8. Lateral eye movement is controlled by the trigeminal nerves.

T / F ....

9. The vagus nerves control breathing.

T / F ....

10. Hearing and equilibrium are controlled by the acoustic nerves.

T / F ....

11. After a spinal nerve is formed, it branches off into rami.

    T / F   ....

12. The grouping together of several rami to form nerve networks is known as ramification.

    T / F   ....

13. Chains of neurons conducting impulses toward or away from the brain are linked to form neural pathways.

    T / F   ....

14. Another name for an external stimulus is an enteroceptive stimulus.

    T /F   ....

15. Descending neural pathways are afferent pathways.

    T / F   ....

16. A reflex is a voluntary response to a stimulus.

    T / F   ....

17. Clinically reflexes are important because their absence indicates neurological damage.

    T / F   ....

18. Another name for the autonomic nervous system is the visceral nervous system.

    T / F   ....

19. The autonomic nervous system is an afferent system.

    T / F   ....

20. The vertebral ganglia of the ANS are housed in the vertebrae.

    T / F   ....

21. The sympathetic and parasympathetic divisions of the ANS maintain homeostasis by keeping one another in check.

    T / F   ....

VI. Fill in the blanks for each of the following statements.

1. Nerves originating from the brain and spinal cord constitute the ....

   .... system.

2. Those nerves and nerve cells coordinated by both the CNS and PNS constitute the

    .... system.

3. The brain is divided into the ...., ..., and ....

4. A collection of nerve cell bodies within the CNS is called a ....

5. A collection of nerve cell bodies outside the CNS is called a ....

6. The area of the brain that controls the rate of breathing is called the ....
    center.

7. Two other names for the sympathetic and parasympathetic divisions of the ANS are

    .... and ....

8. The .... are the protective membranes that cover the brain and spinal cord.

9. The thick outside membrane covering the brain and spinal cord is called the ....

    ....

10. The thin, weblike cover of the brain and spinal cord is known as the ....

    ....

11. The very thin, delicate cover of the brain and spinal cord is called the ....

    ....

12. .... circulates between the inner two membranous
    covers of the brain and spinal cord.

13. From the second cover of the brain and spinal cord, processes called ....

    .... or .... protrude into the blood sinuses.

14. Four .... inside the brain allow for the formation and circulation of fluid.

15. Deep grooves in the surface of the cerebrum are called ....

16. Minor grooves or depressions in the brain's surface are termed ....

17. The ridges of the folds on the surface of the cerebrum are known as ....

18. The .... is the outer layer of gray matter covering the

surfaces of the cerebrum and cerebellum.

19. The gap where the optic tract becomes the optic nerve is called the ....

....

20. .... are the sensory nerves of the skin.

   VII.   Multiple choice: Circle the correct letter.

1. The inability to perform certain body movements is known as
    (a) agnosia
    (b) aphasia
    (c) apraxia
    (d) apoplexy

2. The medical word for stroke is
    (a) agnosia
    (b) aphasia
    (c) apraxia
    (d) apoplexy

3. A blood clot that leaves its original site and blocks an artery is called
    (a) hemorrhage
    (b) embolism
    (c) thrombosis
    (d) none of the above

4. An abnormal deep sleep is called
    (a) coma
    (b) apoplexy
    (c) agnosia
    (d) epilepsy

5. The more serious form of epileptic seizure is referred to as
    (a) petit mal
    (b) grand mal
    (c) epileptic coma
    (d) comatose mal

6. The medical word for an excessive amount of cerebrospinal fluid in the ventricles of the
    brain is
    (a) hydrocerebrum
    (b) hydroencephalus
    (c) hydrocephalus
    (d) hydroventriculus

7. A sympathectomy is performed to relieve
    (a) neuritis
    (b) subdural hematoma
    (c) spina bifida
    (d) hypertension

8. A general feeling of muscular weakness and fatigue resulting from a lack of acetylcholine
   (a) meningitis
   (b) myasthenia gravis
   (c) multiple sclerosis
   (d) neuritis

9. A condition in which the myelin coverings of the brain and spinal cord are destroyed and the gray and white matters become hard
   (a) myasthenia gravis
   (b) scoliosis
   (c) multiple sclerosis
   (d) sclerosis

10. A viral infection characterized by blisterlike sores on the skin
    (a) Parkinson's disease
    (b) shingles
    (c) neuritis
    (d) meningitis

11. A congenital defect characterized by a protruding sac containing cerebrospinal fluid
    (a) spina bifida
    (b) spina bifida occulta
    (c) poliomyelitis
    (d) meningiomas

12. A blood clot originating in one of the membranes covering the brain
    (a) thrombosis
    (b) subdural hematoma
    (c) ischemia
    (d) embolism

13. The medical word indicating the obstruction of a blood vessel
    (a) hematoma
    (b) thrombosis
    (c) ischemia
    (d) syncope

14. Malignant tumors originating from the supportive nerve cells
    (a) gliomas
    (b) meningiomas
    (c) hematomas
    (d) sarcomas

15. The medical word indicating the spread of malignant tumors to other areas of the body
    (a) ischemia
    (b) meatus
    (c) metastasis
    (d) syncope

ANSWERS TO EXERCISES

I.

1. excision of a ganglion, ganglion/ectomy
2. pertaining to the neuroglia, neur/o/gli/al
3. the suturing of a nerve, neur/o/rrhaphy
4. having a medium-sized head, mes/o/cephal/ic
5. hemorrhage in the meninges, mening/o/rrhagia
6. process of forming branches, ram/i/fic/a/tion
7. conducting impulses away from the CNS, ef/fer/ent
8. increased tension of the sympathetic division of the ANS accompanied by vascular spasms and high blood pressure sym/pathic/o/tonia
9. self-producing, aut/o/gen/ic
10. insufficient quantity of blood in the body, olig/emia
11. any disease of the brain, cerebr/o/pathy
12. cogenital absence of all or part of the brain, an/encephal/us
13. visual examination of the ventricles of the brain, ventricul/o/scopy
14. producing myelin, myelin/o/gen/etic
15. general feeling of weakness of neurological origin, neur/asthenia
16. inflammation of two or more nerves, poly/neur/itis
17. softening of the cerebrum, cerebr/o/malacia
18. inflammation of the brain and its protective membranes, mening/o/encephal/itis
19. pertaining to the cerebellum and spinal cord, cerebell/o/spin/al
20. inflammation of a ganglion, ganglion/itis

II.

1. astroglial or astrocyte; 2. ganglioblast; 3. cerebrotomy; 4. cerebellar;
5. neuroanastomosis; 6. thalamotomy; 7. meningomyelocele;
8. corticospinal; 9. sympathectomy; 10. myelinic; 11. gliomata or gliomas;
12. microcephalic; 13. cerebrospinal; 14. ventriculography;
15. encephalitis.

III.

1. (b); 2. (a); 3. (d); 4. (c); 5. (b).

IV.

1. d; 2. i; 3. m; 4. f; 5. a; 6. k; 7. p; 8. g; 9. l;
10. b; 11. n; 12. e; 13. q; 14. o; 15. c; 16. h; 17. j.

V.

1. T
2. F, efferent
3. F, sensory and motor
4. T

5. T
6. F, hypoglossal nerves
7. T
8. F, abducens
9. F, controls heartbeat and movements, also larynx and digestive organs
10. T
11. T
12. F, plexus
13. T
14. F, exteroceptive stimulus
15. F, efferent pathways
16. F, an involuntary response
17. T
18. T
19. F, efferent system
20. F. They run parallel to the vertebral column.
21. T

VI.

1. peripheral nervous;   2. autonomic nervous;   3. cerebrum, cerebellum, brainstem;
4. nucleus;   5. ganglion;   6. pneumotaxic;   7. thoracolumbar, craniosacral;
8. meninges;   9. dura mater;   10. arachnoid mater;   11. pia mater;
12. cerebrospinal fluid;   13. arachnoid villi, granulations;   14. ventricles;
15. fissures;   16. sulci;   17. gyri;   18. cerebral cortex;   19. optic chiasm;
20. dermatomes.

VII.

1. (c);   2. (d);   3. (b);   4. (a);   5. (b);   6. (c);   7. (d);   8. (b);
9. (c);   10. (b);   11. (a);   12. (b);   13. (c);   14. (a);   15. (c).

10 The Special Senses

COMBINING FORMS: SIGHT

	Meaning	Example
THE EYE		
OPHTHALM/O (of-thal'mo)	eye	OPHTHALMOLOGIST (of-thal-mol'o-jist), one who specializes in the eye and the treatment of its diseases
OCUL/O (ok'you-lo)	eye	OCULAR (ok'you-lar), pertaining to the eye
-opia (op'e-a)	sight, vision	ASTHENOPIA (as-the-no'pe-a), weak vision as a result of fatigue
PHAC/O (fak'o)	lens	PHACOMALACIA (fak-o-ma-lay'she-a), a softening of the lens of the eye
PUPILL/O (pou'pi-lo)	pupil	PUPILLARY (pou'pi-ler'e), pertaining to the pupil
CORE/O (ko're-o)	pupil (sometimes iris)	CORECTOPIA (kor-ek-toe'pe-a), a condition in which the pupil is set on one side of the iris
CORNE/O (kor'ne-o)	horny, the cornea	CORNEAL (kor'ne-al), pertaining to the cornea
KERAT/O (ker'a-to)	horny, the cornea	KERATOMALACIA (ker-a-to-ma-lay'she-a), softening of the cornea due to a vitamin A deficiency

	Meaning	Example
SCLER/O (skle′ro)	the sclera, the white portion of the eye	SCLERECTASIA (skle-reck-tay′ze-a), protrusion (dilatation) of the sclera
IR/O (i′ro)	iris	IRITIS (i-ry′tis), inflammation of the iris
IRID/O (ir′i-do)	iris	IRIDOMALACIA (ir-id-o-ma-lay′she-a), softening of the iris
RETIN/O (ret′i-no)	retina	RETINOSCOPY (ret-in-os′ko-pe), visual examination of the retina by examining the refraction of light projected into the eye
CYCL/O (si′klo)	circle, the ciliary body of the eye	CYCLOPLEGIA (si-klo-ple′ge-a), paralysis of the ciliary muscle
LACRIM/O (lak′rim-o)	tear, tear duct	LACRIMAL (lak′rim-al), pertaining to a tear or tear duct
DACRY/O (dak-re-o)	tear	DACRYOADENITIS (dak-re-o-ad-en-eye′tis), inflammation of a lacrimal gland
CONJUNCTIV/O (kon-junk-tie′vo)	conjunctiva, the membrane lining the eyelids	CONJUNCTIVITIS (kon-junk-te-vie′tis), inflammation of the conjunctiva
PALPEBR/O (pal′pe-bro)	eyelid	PALPEBRAL (pal′pe-bral), pertaining to the eyelid
BLEPHAR/O (blef′ar-o)	eyelid	BLEPHAROPTOSIS (blef-ar-op-toe′sis), drooping of the (upper) eyelid
AQU/O (ak′wo)	water	AQUEOUS (ak′wee-us), watery
EXO- (eks′o)	outside	EXOPHTHALMIA (eks-of-thal′me-a), abnormal protrusion of the eyeball

SIGHT

Seeing depends on the eye's sensitivity to different degrees of light and dark and to different colors.

Anatomy of the Eye

The eyeball is a movable sphere containing fluid. It is connected to the *optic nerve* over which visual impulses travel first to the *optic tract* and then to the cortex of the brain. (See Figure 10-1). The wall of the eye consists of three layers. The outer layer is made up of two fibrous coats—the *cornea* and the *sclera*. The middle layer is a vascular layer composed of the choroid (kor'oyd, CHORI/O, skin, membrane), the iris, and the ciliary body. The third and innermost layer is the *retina*, which contains the sight receptors. Internally, the eye is composed of three cavities, each containing fluid. The *anterior chamber*, located between the cornea and the iris, and the *posterior chamber*, located between the iris and the lens, both contain *aqueous humor*, a watery substance. The third cavity, the *vitreous* (vit're-us, VITRE/O, glassy) *chamber*, is a rather large cavity located between the lens and the retina; it contains a jellylike substance, *vitreous humor*. (The entire mass of vitreous humor is called the *vitreous body*.) The *hyaloid canal*, which passes through the vitreous body, develops anteriorly into the *hyaloid fossa*, which houses the lens; posteriorly, the hyaloid canal opens up to the area on the retina called the *optic disc*, which is set over the anterior end of the optic nerve. The *crystalline lens* is located in front of the vitreous body. An opening in the iris, the *pupil*, is located in front of the lens and gauges the amount of light entering the lens. The lens (Figure 10-2), enclosed in a lens capsule, is convex on both sides and consists of layers (*lammellae*, la-mel-lie) of fibrous protein. It is held in place by the *suspensory ligament*, an extension of the *ciliary muscle*. The iris, the colored portion of the eye, is made up of two layers of muscle—the *sphincter layer*, which contracts the pupil, and the *dilator layer*, which expands the pupil.

The retina, the inner layer of the eye wall, has two layers: the outer pigmented layer and an inner nervous layer, the retina proper. The retina proper contains three layers of neurons: (a) *visual receptor neurons*, which are the rods and cones, (b) *bipolar neurons*, which receive the initial impulses of the rods and cones, and (c) *ganglion neurons*, which are attached to the optic nerve fibers.

Aqueous Humor

Aqueous humor is a watery, transparent fluid that circulates from the posterior chamber of the eye to the lens, iris, and pupil, and, finally, into the anterior chamber through the *canal of Schlemm*. If this canal becomes blocked, the aqueous humor is unable to drain and pressure builds up in the anterior chamber, thereby resulting in *glaucoma* and perhaps blindness.

Accessory Structures of the Eye

The *eyebrows, eyelids, eyelashes, conjunctiva,* and *lacrimal apparatus* constitute the eye's accessory structures. All the accessory structures, in one way or another, help to

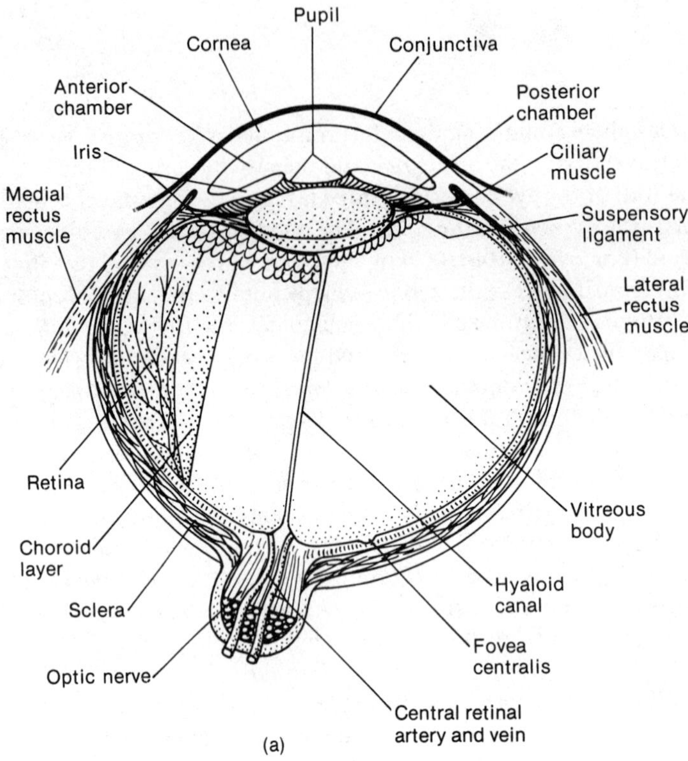

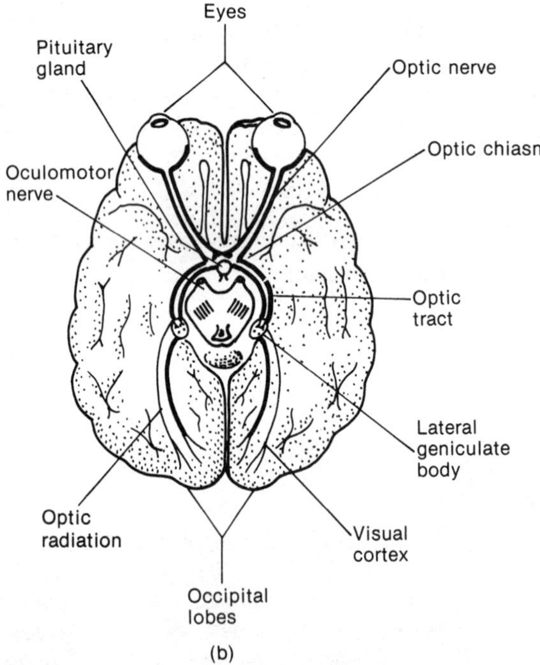

Figure 10-1 The visual apparatus. (a) Structure of the eyeball. (b) Relationship of the eyeballs, optic nerves, and optic tracts to the brain.

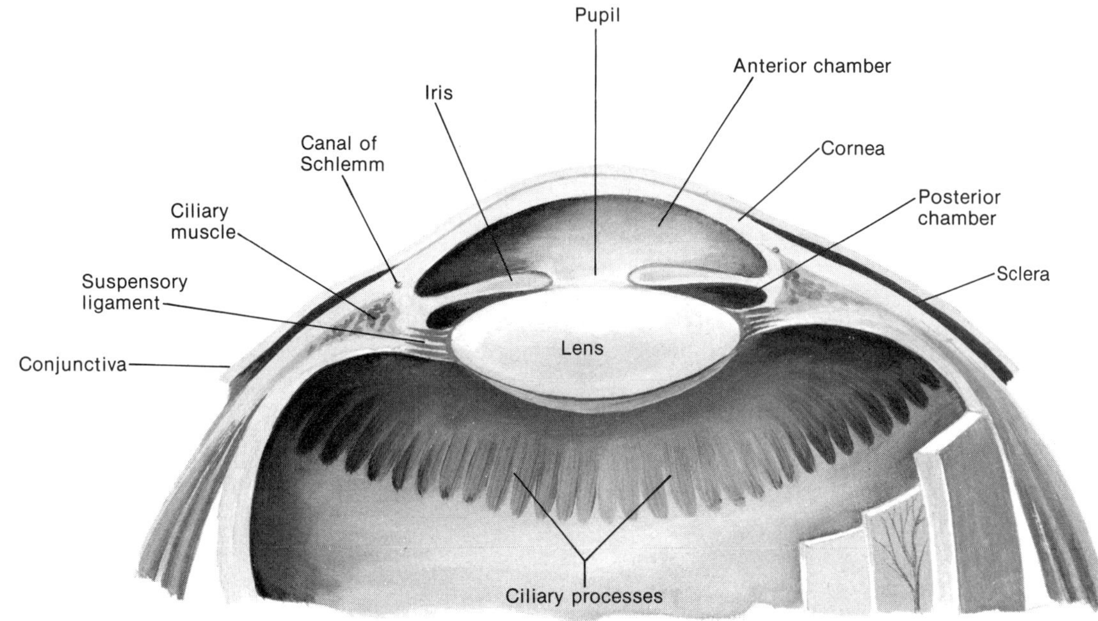

Figure 10-2   The lens and related structures.

protect the eye. The *palpebrae* (eyelids) protect the anterior portion of the eye. They consist of skin and striated muscle and on their inner surface are covered by a mucous membrane, the *conjunctiva*, which folds over part of the eyeball. The *palpebral fissure* is the name given to the slitlike opening between the upper and lower lids. At each end of the palpebral fissure there is an angular portion of the eyelid called the *canthus* (kan'thus). The *caruncle* (kar'un-kel), a small, red protrusion, is located in each medial canthus.

The *lacrimal apparatus* (Figure 10-3) both cleanses and moistens the eye. Every lacrimal apparatus is made up of a *lacrimal gland*, which secretes tears through a dozen *excretory ducts;* and a *lacrimal sac*, which has two *lacrimal ducts* and a *nasolacrimal duct* that empties into the nasal cavity. When the mucous lining of the lacrimal *papillae* (pa-pil'ay, PAPILL/O, nipple, opening of the lacrimal duct) and the nasolacrimal duct become inflamed due to a cold or allergy, tear secretion overflows, resulting in watery eyes.

How the Eye Functions

The retina has two types of light-sensitive cells, *rods* and *cones*. When lighting is poor, rods through the pigment rhodopsin (ro-dop'sin, RHOD/O, rose, visual purple) enable us to see outlines and notice movements. In good lighting the cones enable us to observe details and distinguish colors. The cones are concentrated in a small

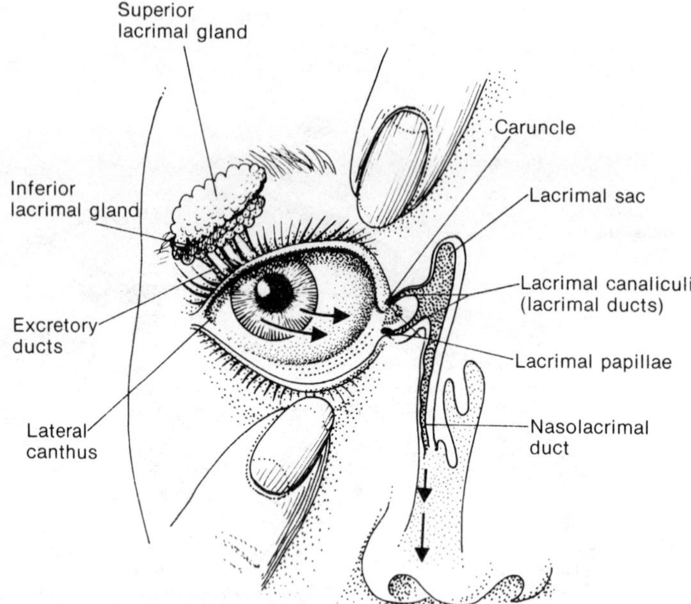

Figure 10-3 The lacrimal apparatus.

indentation in the posterior part of the center of the retina known as the *fovea centralis* (fo've-a sen-tra'lis). Outside the fovea centralis only a few cones exist and the number of rods increases.

When light hits either rods or cones, chemical changes occur. In the rods, rhodopsin becomes *lumirhodopsin*, which, in turn, becomes *scotopsin* (SKOT/O darkness) and retinene (ret-i-nean). Light stimulates the pigment of the cone cells, *iodopsin* (i'o-dop-sin, IO/, violet) and also causes it to break down. After a visual image has been formed on the retina, impulses travel over the optic nerve and tract to the *optic radiation* and visual cortex, where they are interpreted as sight. Those nerve fibers that originate in the median half of each retina cross over to the opposite side in the optic chiasm whereas fibers originating in the temporal half of the retina do not cross over.

Light entering the eye must be regulated and eyeballs must be adjusted for looking at near or distant objects. This process is known as *accommodation*. In accommodation the pupil becomes larger or smaller, depending on the distance of the object being viewed. Focusing is done by the *lens*, which is flattened for distant objects but becomes convex for close objects. The shape of the lens is changed by the relaxing or contracting of the ciliary muscle. Before light rays entering the eye converge on the retina, they are bent (called *refraction*) as they pass through the cornea, aqueous humor, lens, and vitreous humor, which represent the eye's *refraction medium.*

CLINICAL AND PATHOLOGICAL CONDITIONS

Strabismus (stra-biz'mus)
Strabismus is a condition characterized by one eye moving more medially or laterally than the other due to a lack of muscular coordination. As a result, the individual cannot focus on one object. A strabismus present in one eye is called *unilateral* (cockeye), in two eyes *bilateral* (cross-eye).

Myopia (my-o'pe-a, MY/O closed)
Myopia means nearsightedness. The image does not reach the retina and focuses in front of it. It is caused by an elongated eyeball or a lens that does not adjust to near vision and can be corrected with glasses having a *biconcave lens* (concave on both surfaces).

Hyperopia (also called hypermetropia (hy-per-me-trop'e-a))
In hyperopia or farsightedness a blurred image reaches the retina because the eyeball is too short or the lens too flat for normal vision. *Biconvex lenses* are used to correct this condition. Farsightedness commonly occurs in old age (called *presbyopia*, prez-be-o'-pe-a, PRESBY/O, old) as a result of the lens losing its elasticity.

Astigmatism (a-stig'ma-tizm, STIGMAT/O, point)
Due to an abnormally curved lens or cornea the light rays improperly refract and fall on separate areas of the retina, causing blurred vision.

Color blindness
A lack of cones sensitive to some colors of the spectrum—for instance red–green—produces color blindness.

Blindness
Partial or complete blindness results from a number of diseases or injuries. Several injuries are listed below.

1. Injured optic nerve, which produces partial or complete blindness on the affected side.
2. Injury of the optic chiasm, which causes blindness in the lateral half of the external visual field or in the medial half of the internal visual field of both eyes.
3. An injured optic tract.
4. An injured retina.

If one half the visual field is affected, the condition is termed *hemianopia* (or *hemianopsia*). Hemianopia in one eye is called *unilateral hemianopsia*, in both eyes *bilateral hemianopsia*.

Scotoma (sko-toe'ma, SCOT/O, dark)
Scotomas are patches of blind spots in the visual field.

Cataract
The lens becomes clouded because of the breakdown of the lens protein as a result of diabetes, infection, or trauma. The lens is usually removed.

Glaucoma
A blockage of the canal of Schlemm causes a buildup of intraocular pressure. Treatment is with drugs or by surgery to release the pressure.

Conjunctivitis
The conjunctiva, the membrane lining the eyelids, becomes inflamed. *Trachoma* (tra-ko'ma) is a viral conjunctivitis that affects both eyes.

Blepharitis
The hair follicles and glands of the eyelids become inflamed as a result of a bacterial infection.

Keratitis
A bacterial infection causes the cornea to become inflamed.

Sty (also called *hordeolum,* hor-de'o-lum)
The sebaceous glands of the eyelid become inflamed as a result of a bacterial infection.

Endophthalmos and exopthalmos
In endophthalmos the eyeball is sunk deep within its socket as a result of old age, disease, or malnutrition. In exophthalmos the eyeballs protrude abnormally. This condition frequently indicates hyperthyroidism.

Nystagmus (nis-tag'mus, NYSTAGM/O, nod)
This condition refers to the spasmodic, involuntary movement of the eye in any direction.

Nyctalopia (nik-ta-lo'pe-a, NYCT/O, night, AL/O, blindness)
Night blindness usually results from a lack of vitamin A, which is needed for the manufacture of rhodopsin.

Amblyopia (am-ble-o'pe-a, AMBLY/O, dull)
The vision becomes dull or dim but not as a result of anatomical injury or refractive error. Diabetes, alcohol, toxemia, and certain drugs can cause amblyopia.

Mydriatic (mid-ri-at'ik) and miotic (mi-ot'ik) drugs
Certain drugs, such as epinephrine, atropine, and cocaine, are called *mydriatic* because they cause the pupil to dilate. Other drugs like morphine, pilocarpine, and

physostigmine are called *miotic* because they cause the pupil to constrict. Both types of drugs are used to examine the eyes and to treat certain diseases.

TASTE AND SMELL

Both taste and smell are chemical senses. This means that substances must be dissolved in liquid (for taste) or air (for smell) before they can be tasted or smelled.

The *tongue* (Figure 10-4) is the chief organ of gustation (GUST/O, taste). The tongue's surface is covered with numerous protrusions or bumps called *papillae* (pa-pil′ay PAPILL/O, nipple). On the posterior portion of the tongue the largest papillae, the *vallate* (VALLAT/O, walled) *papillae*, are arranged in a V shape. The two smaller types of papillae, the *filiform* (thread shaped, FIL/O, thread) and *fungiform*, make up the rest of the tongue's surface. Each area of the tongue is sensitive to a specific taste. Gustatory impulses are transmitted to the brain in the following manner.

Gustatory cells of the taste buds ⎯transmit to⎯→ facial nerves (for the anterior two-thirds of the tongue) or glossopharyngeal nerve (posterior one-third of the tongue) ⎯→ gustatory nucleus of medulla ⎯→ thalamus ⎯→ temporal lobe of cerebral cortex.

The *olfactory sense*, the sense of smell, detects odors when substances, suspended

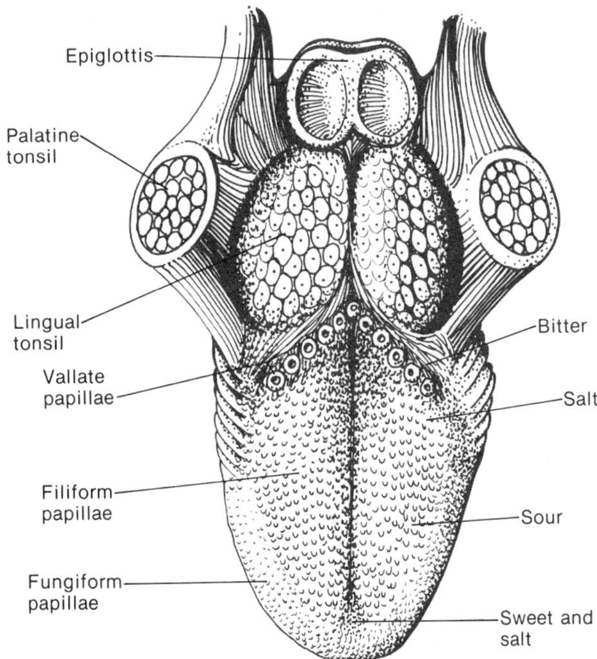

Figure 10-4 The various types of papillae found on the tongue, and the areas of the tongue where the different kinds of tastes are projected.

in air, come in contact with *olfactory* (ol-fak'to-re, OLFACT/O, smell) *cells* located in the mucous membrane of the upper portion of the nasal cavity. Olfactory impulses are transmitted to the brain in the following manner.

Olfactory cells in the mucous membrane ⟶ olfactory bulb ⟶ olfactory tract ⟶ frontal lobe of the cerebrum.

EXERCISES: THE EYE

I. Give the meaning for each of the following medical words. Divide each word into base(s), prefix, and suffix; underline the letter(s) that has the primary stress. *Example:*

INTRAOCULAR   pertaining to the area within the eyeball   intra/ocul/ar

1. CORECTOMY ....

2. SCLERAL ....

3. KERATOPLASTY ....

4. DACRYOCYSTECTOMY ....

5. LACRIMATION ....

6. XEROTIC (XER/O, ze'ro, dry) KERATITIS ....

7. OPHTHALMODYNAMOMETER (DYNAM/O, dy'na-mo, power)

    ....

8. OCULOMOTOR ....

9. CORNEOUS ....

10. DACRYOADENALGIA ....

11. BLEPHARORRHAPHY ....

12. PUPILLOSTATOMETER (STAT/O, sta'to, halting, standing still)

    ....

13. OPHTHALMIA ....

14. CORNEITIS ....

15. IRIDOPTOSIS ....

> **II.** Make medical words from the following phrases. Indicate the primary stress by underlining the stressed letter(s). *Example:*

incision of a lacrimal duct

lacri<u>mot</u>omy
....

1. diseased condition of the eye due to fungus

....

2. an instrument for measuring the diameter of the pupil of the eye

....

3. horn shaped

....

4. pertaining to the mucus membrane lining the eyelid

....

5. inflammation of the retina

....

6. an abnormal narrowing of the pupil of the eye

....

7. an examination of the cornea

....

8. excision of (part of) the iris

....

9. a lacrimal sac

....

10. paralysis of the iris (iridal sphincter)

....

11. excision of (part of) the ciliary body

....

12. inflammation of the cornea and iris

....

13. inflammation of the gland(s) of the eyelid

....

14. inflammation of a lacrimal sac

....

15. incision of a tear duct

....

    III.   Fill in the blank spaces for each of the following statements.

1. The outermost layer of the wall of the eye is made of two fibrous covers: the ....

and the ....

2. The ...., the ...., and the ....

.... comprise the middle, vascular layer of the eye.

3. The third layer of the wall of the eye is the ...., and it contains the sight receptors.

4. Internally, the eye is given its shape by three fluid-filled cavities:

(a) the .... between the cornea and the iris,

(b) the posterior chamber between the .... and the ....,

(c) the .... between the lens and retina.

The first two cavities contain ...., a thin, watery

substance; the third cavity contains a gelatinous substance called ....

....

5. The lens of the eye is housed in the ..../.........

6. The opening in the iris that gauges the amount of light entering the eye is called the

   . . . .

7. The retina proper contains three layers of neurons:

   (a) . . . . known as rods and cones,

   (b) . . . ., which receive the impulses initiated by the rods and cones,

   (c) . . . ., which communicate with the optic nerve fibers.

8. When the . . . . becomes blocked, the aqueous humor cannot drain and causes pressure to build up in the anterior chamber of the eye, causing the

   disease known as . . . .

9. The inner surface of the eyelids is covered by a mucous membrane known as the . . . .

   . . . .

10. The . . . . refers to the slit between the upper and lower eyelids.

11. The . . . . is a small protrusion located in each medial . . . .

    . . . . or angular portion of the eyelid.

12. Each lacrimal apparatus consists of a . . . ., a . . . .

    . . . ., and a . . . .

13. The light-sensitive cones are concentrated in the center area of the retina called the

    . . . .

14. In the light-sensitive rod light activates the substance . . . .

15. Impulses coming from the retina travel over the . . . . and optic tract on their way to the visual center of the cortex.

16. The process of regulating light entering the eye and adjusting the eye for looking at objects

    is known as . . . .

17. .... refers to the "bending" of light rays as they pass through the cornea, the aqueous humor, the lens, and the vitreous humor.

IV. Multiple choice: Underline the correct letter.

1. A condition in which the individual cannot focus on an object because of one eye moving more medially or more laterally than the other eye
    (a) nystagmus
    —(b) strabismus
    (c) amblyopia
    (d) endophthalmus

2. The medical word for farsightedness
    (a) hyperopia
    (b) myopia
    (c) hypermetropia
    (d) both (a) and (c)

3. A condition in which the lens of the eye becomes clouded
    (a) glaucoma
    (b) trachoma
    (c) cataract
    (d) nyctalopia

4. A bacterial infection of the sebaceous glands of the eyelid
    (a) blepharitis
    (b) conjunctivitis
    (c) sty
    (d) keratitis

5. Blindness in one-half of the visual field
    (a) semiglaucoma
    (b) hemianopsia
    (c) hemikeratitis
    (d) astigmatism

6. A viral form of conjunctivitis that usually affects both eyes
    (a) trachoma
    (b) blepharitis
    (c) nyctalopia
    (d) bilateral conjunctivitis

7. The medical term for night blindness
    (a) nystagmus
    (b) nyctalopia
    (c) amblyopia
    (d) presbyopia

8. The name given to drugs that cause the pupil of the eye to dilate
    (a) miotic
    (b) exophthalmic
    (c) mydriatic
    (d) enophthalmic

9. A spasmodic, involuntary movement of the eye
   (a) nystagmus
   (b) nyctalopia
   (c) astigmatism
   (d) hordeolum

10. A bacterial inflammation of the cornea
    (a) blepharitis
    (b) sty
    (c) conjunctivitis
    (d) keratitis

COMBINING FORMS: HEARING

	Meaning	*Example*
THE EAR		
AUDI/O (au'dee-o)	hearing	AUDIOMETER (au-dee-om'e-ter), instrument for testing
ACOU/O (a-kou'o)	hearing	ACOUSTIC (a-kou'stik), pertaining to the sense of hearing
AUR/O (o'ro)	ear	AURAL (o'ral), pertaining to the ear
OT/O (o'to)	ear	OTITIS (o-tie'tis), inflammation of the ear
CERUMIN/O (se-rou'men-o)	cerumen, wax	CERUMINOSIS (se-rou-mi-no'sis), abnormal amount of wax formation
TYMPAN/O (tim'pan-o)	tympanum, eardrum, middle ear	TYMPANOTOMY (tim-pan-ot'o-me) incision of the eardrum
MYRING/O (mir-in'go)	eardrum, tympanic membrane	MYRINGOSCOPE (mir-in'go-skope), instrument for examining the eardrum
MALLE/O (mal'e-o)	malleus, hammer, the first of the three ossicles of the middle ear	MALLEOINCUDAL (mal-e-o-in'ku-dal), pertaining to the malleus and the incus
INCUD/O (in'ku-do)	incus, anvil, (second ossicle)	INCUDECTOMY (in-ku-dek'toe-me), excision of the incus

	Meaning	*Example*
STAPED/O (sta'pe-do)	stapes, stirrup (third ossicle)	STAPEDECTOMY (sta-pe-dek'toe-me), excision of the stapes
SALPING/O (sal-pin'go)	tube, especially the eustachian or fallopian tube	SALPINGEMPHRAXIS (sal-pin-jem-frak'sis), obstruction of the eustachian tube resulting in deafness
EUSTACHI/O (you-stay'key-an)	eustachian tube	EUSTACHIAN (you-stay'key-an) pertaining to the eustachian tube
COCHLE/O (kok'lee-o)	cochlea, the snail-shaped portion of the inner ear	COCHLEAR (kok'lee-ar), pertaining to the cochlea
LABYRINTH/O (lab-i-rin'tho)	labyrinth, intricate winding path of the inner ear	LABYRINTHINE (lab-i-rin'thyn), pertaining to the labyrinth
VESTIBUL/O (ves-tib'you-lo)	a cavity at the entrance of a canal, the middle portion of the middle ear	VESTIBULAR (ves-tib'you-lar), pertaining to a vestibule
UTRICUL/O (ou-trik'you-lo)	a sac, the utricle: a sac of the membranous labyrinth located in the vestibule of the bony labyrinth	UTRICULITIS (ou-trik-you-lie'tis), inflammation of the utricle
SACCUL/O (sak'you-lo)	a small bag or sac, the saccule: a small bag of the membranous labyrinth located in the vestibule of the bony labyrinth and containing maculae	UTRICULOSACCULAR (ou-trik-you-lo-sak'you-lar), pertaining to the utricle and saccule
AMPULL/O (am-pul'lo)	a baglike protrusion of a canal or duct, a protrusion at the end of a semicircular canal	AMPULLITIS (am-pul-eye'tis), inflammation of an ampulla
ANKYL/O (ang'ki-lo)	bent, crooked, the fusion of two parts	ANKYLOSIS (ang-ki-lo'sis), the fusion of a joint

HEARING

Hearing is the perception of sound that results from waves produced by the vibration of an object. Sound waves have three qualities: (a) *pitch* or *frequency*, the number of vibrations in a given period of time, (b) *intensity*, the strength of the sound wave, and (c) *timbre*, the quality of the overtones produced by a sound.

Hearing or *audition* depends on a mechanical action for the production of a nerve impulse (Figure 10-5). Sound waves are picked up by the earflap, called the *pinna*

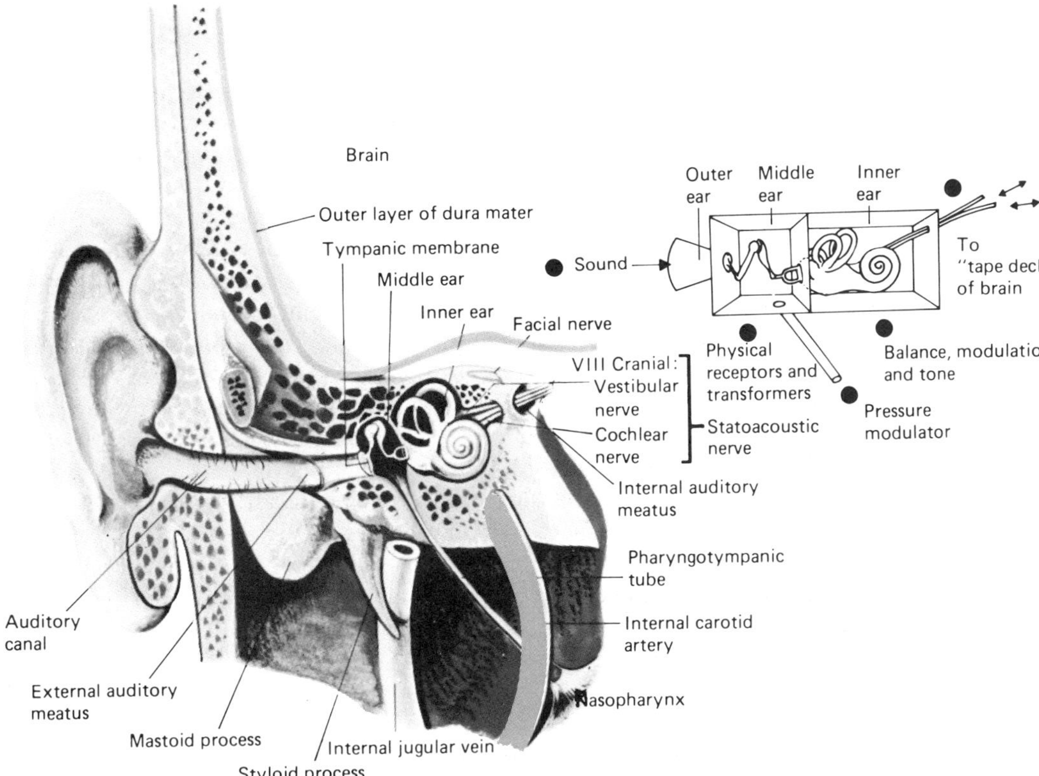

Figure 10-5 The auditory apparatus and its anatomical relationships.

(pin′a) or *auricle* (o′ri-kel) and travel through the auditory canal, which is lubricated with a protective covering of wax called *cerumen*, to the *external auditory meatus* (me-ay′tus, MEAT/O, opening, a *meatus* is an opening or passage), which leads to the *eardrum*, the *tympanic membrane* (the first structure of the middle ear). The vibration produced by the effect of the sound waves on this membrane is passed along to the *malleus*, the first of three small bones called *ossicles*. The malleus, in turn, vibrates the *incus* or anvil, which then activates the *stapes* (stirrup). The stapes is attached to the *oval window*, the opening leading to the cochlea, the outer structure of the inner ear. The middle ear, located in the temporal bone of the skull, is also joined to the *eustachian tube* (also called the *pharyngotympanic tube*), which enables us to equalize the pressure on both sides of the eardrum.

After the vibrations have been passed along from the stapes to the oval window, they are then sent through the *perilymph*, a fluid located in the area of the cochlea called the *scala vestibuli* (skay′la ves-tib′you-lie). Next, the vibrations pass through the vestibular membrane, the roof of the cochlear duct, to the *endolymph*, which fills this duct. Finally, in the *organ of Corti*, where dendrites of the acoustic nerve are set around the hair cells, the vibrations cause the hairs to move and stimulate the *tectorial membrane*, a gelatinous membrane embedded with the dendrites of the acoustic nerve.

From here the nerve impulses (formerly vibrations) travel to the cerebrum via the various portions of the brainstem.

Besides hearing, the winding pathways of the inner ear or *labyrinth* also maintain our sense of balance and equilibrium. The labyrinth is composed of two parts: the *membranous labyrinth* and the *bony labyrinth*, which covers the former. The membranous labyrinth is bathed in *perilymph* and contains its own fluid, *endolymph*. The canals of the membranous labyrinth—the superior, lateral, and posterior *semicircular canals*—are connected to the cochlea by the *vestibule*, an oval-shaped cavity. In this vestibule there are two structures, the *utricle* and the *saccule*, which are enlarged portions of the canals. The utricle and semicircular canals enable us to maintain our sense of balance and proprioceptive sense (awareness of the position of the body and body parts in space). Groups of hairs (called *cristae*) contained in enlarged portions of the canals (called *ampullae*) that connect with the utricle are moved by endolymph, resulting in impulses being sent to the acoustic nerve. In this manner, our sense of dynamic equilibrium is maintained.

Within the utricle and saccule there are structures called *maculae* (mak'you-lie, spots). The maculae are composed of hair cells and a gelatinous membrane containing bits of calcium carbonate known as *otoliths* or earstones. A change in the movement of the head causes the otoliths to exert pressure on the hair cells that send impulses to the acoustic nerve. In this manner, static equilibrium is maintained. The saccule may perform a similar function.

CLINICAL AND PATHOLOGICAL CONDITIONS

Deafness

Hearing is measured by an *audiometer* that measures pitch and amplitude. Both a partial and a total loss of hearing can be attributed to one of three causes: conduction deafness, nerve deafness, or central deafness. In *conduction deafness* the ossicles of the ear become stiff (called *ankylosis*) at the joints or pressure on both sides of the tympanic membrane can't be relieved by the eustachian tube. *Nerve deafness* occurs when the cochlea or cochlear portion of the acoustic nerve is damaged. There is no cure for this form of deafness, which is commonly associated with loss of hearing in old age (*presbyacusia*, prez-be-a-ku'ze-a). *Central deafness* is a destruction of the acoustic center in the temporal lobe of the cerebral cortex. There is no cure for this form of deafness.

Otitis

There are three types of this inflammation: otitis externa, media, and interna. Each type affects a different area of the ear and each type is *suppurative*.

Tinnitus (tin'e-tus)

A ringing sound develops as a result of a buildup of wax, damage to the acoustic nerve, or a side effect of a drug (e.g., aspirin).

Otosclerosis
Deafness is the result of the hardening of the labyrinthine tissue and the formation of spongy bone around the oval window. The stapes anlylosizes.

Vertigo (ver'te-go)
This disorder of equilibrium produces a feeling of moving around in space (called subjective vertigo) or a feeling that objects are moving around (objective vertigo). Vertigo is caused by many diseases, including diseases of the ear and general body toxemia.

Ménière's (men-ee-ayr') disease
This is a degeneration of the structures of the vestibule. These structures become dilated, producing tinnitus, vertigo, and deafness.

Motion sickness
This general sick feeling (*malaise*, ma-layz') is accompanied by nausea and frequently vomiting. Equilibrium is affected as a result of riding in a car, ship, and so on.

EXERCISES: THE EAR

I. Give the meaning for each of the following medical words. Divide each word into base(s), prefix, and suffix; underline the letter(s) that has the primary stress. *Example:*

OTOMYCOSIS   a fungus infection of the ear   ot/o/myc/osis

1. TYMPANOPLASTY

2. INCUDAL

3. COCHLEOPALPEBRAL

4. AUDITORY

5. OTOPYORRHEA (PY/O, pus)

6. ANKYLOBLEPHARON

7. ACOUMETER

8. MYRINGODECTOMY

9. LABYRINTHOTOMY

10. OTORHINOLOGY

11. EUSTACHITIS ....

12. INCUDOSTAPEDIAL ....

13. TYMPANITIS ....

14. STAPEDIOVESTIBULAR ....

15. COCHLEITIS ....

II. Make medical words from the following phrases. Indicate the primary stress by underlining the stressed letter(s). *Example:*

pertaining to the middle ear

tym<u>pan</u>ic
....

1. instrument for examining the eustachian tube

....

2. instrument for examining the ear

....

3. inflammation of the labyrinth

....

4. pertaining to both the vestibule and cochlea

....

5. pertaining to the utricle

....

6. the sense of hearing

....

7. pertaining to both the ear and the pharynx

....

8. having/pertaining to the waxlike substance of the ear

....

9. inflammation of the eardrum and mastoid process

....

10. instrument for cutting the tympanic membrane

....

III. Match the medical words with their common names or descriptions.

1. the earflap ....

2. the waxlike substance coating the auditory

   canal ....

3. a medical term meaning opening or passage ....

4. the eardrum ....

5. the earbones ....

6. hammer ....

7. anvil ....

8. stirrup ....

9. the structure leading to the inner ear ....

10. eustachian tube ....

11. a snail-shaped structure in the middle ear ....

12. the winding pathways of the inner ear ....

13. dendrites of the acoustic nerve are located

    here ....

14. the fluid of the bony labyrinth ....

15. the fluid of the membranous labyrinth ....

a. incus

b. utricle

c. pharyngotympanic
   tube

d. organ of Corti

e. ampullae

f. maculae

g. pinna

h. labyrinth

i. endolymph

j. cerumen

k. saccule

l. tympanic membrane

m. perilymph

n. oval window

o. meatus

p. proprioception

16. awareness of the position of the body parts   q. stapes

     in space ....   r. cochlea

17. enlarged portions of the semicircular canals ....   s. ossicles

18. two saclike structures located in the vestibule of the
                                                                    t. malleus
     bony labyrinth (two letters) ....

19. structures containing hair cells and otoliths ....

     IV. Complete the following statements by filling in the blank spaces.

1. The abnormal stiffening of a joint is called ....

2. In .... the acoustic center in the temporal lobe of
    the brain is damaged.

3. Sometimes aspirin produces a side effect called ...., which is characterized
    by a ringing sensation.

4. An .... is an instrument for measuring pitch and amplitude.

5. .... is a suppurative inflammation of the external, middle, or inner ear.

6. .... is a disorder affecting equilibrium in which the individual feels that he
    is constantly moving.

7. .... is a form of deafness in which the ossicles
    become stiff and can no longer transmit vibrations.

8. .... is a general sick feeling, including nausea, and frequently accom-
    panies motion sickness.

9. .... is a form of deafness caused by the formation of spongy bone
    around the oval window and the hardening of labyrinthine tissue.

10. Deafness in old age, called ...., is often the result of nerve deafness.

ANSWERS TO EXERCISES: THE EYE

     I.

1. excision of the iris, cor/ectomy

2. pertaining to the sclera, scler/al
3. surgical restructuring of the cornea, kerat/o/plasty
4. excision of a lacrimal sac dacry/o/cyst/ectomy
5. the process of forming and secreting tears, lacrim/a/tion
6. inflammation of the cornea resulting from dry conjunctiva, xer/o/tic kerat/itis
7. instrument for measuring the pressure exerted by the arteries of the eyes, ophthalm/o/dynam/o/meter
8. pertaining to the eye movements, ocul/o/motor
9. possessing horns, horny, corne/ous
10. painful lacrimal gland, dacry/o/aden/algia
11. suture of an eyelid, blephar/o/rraphy
12. instrument for measuring the distance between the centers of the pupils, pupill/o/stat/o/meter
13. serious inflammation of the eye, ophthalmia
14. inflammation of the cornea, corne/itis
15. drooping (prolapse) of the iris, irid/o/ptosis

II.

1. oculomycosis;   2. pupillometer;   3. keratoid;   4. conjunctival;
5. retinitis;   6. corestenoma;   7. keratoscopy;   8. iridectomy;
9. dacryocyst;   10. iridoplegia;   11. cyclectomy;   12. corneoiritis;
13. blepharadenitis;   14. dacryocystitis;   15. lacrimotomy.

III.

1. cornea, sclera
2. choroid layer, iris, ciliary body
3. retina
4. anterior chamber, iris, lens, vitreous chamber, aqueous humor, vitreous humor
5. hyaloid fossa
6. pupil
7. visual receptor neurons, bipolar neurons, ganglion neurons
8. canal of Schlemm, glaucoma
9. conjunctiva
10. palpebral fissure
11. caruncle, canthus
12. lacrimal gland, lacrimal sac, nasolacrimal duct
13. fovea centralis
14. rhodopsin
15. optic nerve, optic tract
16. accommodation
17. refraction

IV.

1. (b);   2. (d);   3. (c);   4. (c);   5. (b);   6. (a);   7. (b);   8. (c);
9. (a);   10. (d).

ANSWERS TO EXERCISES: THE EAR

I.

1. surgical restructuring of the eardrum, tympan/o/plasty
2. pertaining to the ear's anvil, incud/al
3. pertaining to the cochlea and eyelid, cochle/o/palpebr/al
4. pertaining to the sense of hearing, audit/ory
5. purulent discharge from the ear, ot/o/py/o/rrhea
6. fusion of the eyelids, ankyl/o/blephar/on
7. instrument for measuring the sharpness of hearing, acou/meter
8. excision of all or part of the tympanic membrane, myring/o/(d)ectomy
9. incision of the labyrinth, labyrinth/otomy
10. the branch of medicine dealing with the ear and nose and their diseases, ot/o/rhin/o/logy
11. inflammation of the eustachian tube, eustach/itis
12. pertaining to the incus and stapes, incud/o/staped/ial
13. inflammation of the eardrum, tympan/itis
14. pertaining to the stapes and vestibule, stapedi/o/vestibul/ar
15. inflammation of the cochlea, cochle/itis

II.

1. salpingoscope;   2. auriscope;   3. labyrinthitis;   4. vestibulocochlear;
5. utricular;   6. audition;   7. otopharyngeal;   8. ceruminous or ceruminal;
9. tympanomastoiditis;   10. myringotome.

III.

1. g;   2. j;   3. o;   4. l;   5. s;   6. t;   7. a;   8. q;   9. n;
10. c;   11. r;   12. h;   13. d;   14. m;   15. i;   16. p;   17. e;
18. b and k;   19. f.

IV.

1. ankylosis;   2. central deafness;   3. tinnitus;   4. audiometer;   5. otitis;
6. vertigo;   7. conduction deafness;   8. malaise;   9. otosclerosis;
10. presbyacusia.

11 The Cardiovascular System; Blood and Lymph

COMBINING FORMS

	Meaning	Example
CARDI/O (kar′de-o)	heart	ELECTROCARDIOGRAM (e-lek-tro-kar′de-o-gram), a record of the electrical impulses of the heart
CORON/O (ko-ro′no)	crown, the heart	CORONARY (kor′o-na-re), pertaining to the heart
AORT/O (ay-or′to)	aorta	AORTIC (ay-or′tik), pertaining to the aorta
ATRI/O (ay′tre-o)	cavity, atrium	ATRIOVENTRICULAR (ay-tre-o-ven-trik′you-lar), pertaining to the atrium and ventricle
VALV/O (val′vo)	valve	VALVOTOMY (val-vot′o-me), incision of a valve
-L /O	suffix indicating *small* (*-le* ending)	VALVULITIS (val-vu-ly′tis), inflammation of a (small) valve
SIN/O (sy′no)	cavity, sinus	SINOATRIAL (sy-no-ay′tre-al), pertaining to the venous sinus and the atrium
ANGI/O (an′je-o)	vessel	ANGIOGRAM (an′je-o-gram), x ray of a blood vessel that is injected with a substance that appears opaque on the x ray
VAS/O (vas′o)	a vessel	VASOCONSTRICTOR (vas-o-kon-strik′tor), that which constricts a blood vessel

	Meaning	*Example*
ARTERI/O (ar-tee're-o)	artery	ARTERIOSTENOSIS (ar-tee-re-o-ste-no'sis), narrowing of an artery
ARTERIOL/O (ar-tee-re-o'lo)	small artery, arteriole	ARTERIOLAR (ar-tee-re-o'lar), pertaining to an arteriole
VEN/O (ve-no)	vein	VENOUS (ve'nus), pertaining to a vein or the veins
VENUL/O (ven'u-lo)	small vein, venule	VENULAR (ven'u-lar), pertaining to a venule
PHLEB/O (fleb'o)	vein	PHLEBITIS (fleb-eye'tis), inflammation of a vein
CAPILL/O (kap'i-lo)	very small blood vessel	CAPILLARY (kap'i-la-re), very small blood vessel
STETH/O (steth'o)	chest	STETHOSCOPE (steth'o-skope), instrument for listening to sounds produced in the chest or body in general
SPHYGM/O (sfig'mo)	pulse	SPHYGMOMANOMETER (sfig-mo-man-om'et-er), instrument for measuring arterial blood pressure
OX/O (oks'o)	oxygen	ANOXIA (an-oks'e-a), lack of oxygen
OXY- (ok'se)	oxygen	OXYHEMOGLOBIN (ok-si-he-mo-glo'bin), oxygenated blood
HEM/O (he'mo)	blood	HEMORRHAGE (hem'o-rij), discharge of blood from a blood vessel
HEMAT/O (he'ma-to)	blood	HEMATURIA (he-ma-tu're-a), presence of blood in the urine
-EMIA (-ee'me-a)	suffix meaning *blood*	ANEMIA (a-nee'me-a), reduction of red blood cells or hemoglobin
BAS/O (ba'so)	base (in contrast to an acid)	BASOPHIL (ba'so-fil), a type of white blood cell whose granules stain with a base dye
PHIL/O (fi'lo)	love, affinity for, frequently a suffix	EOSINOPHIL (e-o-sin'o-fil), a type of white blood cells whose granules stain with an acid dye

	Meaning	*Example*
GRANUL/O (gran'you-lo)	granule	AGRANULOCYTE (a-gran'you-lo-syt), a white blood cell not containing granules
PLASM/O (plaz'mo)	plasma, the liquid portion of blood	PLASMAPHERESIS (plaz-ma-fer-ee'sis, -PHERESIS removal), separation of plasma from the formed elements of the blood by means of a centrifuge
THROMB/O (throm'bo)	clot	THROMBOSIS (throm-bo'sis), the formation of a blood clot
-POIESIS (poy-ee'sis)	suffix meaning *production*	HEMOPOIESIS (he-mo-poy-ee'sis), production of blood cells
FIBR/O (fy'bro)	fiber, fibrous tissue	FIBROUS (fy'brus), composed of fiber or fibrous tissue
FIBRIN/O (fy-brin'o)	fibrin, a fibrous protein produced in clotting	FIBRINOGEN (fy-brin'o-jen), a substance that is converted into fibrin.
-IN (in)	suffix indicating a chemical substance	ERYTHROPOIETIN (e-rith-ro-poy'e-tin), a hormone regulating red blood cell production
RETICUL/O (re-tik'you-lar)	network, netlike	RETICULAR (re-tik'you-lar), in a network
SIDER/O (sid'er-o)	iron	HEMOSIDERIN (he-mo-sid'er-in), the iron-containing pigment of hemoglobin
AGGLUTIN/O (a-glou'ti-no)	clumping	AGGLUTINOGEN (a-glou-tin'o-jen), a chemical that stimulates an agglutinin
GLOB/O (glo'bo)	round, globe	GLOBIN (glo'bin), globin, protein
TON/O (to'no)	tension, osmotic pressure	HYPERTONIC (hi-per-ton'ik), having an osmotic pressure greater than that of another solution
SER/O (se'ro)	serum, a liquid coating of serous membranes, liquid exudate of a clot	SEROUS (sir'us), containing serum

	Meaning	*Example*
NUCLE/O (nu-kle′o)	nucleus	MONONUCLEAR (mon-o-nu′kle-ar), having one nucleus
KARY/O (kar′e-o)	nucleus	MEGAKARYOCYTE (meg-a-kar′e-o-syt), a cell with a large nucleus
MEGA- MEGAL/O	large	MEGALOCARDIA (meg-a-lo-kar′de-a), enlargement of the heart
-STASIS (stay′sis)	suffix meaning *halting, stopping*	HEMOSTASIS (he-mo-stay′sis), halting the flow of blood
PHAG/O (fag′o)	eat	PHAGOCYTE (fag′o-syt), a cell that engulfs and destroys particles and microorganisms
IMMUN/O (im-mu′no)	safe, immune	IMMUNOLOGY (im-mu-nol′o-je), the study of immunity to disease
LYMPH/O (lim′fo)	lymph	LYMPHADENITIS (lim-fad-en-eye′tis), inflammation of a lymph gland
NOD/O (no′do)	knot, node, swelling	NODAL (no′dal), having a node
SPLEN/O (splee′no)	spleen	SPLENOMYELOMALACIA (splee-no-my-el-o-ma-lay′she-a), softening of the spleen and bone marrow
THYM/O (thy′mo)	thymus gland	THYMIC (thy′mik), pertaining to the thymus gland
TONSILL/O (ton′sil-o)	tonsil	TONSILLECTOMY (ton-sil-ek′to-me), removal of the tonsils
ATHER/O (ath′er-o)	fatty buildup	ATHEROSCLEROSIS (ath-er-o-skler-o′sis), hardening of the arteries accompanied by a buildup of fatty plaque
NECR/O (nek′ro)	death	NECROSIS (ne-kro′sis), death of an area of tissue surrounded by living tissue
ANGIN/O (an-jy′no)	choking	ANGINAL (an-jy′nal), pertaining to angina or choking

	Meaning	*Example*
TACH/O (ta'ko)	quick	TACHYCARDIA (tak-e-kar'de-a), abnormally rapid heart rate
BRACHY- (brak'e)	short	BRACHYCARDIA (brak-e-kar'de-a), abnormally slow heart rate
ANEURYSM/O (an'you-riz-mo)	widening (abnormal)	ANEURYSMORRHAPHY (an-you-riz-mor'a-fe), suturing of an aneurysm
VARIC/O (var'i-ko)	twisted vein varix	VARICOSE (var'i-kos), twisted (veins)

The *circulatory system* is a network of blood vessels that bring nutrients and other essential elements to the cells throughout the body and carry away wastes. The heart is the pump that circulates the blood throughout this network of blood vessels. Blood enters the two upper chambers of the heart, the *atria*, and leaves through the two lower chambers, the *ventricles*. Blood leaving the left ventricle of the heart travels to all parts of the body (called *systemic circulation*) whereas blood leaving the right ventricle travels to the air sacs of the lungs to be oxygenated (called *pulmonary circulation*, PULM/O lung). As the blood leaves the left ventricle, it passes through the *aorta*, the largest artery in the body. At the aorta the process of branching off into smaller arteries begins almost immediately and continues until every area of the body is reached.

ANATOMY OF THE HEART

The heart, the pump of the cardiovascular system, is located in the center of the thoracic cavity (Figure 11-1) and is positioned so that the right ventricle faces anteriorly and the left ventricle posteriorly. The heart itself is contained in a sac, the *pericardium*, which has two layers. The *visceral pericardium* (also called the epicardium) is directly attached to the heart; the outer membrane, the *parietal pericardium*, is separated from it by a fluid-filled pericardial space. Thick muscle called *myocardium* which is lined with epithelial tissue (*endocardium*) constitutes the entire heart. The *trabeculae carneae* (tra-bek'you-lie kar'ne-eye) are the muscles of the walls of the ventricles; the *musculi pectinati* (mus'kul-eye pek-ti-nat'eye) are the muscles of the walls of the atria.

The heart has four chambers: the *right* and *left atria*, which are closed by an earlike flap called an *auricle*, and the *right* and *left ventricles*. The *interatrial, intraventricular,* and *atrioventricular septa* (fences) separate the atria and ventricles. The *right atrioventricular valve* enables the right atrium and the right ventricle to communicate. The *left atrioventricular valve* (also called the *mitral valve*) joins the left atrium to the left ventricle. In the fetus the right and left atria are joined by the *foramen*

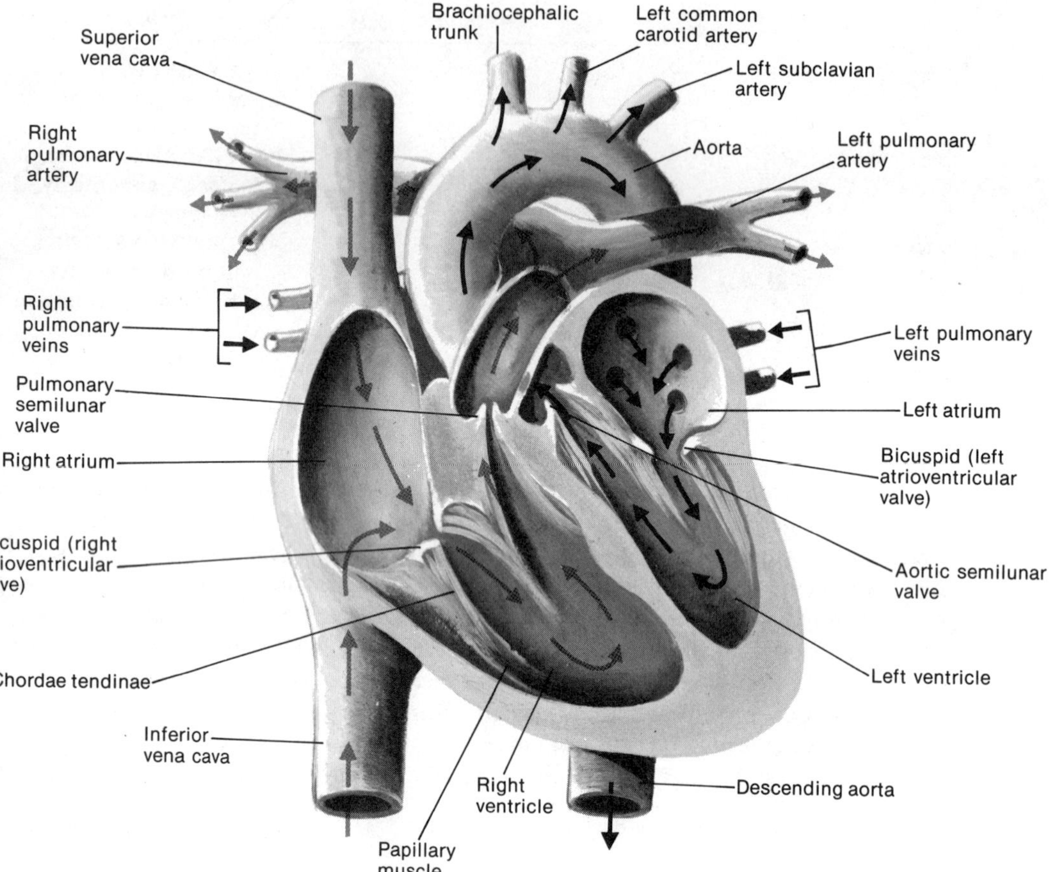

Figure 11-1   Internal structure of the heart.

ovale (for-a′men o-val′e), which closes before birth, leaving a depression called the *fossa ovale*. The same is true for the ventricles of the fetal heart. They are connected before birth by an interventricular foramen. If either foramen doesn't close, a defect in the heart results.

There are two types of heart valves (Figure 11-2). The atrioventricular valves are *flap valves* that are forced shut during contraction of the ventricles. The *semilunar valves* are positioned at the openings of the aorta and pulmonary trunk and prevent blood from flowing back into the ventricles. The aortic and pulmonary semilunar valves open whenever the atria rest whereas the bicuspid and tricuspid valves close. At the end of the contraction of the ventricles, the atrioventricular valves open and the semilunar valves close. The regular opening and closing of these valves produce the heart sounds "lub-dup" heard with a stethoscope. Listening for sounds produced within the body is called *auscultation* (aus-kul-tay′shun, AUSCULT/O listen).

The heart is the first organ to receive oxygenated blood. From the ascending portion of the aorta two *coronary arteries* supply blood to the entire heart.

HEARTBEAT AND CARDIAC CYCLE

Heartbeat is a product of the heart muscle (*myogenic*). It is initiated by an area of cardiac muscle in the wall of the right atrium. This area of cardiac muscle tissue is called the *sinoatrial* (SA) *node* (NOD/O swelling) or pacemaker. A *systole* (sis' to-lee) is the contraction of the heart. This initial contraction spreads to both atria and causes them to contract at the same time. Stimulated by the contraction impulses of the SA node, another special area of cardiac muscle, the *atrioventricular* (AV) *node*, which is located in the wall of the right atrium near the interventricular septum, causes the ventricles to contract. This step is accomplished by impulses that are carried to the ventricles over the cardiac muscle fibers known as the *bundle of His*. This structure's branches cover the ventricular walls with its fibers, the *Purkinje* (per-kin'jee) *fibers*. Once stimulated, the heart produces a maximal contraction. During its systole it cannot be stimulated to contract again. (*Tetanization* is the process of artificially inducing muscular contraction.) The heart's rest period, called a *diastole*, is somewhat longer than that of skeletal muscles.

Heart rate, the number of beats per minute, is controlled by the autonomic nervous system. The sympathetic division of the ANS increases heartbeat through *cardioaccelerator nerves;* the parasympathetic division decreases heartbeat through *cardioinhibitor nerves.*

The electrical impulses originating in the heart can be measured by an *electrocardiograph* whose *electrodes* (metal plates) are attached to an individual's wrists and ankles and to his chest with a suction cup. Common places where electrodes are attached are called *leads*—for instance, the right and left wrists (Lead I) or the right wrist and left ankle (Lead II). The electrocardiogram records a five-wave sequence

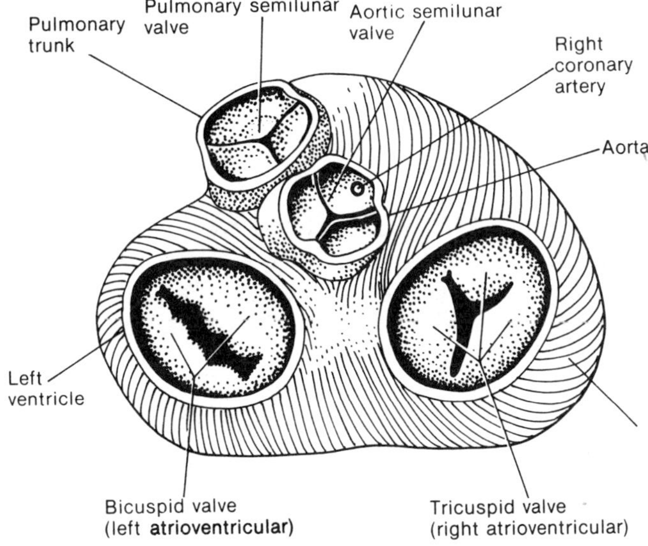

Figure 11-2 The heart valves.

called a *tracing*. The five waves are P wave, Q wave, R wave, S wave, and T wave. Each wave is interpreted in the following manner.

P wave: electrical wave of heartbeat passing along the atria.

Q-R-S complex: electrical wave passing along the ventricles.

T wave: rest period when the heart repolarizes.

Irregular P waves indicate a diseased SA node; a lengthy Q-R-S complex may mean blockage of the bundle of His and its branches. Damage to the myocardium shows up as an inverted T wave.

REFLEXES INFLUENCING HEART RATE

Changes in blood pressure stimulate pressure-sensitive receptors called *baroreceptors* (BAR/O density, pressure) that are located in the carotid sinus, the venae cavae, and right atrium. For example, after vigorous exercise the heart rate is increased as a result of increased blood pressure stimulating the baroreceptors of the venae cavae and right atrium. These receptors relay an impulse to the medulla, which, in turn, acts on the autonomic nervous system to increase heart rate (called the Bainbridge reflex). This condition, however, does not last for long, for higher blood pressure eventually causes the heart rate to slow. This principle is known as *Marey's law of the heart. Cardiac output* is the amount of blood pumped by the left ventricle per minute. It is calculated by multiplying the heartbeat by the amount of blood pumped with each stroke. The *cardiac cycle* is the time between one heartbeat and the next. The entire cycle lasts for 0.8 second and is divided in the following manner: 0.1—atrial systole, 0.3—ventricular systole, 0.4—diastole. Throughout the ventricular rest the heart is in a resting stage called *diastasis*.

THE BLOOD VESSELS

There are three types of blood vessels: artery, vein, and capillary. An *artery* transports blood away from the heart whereas a *vein* brings blood to the heart. A *capillary* is a very fine, microscopic blood vessel that joins both arteries and veins by connecting with very small arteries called *arterioles* and very small veins called *venules*. Gases, nutrients, and wastes are exchanged between the capillaries and the surrounding cells. The arteries of the systemic circulation carry oxygenated blood throughout the body; the arteries of the pulmonary circulation, however, carry deoxygenated blood to the lungs, which send oxygenated blood back to the heart through the veins. Figure 11-3 shows the structure of the blood vessels, Figure 11-4 the major arteries of the body, and Figure 11-5 the major veins of the body.

Blood leaves the heart through the *aorta* (systemic circulation) and through the pulmonary trunk (pulmonary circulation). The *superior vena cava* returns blood to the

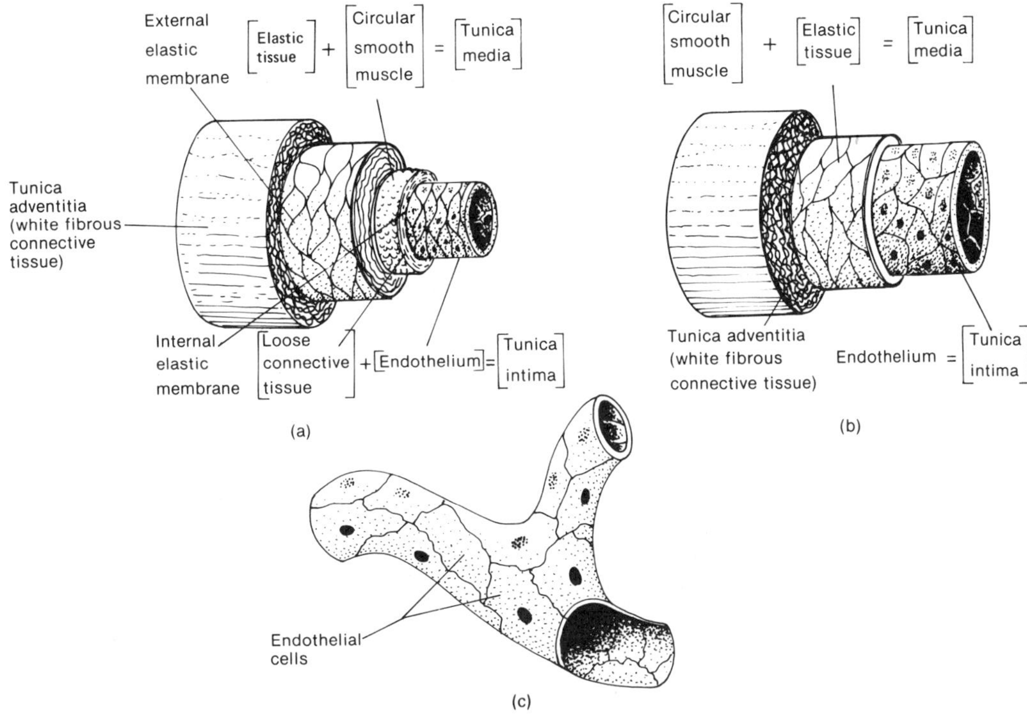

Figure 11-3 Structure of blood vessels: (a) artery; (b) vein; (c) capillary.

heart (enters the right atrium) from the head, neck, and upper extremities; the *inferior vena cava* returns blood from the rest of the body (again through the right atrium). Oxygenated blood from the lungs enters the left atrium through four *pulmonary veins*.

The veins of visceral organs of the abdomen form the *hepatic portal system*. The veins of the stomach, intestines, pancreas, and spleen empty into a large vein called the *portal* (PORT/O carry) *vein*, which carries the blood to the liver. In the liver the venous blood is filtered and detoxified of poisonous substances and leaves the liver by way of the right and left hepatic veins.

FETAL CIRCULATION

The *placenta* (pla-sen'ta) connects the blood vessels of the fetus with those of the mother (Figure 11-6). Nutrients and oxygen are carried to the fetus by way of the *umbilical vein* and wastes leave through the *umbilical arteries*. The entire structure is called the *umbilical cord*. Most of the blood entering the fetus passes through the *foramen ovale* and into the left atrium. The ductus arteriosus (duk'tus ar-teer'e-o-sus), a temporary structure, detours blood away from the lungs to the aorta. Arterial and venous blood are not differentiated until birth.

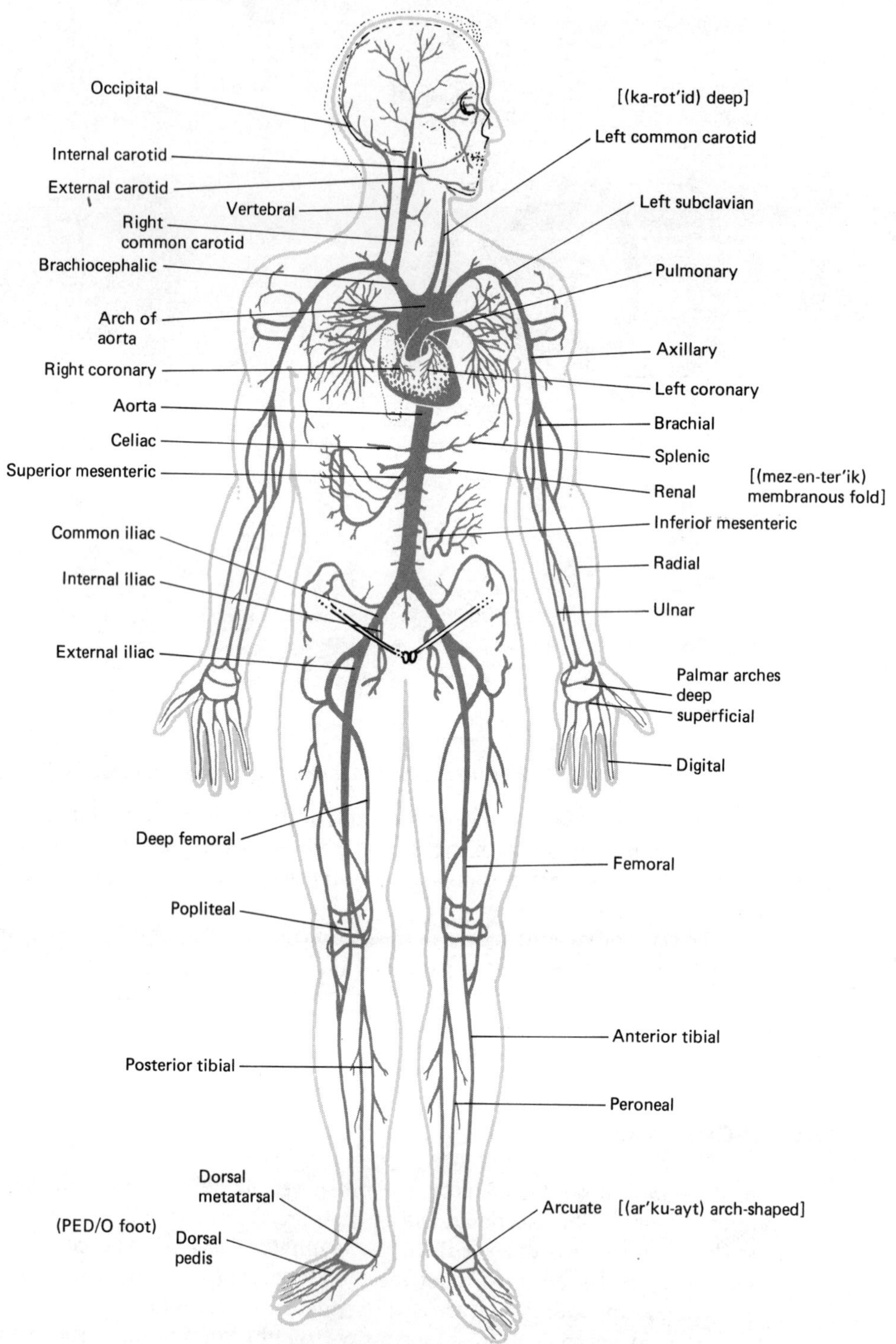

Figure 11-4 The major arteries of the body.

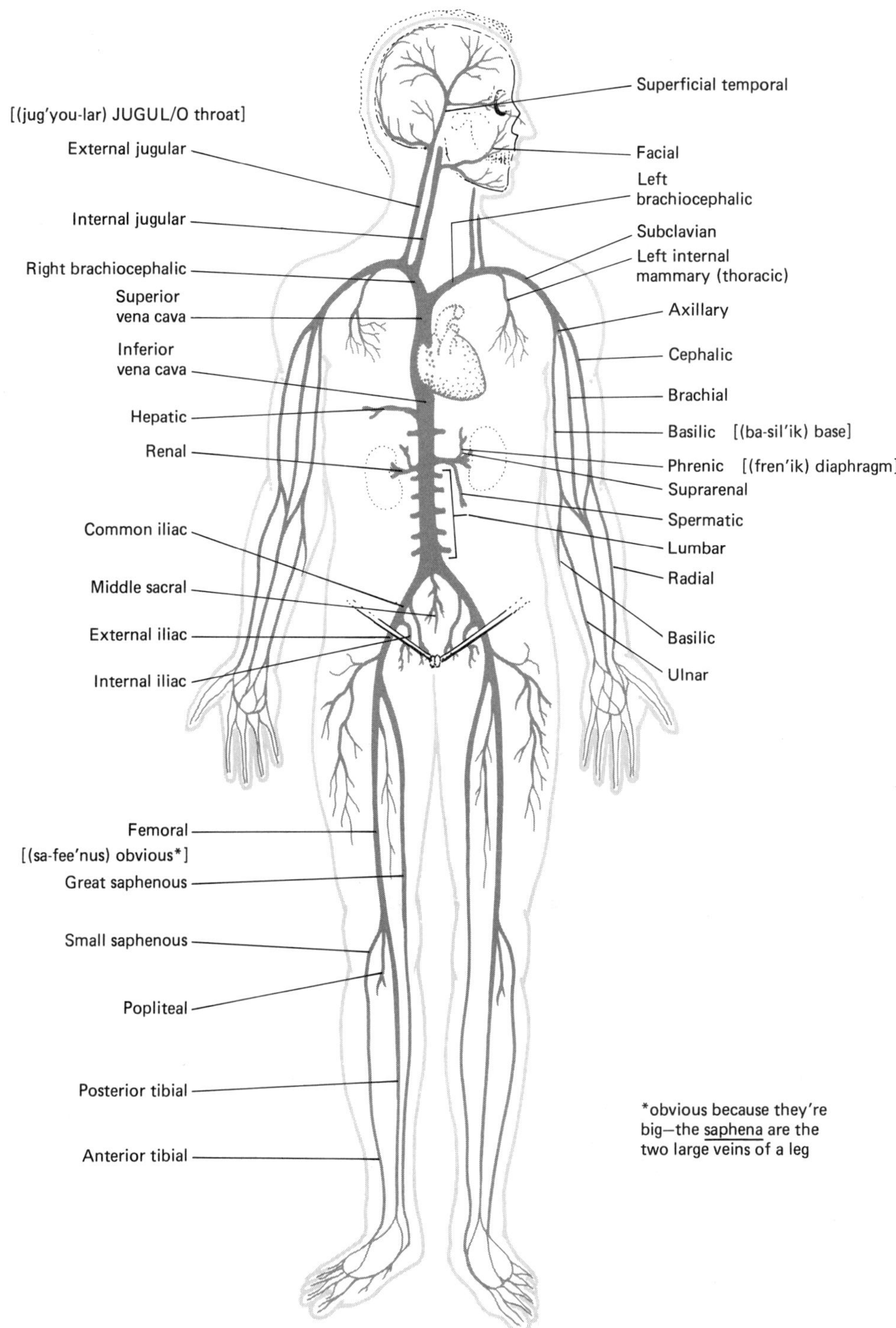

Figure 11-5   Major veins of the body.

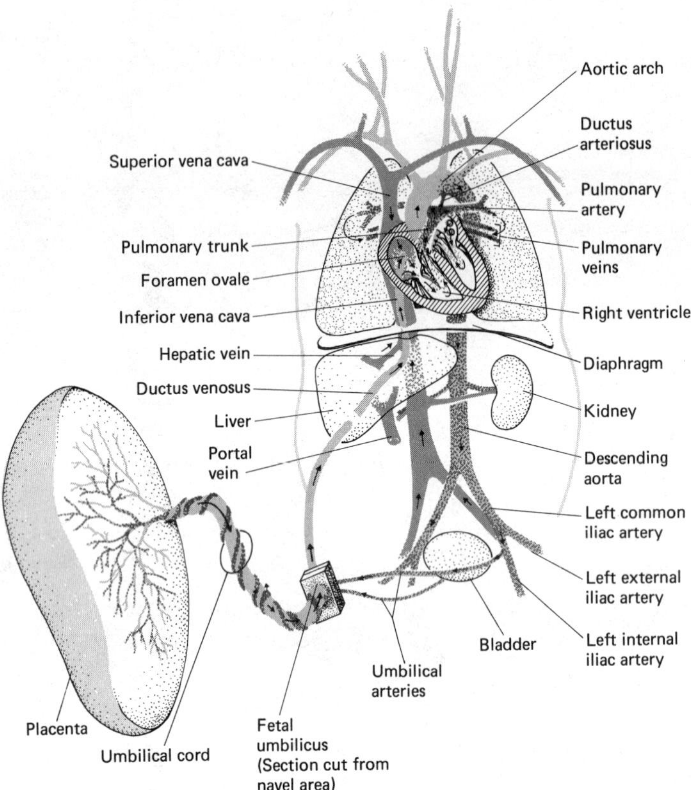

Figure 11-6   The fetal circulation.

ARTERIAL AND VENOUS BLOOD PRESSURES

In the arteries low blood pressure occurs when the blood moves along with little resistance. As arterial resistance increases, so does arterial blood pressure. The diameter of the blood vessels is a major method of controlling blood pressure. The diameter of the *arterioles* is especially important in the control of blood pressure. Monitored by the autonomic nervous system, the arterioles can constrict to increase resistance, thereby raising blood pressure, or can dilate to reduce resistance with a corresponding reduction in blood pressure. Arteriole effect on blood pressure is know as *peripheral resistance*. The diameter of the arterioles is controlled by a *vasomotor control mechanism* that consists of three types of reflexes:

Vasomotor pressoreflexes

Pressoreceptors (also called baroreceptors) in the carotid and aortic sinuses stimulate the vasomotor center of the medulla, which, in turn, causes the arterioles of the skin and abdominal organs to dilate, resulting in a decrease in peripheral resistance.

Vasomotor chemoreflexes
Chemoreceptors in the carotid and aortic arteries are activated by low blood oxygen levels (*hypoxia*), high blood levels of carbon dioxide (*hypercapnia*), and low blood pH. Any of these conditions will cause the vasoconstrictor center in the medulla to constrict the arterioles.

Medullary ischemic reflexes
Because of the reduced flow to the medulla resulting in hypoxia, the vasoconstriction center of the medulla causes the arterioles to constrict.

Peripheral resistance through the constriction or dilation of the arterioles is the primary method of controlling arterial blood pressure. Several other factors that contribute to arterial blood pressure are cardiac output, the ability of the arteries themselves to contract and expand, the volume and viscosity (density) of the blood, and the velocity of the blood.

Blood pressure is measured by a *sphygmomanometer* (sfig-mo-man-om′e-ter, MAN/O thin). Pressure is put on an artery, for instance, in the upper arm by an inflated cuff, resulting in the occlusion of that artery. As the pressure is slowly removed and the pulse returns, the level of the mercury column on the sphygmomanometer is noted. It gives the *systolic pressure*. Because the pressure is being relieved, the pulse returns to a normal, fainter beat. This reading is the *diastolic pressure*. What we refer to as the "pulse" is the throbbing of the arteries as newly pumped blood passes through an artery. The pulse indicates the number of times that the left ventricle contracts per minute. Although the wrists are most frequently used in taking the pulse, areas like the ankle and temple can also be used.

Unlike the arteries, the veins, which contain about 60% of the body's total blood volume, don't have the direct help of the heart. Several factors contribute to venous flow. Vein diameter prevents blood from building up or pooling. The skeletal muscles facilitate venous blood flow by their movements. Blood is drawn up into the thorax by the action of the diaphragm in respiration. The venous valves (Figure 11-7) prevent blood from flowing back.

THE COMPOSITION OF BLOOD

Blood, the substance that flows through the vessels of the cardiovascular system, is composed of cells or cell-like structures and an extracellular fluid called *plasma* (plaz′ma, PLASM/O formed). Blood has two functions: transportation and the maintenance of homeostasis. Besides transporting nutrients, wastes, and gases, the blood also transports various substances, such as hormones and antibodies. The blood helps to maintain homeostasis by regulating pH (blood pH is 7.4), tissue-water content (through *osmosis*, oz-mo′sis, absorption), body temperature and by protecting the body through phagocytosis, coagulation, and the production of antibodies.

The extracellular fluid of the blood, the *plasma*, constitutes about 55% of the blood volume. The remaining blood volume is composed of *formed elements* (Figure

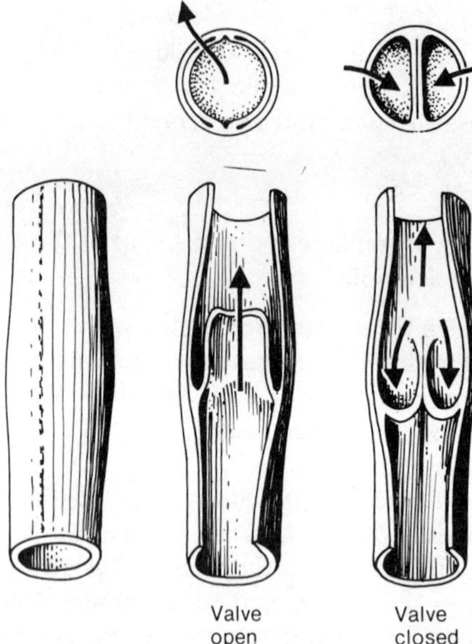

Figure 11-7 Venous valves and their actions.

11-8), which are *erythrocytes* (red blood cells—RBCs), *leukocytes* (white blood cells—WBCs), and *thrombocytes*, also called *platelets* (plate'lets), which are pieces of cells. By placing blood into a special tube called a Winthrobe tube and adding an anticoagulant, the formed elements will settle to the bottom of the tube after awhile. The time that it takes for the formed elements to settle is called the *sedimentation rate.* Certain infections cause the sedimentation rate to increase. When the tube is placed into a centrifuge, the *hematocrit* (-crit means separate), which is the volume of formed elements, especially erythrocytes, can be obtained.

Red Blood Cells (RBCs)

Red blood cells (also called *erythrocytes* or *red corpuscles;* corpuscle is an older term meaning any blood cell) are flat, biconcave discs lacking a nucleus. They have very flexible membranes that enable them to move easily through capillary networks. A mature male has about five million RBCs per cubic centimeter of blood. A *hemacytometer* is used to count the number of erythrocytes in a cubic millimeter of blood.

Hemoglobin, the pigment of erythrocytes, is capable of carrying oxygen or carbon dioxide. For this reason, it is called a *respiratory pigment*. Hemoglobin has a protein and lipid *stroma* (internal composition) and, along with the cell's membrane, constitutes the entire erythrocyte. Hemoglobin takes on oxygen in the microscopic air sacs (*alveoli*, al-vee'o-lie) of the lungs. Oxygen-carrying hemoglobin called *oxy-*

hemoglobin is a bright red, whereas *reduced* or *deoxygenated* hemoglobin is a dark red.

A red blood cell, which has a lifespan of about 120 days, is produced in an adult in the membranous bones (e.g., the skull) and in the proximal areas of the femur and humerus. All blood cells begin as *hemocytoblasts*, also called *stem cells* (Figure 11-9). Before the red blood cell enters the blood, it loses its nucleus. Forming red blood cells is called *erythropoiesis; hemopoiesis* is the formation of all blood cells. The materials necessary for erythrocyte production are iron and amino acids, and such catalysts as copper and vitamin B compounds. Exhausted erythrocytes break down and their parts are consumed by phagocytes called *reticuloendothelial cells* in the liver, spleen (stores RBCs and destroys those that are exhausted), and bone marrow. The iron is saved in the form of *hemosiderin*, an iron-protein pigment, and the remainder of hemoglobin is formed into the bile pigment *bilirubin*, which is excreted in the bile.

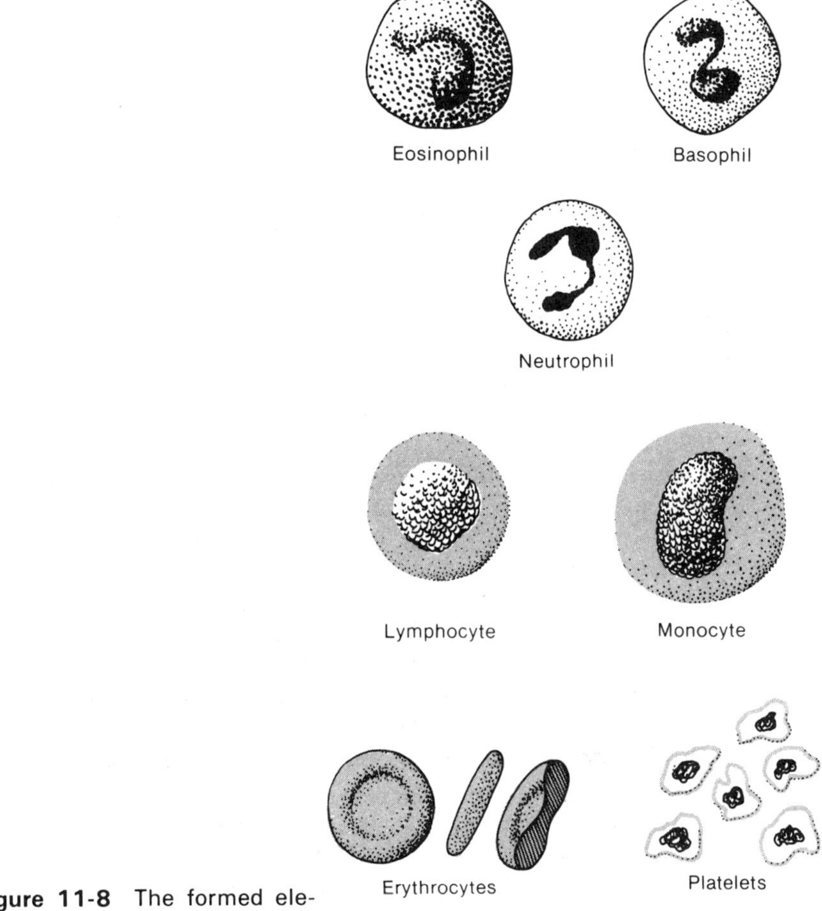

Figure 11-8 The formed elements of blood.

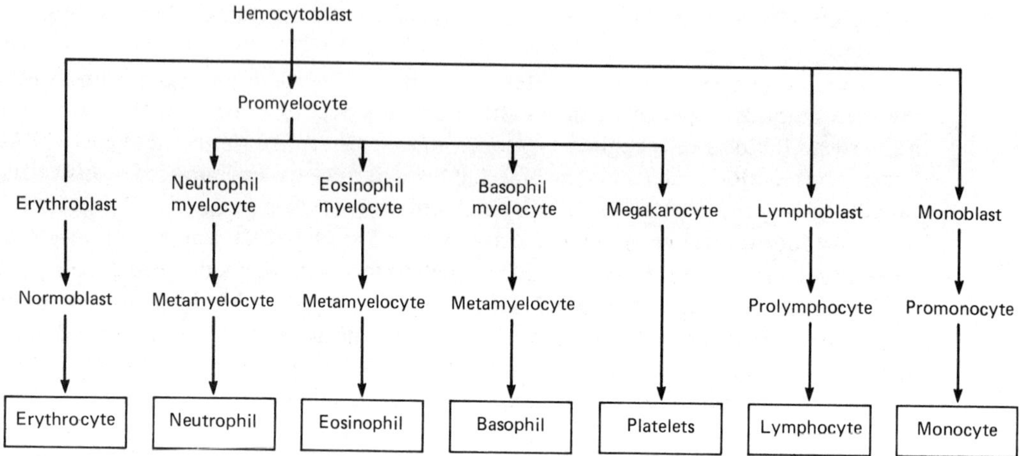

Figure 11-9   Diagram of blood cell formation.

White Blood Cells (WBCs)

Unlike erythrocytes, all *leukocytes* have nuclei. There are two groups of leukocytes: *granulocytes* and *agranulocytes*. The granulocytes contain granules that appear dark when stained. *Neutrophils*, which stain well with neutral dyes, *eosinophils* (EOSIN/O rosy red), which stain well with acidic dyes, and *basophils*, which stain well with alkaline dyes are all types of granulocytes. Neutrophils account for nearly 70% of all white blood cells and have elongated nuclei that appear as *lobes. Lymphocytes* and *monocytes* are examples of agranulocytes. There are both large and small lymphocytes and they develop in the tonsils, spleen, and lymph nodes. Monocytes develop from lymphoid tissue and bone marrow and have large nuclei. Leukocytes live for only a few days; lymphocytes, however, can live for much longer, sometimes as much as 300 days. The number of white blood cells in the blood varies from 5 to 10,000 per cubic centimeter of blood.

The primary function of white blood cells is to engulf and destroy foreign substances. This function is known as *phagocytosis*. White blood cells are attracted to infected tissue as a result of a chemical message sent by the tissue (a process called *chemotaxis*, key-mo-taks'is). The white blood cells pass through the capillary walls and infiltrate the infected tissue by a process called *diapedesis* (di-a-pe-dee'sis). *Pus* is a mixture of pathogenic organisms, white blood cells, dead bacteria and white blood cells, and their by-products. The agranulocytes contribute to tissue repair and produce *antibodies*, chemical substances used to offset specific substances (*antigens*) that have entered the body.

Platelets are fragments of *megakaryocytes*, which are large bone marrow cells. The platelets seal holes in small blood vessels. When platelets rupture at the site of a wound, a chemical initiating coagulation is released.

Plasma, the blood fluid, is about 90% water and 10% protein. Plasma provides a suspension medium for the formed elements of the blood. Sometimes the osmotic relationship between the plasma and formed elements can become unbalanced. If the plasma becomes *hypotonic*, hemoglobin mixes with the water that has diffused into the cells from the surrounding plasma, causing *hemolysis*. In a *hypertonic* plasma the red blood cells shrink as a result of water leaving the cell body. This shrinkage is called *crenation*. Several substances are contained in plasma. One protein, *albumin* (al-bu'min), maintains the osmotic balance between plasma and tissue and between plasma and formed elements. Both *fibrinogen* and *prothrombin*, substances necessary for clotting, are contained in plasma. Plasma also contains the protein *gamma globulin* (GLOBUL/O round body), which is important in immunizing the body against disease. Body nutrients are transported by plasma, and the level of calcium, sodium, and potassium salts in plasma helps to maintain the body's electrolyte balance. Plasma transports waste products to the kidneys, and such substances as hormones, enzymes, and antibodies travel throughout the body as substances within plasma.

A series of reactions occurs to halt the loss of blood (*hemostasis*) when a blood vessel is damaged. The blood vessels narrow (*vasoconstriction*), a *platelet plug* forms, and blood begins to *coagulate*. *Coagulation*, the sealing of a wound by a blood clot, is accomplished by the conversion of *prothrombin* to *thrombin* and *fibrinogen* to *fibrin*. Vitamin K is essential to clotting, for it contributes to the formation of prothrombin. The actual clot initially appears as a gelatinous cover that later shrinks into a harder cover surrounded by a pale yellow fluid called *serum* (plasma without its protein constituents). The clot itself is a meshwork (*reticulum*) of fibrin and some trapped blood cells.

A *hemorrhage* refers to excessive bleeding or to minor bleeding in an important part of the body—for instance, cerebral hemorrhage. There are several methods for controlling a hemorrhage. The most common are *litigation* or tying them, clamping them with *hemostats*, applying tourniquets, and applying direct pressure over the wound. By applying pressure to arteries near the surface or to those arteries lying over a bone, hemorrhage can be controlled. The six major pressure points of the body are

1. The skull in front of each temporal artery.
2. The lower jaw (facial arteries).
3. The thyroid cartilage or vertebral column (common carotid artery).
4. The first rib (subclavian artery).
5. A few inches above the elbow above the inner side of the arm (brachial arteries).
6. The central area of the groin against the pubic bone (femoral artery).

BLOOD TYPING

Blood can be grouped into four types according to the presence or absence of certain antigens producing antibodies that cause *aggultination* (causes harmful micro-organism to clump together, thus destroying them). The blood types are

A   Antigen A is present.

B   Antigen B is present.

AB   Both antigens are present.

O   Neither antigen is present.

In addition, each blood type contains *agglutinins* or antibodies that will cause the red blood cells to clump if an incompatible antigen and antibody are mixed (Table 11-1). Another protein in blood grouping to be considered is the *Rh factor* or D antigen. The Rh (Rh from rhesus monkey, where it was first discovered) antigen is present in the blood of most people. A person having the Rh protein is called Rh positive, whereas an individual lacking it is called Rh negative. The mixing of Rh positive and Rh negative blood will cause agglutination and hemolysis.

Table 11-1   Blood Typing or Grouping

Type or group*	Percentage occurrence	Antigens (agglutinogens) in red cells	Antibodies (agglutinins) in plasma	Agglutination when mixed?			
				A	*B*	*AB*	*O*
A	41	A	Anti-B	No	Yes	No	Yes
B	10	B	Anti-A	Yes	No	No	Yes
AB	4	A and B	None	Yes	Yes	No	Yes
O	45	none	Anti-A & Anti-B	No	No	No	No

*Where mixing is concerned, the type or group in the left-hand column is that of the donor; the type or group at the upper right is that of the recipient.

BLOOD BUFFERS

Blood buffers are substances that maintain the pH of the blood close to 7.4 (slightly alkaline). Most of the buffers form a *buffer pair*, an acid and a salt of that acid. An example of a buffer pair is the bicarbonate buffer (carbonic acid and sodium bicarbonate).

THE LYMPHATIC SYSTEM

Lymph is a plasmalike fluid that circulates throughout the body. It surrounds the cells (intercellular) and the tissues (interstitial, in-ter-stish′e-al). Lymph is the portion of plasma that leaves the blood and passes through the capillary walls by a process called *transudation* (tranz-ou-day′shun). Lymph contributes to homeostasis by moving water and substances from the spaces between the tissues to the blood. It is returned to the circulation after passing through the several structures that constitute the *lymphatic system*. Throughout the body, lymph is collected in the *lymph capillaries* (called *lacteals* in the intestinal lining) and passes through the *lymph vessels* to the *lymph nodes*, which occur along the lymph vessels (Figure 11-10). The lymph nodes are like tiny capsules with many compartments. In these compartments microorganisms and foreign particles are filtered from the lymph. The *lymph nodules* of the lymph nodes produce *lymphocytes*. Lymph from the upper right side of the body (above the diaphragm) drains into the *right lymph duct;* lymph from the rest of the body drains into the *thoracic duct* (Figure 11-11).

Other lymphatic structures are Peyer's patches, the thymus gland, the spleen, and the tonsils. *Peyer's patches* are nodules of lymphoid tissue in the ileum (lower section of the small intestine). The *thymus* is a double-lobed gland located in the thorax above the heart and is mainly composed of lymphoid tissue. The thymus aids in the development of immune response and atrophies soon after puberty. The *spleen*, in addition to serving as a blood bank for the body, produces antibodies. The *tonsils* are three pairs of lymphoid tissue that act to prevent bacteria from invading the upper respiratory and digestive tracts. The pharyngeal tonsils (also called adenoids) are located in the posterior wall of the nasopharynx, the palatine tonsils in the posterior side walls of the throat, the lingual tonsils on the posterior part of the tongue. Frequently, the palatine tonsils are removed in childhood. Like the thymus, the tonsils contribute to the body's development of immune response.

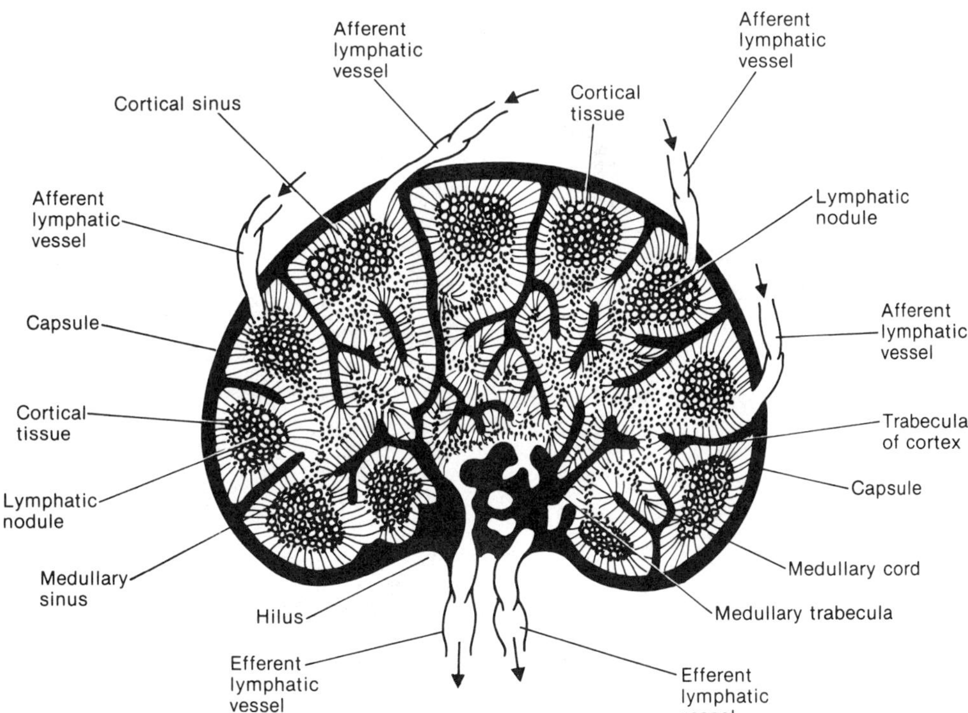

Figure 11-10 Structure of a lymph gland or node.

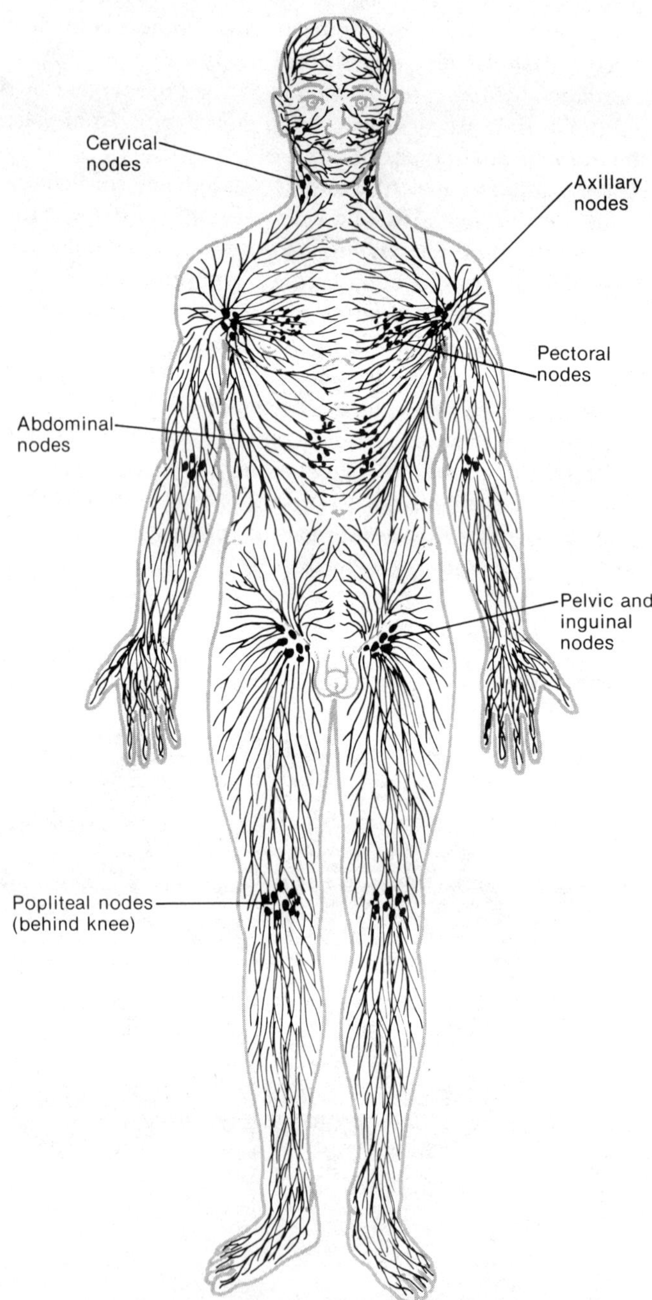

Figure 11-11 The major lymphatics of the body.

CLINICAL AND PATHOLOGICAL CONDITIONS

Pericarditis
The visceral membrane of the pericardium becomes inflamed, the amount of the pericardial fluid decreases, and painful adhesions of the membrane may develop.

Cardiac tamponade (tam-pon-ayd')
The accumulation of pericardial fluid in the pericardial cavity interferes with heartbeat.

Coronary thrombosis
An intravascular clot that remains in one place is called a *thrombus*. When an intravascular clot moves from its original place to another area of the body, it is called an *embolus*. In *coronary thrombosis* a coronary artery is *occluded* (blocked) by a blood clot. Because blood is prevented from reaching the myocardium, myocardial tissues begin to die. This process is referred to as a *myocardial infarction* (in-fark'shun; infarction is the *necrosis* or the death of an area of tissue resulting from the lack of blood). Sometimes a blocked artery can be bypassed by anastomosing vessels.

Angina pectoris (an-jy'na pek'tor-is)
Literally, angina pectoris means a choking of the chest. It is a pain in the chest in the heart area resulting from a lack of blood.

Cardiac arrest
Circulation of blood stops as a result of a coronary thrombosis.

Arrhythmia (a-rith'me-a)
Arrhythmia is an irregular heart rhythm. There are several types.
   Variation of SA node activity.   In *tachycardia* the heart rate increases; in *bradycardia* the heart rate decreases. Drugs such as caffeine and epinephrine increase heart rate; drugs such as alcohol and nitroglycerine slow heart rate.
   Heart block.   Electrical impulses from the atria to the ventricles are obstructed. Two types of heart block are *AV block*, which occurs in the atrioventricular node, and *bundle-branch block*, in which one of the branches in the bundle of His is blocked. There are three degrees of heart block.

1. First degree: a delayed impulse causes the ventricular contraction to occur abnormally late.
2. Second degree: the ventricles contract less than the atria as a result of missing some sinoatrial impulses.
3. Third degree: complete separation of the atrial and ventricular beats.

An *artificial pacemaker* leading to the right ventricle may be implanted in the axilla to correct heart block.

Fibrillation and flutter. *Fibrillation* refers to rapid and incomplete atrio-ventricular contractions; *flutter* refers to very rapid atrial contractions. Several areas of the heart act as pacemakers and heartbeat is weak and uncoordinated. Usually the use of external shock (called *defibrillation*) can return normal coordination.

Heart murmur

Heart murmurs are abnormal heart sounds produced as a result of heart valves not closing completely. Not all murmurs are pathological. For example, *functional murmurs* occur in children during vigorous exercise and are usually outgrown. Pathological conditions can cause the opening between the valve parts to become narrow (e.g., aortic and mitral stenoses) or may cause the blood to flow backward (*regurgitation*) as a result of an incompletely closed valve.

Heart disease resulting from bacteria

Rheumatic carditis. As a result of rheumatic (RHEUM/O discharge) fever, all areas of the heart tissue may become inflamed (carditis), causing the heart valves to be deformed. Either stenosis of the valve or regurgitation occurs.

Bacterial endocarditis. The membrane lining the heart becomes inflamed, especially the lining of the valve. Infection, irregular heart murmur, and embolization of pieces of heart valve accompany this disease.

Congenital malformations

Septal cardiac defects. When the partitions (septa) between the atria and ventricles do not form properly, septal defects, such as a hole in the septum, form. Ventricle septal defects occur more often than atrial septal defects and are more damaging because blood in the left ventricle can pour into the right ventricle, damaging the lungs.

Tetralogy of Fallot (te-tral'o-je of Fa-lo'). A set of four congenital defects: (a) pulmonary stenosis, (b) ventricular septal defect, (c) aorta leaning too far to the right, and (d) hypertrophy (thickening) of the right ventricle.

Patent ductus arteriosus (pa'tent duk'tus ar-teer-e-o'sus) ***and patent foramen ovale*** (for-a'men o-va'le). In patent ductus arteriosus the blood vessel in the fetus that connects the pulmonary trunk with the aorta does not atrophy but remains open. In patent foramen ovale the opening that connects the two atria of the fetal heart remains open. The result is that both oxygenated and deoxygenated blood mix, thus causing the mucous membranes of the baby to have blue coloration—hence the name "blue baby" (cyanosis). Both conditions are corrected surgically.

Diseases of the blood vessels

Hypertension or high blood pressure. Systolic, diastolic, or both blood pressures are above what is considered normal pressure. As systolic pressure rises, the danger of a ruptured blood vessel, especially a cerebral blood vessel, increases. High diastolic pressures can damage several delicate organs, such as the liver, kidneys, brain, and retina, by causing their blood vessels to become both sclerotic and stenotic. Diastolic hypertension is caused by peripheral vasoconstriction. (a) A kidney suffering from renal ischemia will produce *renin*, which ultimately causes a powerful vasoconstrictor, angiotensin II, to be produced by the plasma. The result is *renal hypertension* (hypertension caused by the kidney). (b) Sodium retention by the kidneys also causes hypertension, since water retention and a corresponding increase in blood volume and pressure occur. (c) Vasodilating chemicals called *prostoglandins* (produced by many organs, such as the brain, kidneys, and lungs) are not activated during renal ischemia.

Arteriosclerosis. The arterial wall becomes thick and loses its elasticity and resiliency. Blood flow is reduced; blood pressure is increased. *Atherosclerosis*, the buildup of fatty substances along the arterial wall, frequently accompanies arteriosclerosis.

Atherosclerosis. Fatty substances (atheromas) build up on the interior portions of the vessel wall, causing them to become thick, narrow, and stiff and resulting in a decreased blood flow. Atherosclerosis, considered a normal affliction of aging, can be hastened or worsened by a lack of exercise, a high fat diet, and cigarette smoking. Hypertension and thrombosis accompany ateriosclerosis and atherosclerosis. Sometimes a *thromboendarterectomy* can be performed to clear out the fatty accumulation from the artery. Arterial bypasses can bring blood to an organ with sclerotic vessels.

Aneurysm (an'you-rizm, a widening). The pressure of blood against a vessel wall weakened by arteriosclerosis causes a portion of that wall to expand like a balloon, which may burst into the surrounding tissue.

Thrombophlebitis. Inflammation of the wall of a vein with the subsequent development of a clot is most frequently caused by poor venous circulation (*venous stasis*). This poor circulation of blood provides ideal conditions for clot formation.

Varicose veins. As a result of the pooling of blood in the superficial veins of the legs, the veins are abnormally enlarged. The valves in these veins become incompetent and the condition worsens. These veins turn into a twisted mass that frequently must be removed surgically.

Cardiac Catheterization

Catheterization is the process by which a hollow tube is inserted into a passageway or cavity for the purpose of withdrawing or depositing fluid. *Cardiac catheterization* is a procedure in which a catheter, by way of a peripheral artery, is introduced into a chamber of the heart or one of the major vessels so that the anatomy of the heart can be visualized and specific function tests performed. In addition, an *angiocardiography*, the injection of a special dye into the heart for further testing of function and possible occlusion, can also be performed during cardiac catheterization.

Cardiac catheterization is a sterile procedure performed in the cardiac catheterization laboratory or the x-ray department. The patient, who has not eaten for about 8 hours prior to the procedure, is tranquilized and must remain lying flat for the duration of the tests (about 3 or more hours); he or she is constantly monitored by an

Table 11-2 Cardiac Catheterization Procedures

Area catheterized	Procedure	Information from this procedure	Disorders detected
Right-heart catheterization	Catheter is inserted into the right brachial artery. From here it is advanced into the right atrium across the tricuspid valve and into the right ventricle. It can then be moved into the pulmonary artery. A second catheter containing a dye is inserted.	Pressures produced by the right atrium and right ventricle Pulmonary wedge pressure (indicates pressure produced by the left atrium) Cardiac output (measured by an instrument called a *thermodilution computer*)	Mitral stenosis Mitral incompetency Left-to-right shunt (A *shunt* is an abnormal opening in the septum of one of the chambers of the heart, causing blood to flow into this chamber.) See also p. 361.
Left-heart catheterization	The catheter is inserted into the brachial or femoral artery.	Pressure produced by the left ventricle Condition of the mitral and aortic valves Functioning of the left ventricle muscle	Mitral and aortic incompetency Elevated pressure caused by a stenosed valve
	Left-heart *ventriculography*. A dye is injected into the apical region of the left ventricle.	Measurement of the contractions of left ventricle	Condition of the cardiac muscle

electrocardiograph (EKG). The catheter is usually inserted into the right or left brachial artery at the antecubital fossa. From this point it is moved through the artery until it reaches the heart. Table 11-2 lists the procedures and information derived from each procedure. The following side effects of cardiac catheterization have been grouped according to the degree of seriousness.

1. Skin irritation, vomiting, nausea, the production of a thrombus near the area where the catheter was inserted
2. Ventricular tachycardia, premature ventricular contractions, ventricular fibrillation
3. The following items are considered life-threatening complications: arrhythmia, pneumothorax (air in the thoracic cavity), arterial occlusion, myocardial infarction.

Diseases of the blood

Anemia. A decrease in the available hemoglobin causes a proportionate decrease in the amount of oxygen being carried to body tissues. Anemia is characterized by a general paleness and increased heart and respiratory rates. Anemias are classified according to erythrocyte morphology (shape and size) or according to the cause of the disease. A loss of red blood cells, the hemolysis of red blood cells, and insufficient production of red blood cells produce anemia. Different types of anemia are listed below.

1. *Nutritional deficiency anemias* result from the lack or depletion of essential nutritional elements. *Iron-deficiency anemia* and *vitamin B12 deficiency anemia* are examples of nutritional-deficiency anemias. *Pernicious anemia* is caused by the lack of the substance *intrinsic factor*, which is necessary for the absorption of vitamin B12
2. There are several types of *hereditary anemias*. In *sickle cell anemia* the erythrocytes take on a sickle shape when exposed to low oxygen levels. Thalassemia (THALASS/O sea) occurs most frequently among individuals of Mediterranean ancestry. There is a defect in the rate of hemoglobin chain production.
3. *Aplastic* (PLAS/O development) *anemia* is usually a chemically induced anemia. Hemopoiesis stops due to a decrease in the amount of hemopoietic cells in the bone marrow.

Individuals with aplastic anemia develop infections and hemorrhages easily and require frequent blood transfusions.

Polycythemia (pol-e-sy-thee′me-a).   An excessive number of red blood cells is produced frequently as a response to hypoxia. In *polycythemia vera* (true) increased bone marrow activity produces excessive numbers of erythrocytes, leukocytes, and platelets. Blood volume is increased and the incidence of thrombosis is greater. Also, leukemia may develop. Patients with this disease are bled and given drugs to reduce bone marrow activity.

Infectious mononucleosis.   An excessive number of abnormal mononuclear leukocytes is produced as a result of a viral infection. Fever, sore throat, enlarged lymph glands, and general fatigue occur.

Leukemia.   This is a form of blood cancer in which the white blood cells multiply uncontrollably. Leukemias are classified according to the white blood cell involved. For example, lymphocystic leukemias develop from lymph cells.

Inherited plasma-clotting disorders.   *Hemophilia* is an hereditary blood disease in which the blood fails to clot. It is a recessive X-chromosome-linked disorder causing the male offspring to be a hemophiliac and the female offspring to be a carrier. *Hemophilia A* is caused by a deficiency of factor VIII in the plasma. In *hemophilia B* factor IX is deficient. Another clotting disorder, *Von Willebrand's syndrome*, is an inherited bleeding disorder affecting both males and females. It is caused by a lack of factor VIII. Bleeding disorders are treated by administering blood-clotting factors.

Erythroblastosis fetalis.   This disorder occurs when the fetus is Rh^+ and the mother is Rh^-. The mother's blood has built up anti-Rh agglutinins as a result of a previous pregnancy. The antiagglutinins cause the fetal red blood cells to clump and block blood vessels. As the red blood cells break up, hemoglobin is converted to bilirubin, a yellow bile pigment. A transfusion of Rh⁻ blood is necessary to save the baby.

Lymphatic disorders

Lymphomas are malignant tumors arising in lymphoid tissue. There are basically two types of lymphomas: Hodgkin's disease and non-Hodgkin lymphoma. *Hodgkin's disease* is characterized by the enlargement of the lymphoid tissue, the spleen, and the liver. Both types of lymphomas progress in the following manner. Lymph nodes of one body area become affected ――$\xrightarrow{\text{spread to}}$ several areas on the same side of the diaphragm ――$\xrightarrow{\text{spread to}}$ other side of the diaphragm and to the spleen ――$\xrightarrow{\text{spread to}}$ bone marrow and other body organs.

EXERCISES

I. Give the meaning for each of the following medical words. Divide each word into base(s), prefix, and suffix; underline the letter(s) that has the primary stress. *Example:*

ARTERIOTOMY incision of an artery arteri/<u>ot</u>omy

1. METARTERIOLE (MET(A) after) ....

2. ANGIOMA ....

3. STETHOMETER ....

4. SEPTICEMIA (SEPTIC refers to pathogenic organisms and their toxins)

....

5. PLASMOCYTOMA ....

6. UREMIA ....

7. SPHYGMIC ....

8. ANGIOSCOPE ....

9. CARDIOGENIC ....

10. ARTERIOLITIS ....

11. VASOGRAPHY ....

12. HEMOTROPHIC ....

13. BASOCYTOPENIA ....

14. AGRANULOCYTOSIS ....

15. ANOXIC ....

16. ANGIOSTENOSIS ....

17. VASCULAR ....

18. VENULITIS ....

19. INTERVENTRICULAR ....

20. VASOMOTOR ....

21. HEMOCYTOBLAST ....

22. INTRAVASCULAR ....

23. NEUTROPHILIA ....

24. ARTERIONECROSIS ....

25. CARDIOPULMONARY ....

26. AGGLUTININ ....

27. RETICULOENDOTHELIAL ....

28. PROTHROMBIN ....

29. SPLENOKERATOSIS ....

30. TACHYARRHYTHMIA ....

31. THROMBOPHLEBITIS ....

32. ANEURYSMECTOMY ....

33. ANTISERUM ....

34. GAMMA GLOBULIN ....

35. ARTERIOFIBROSIS ....

36. THROMBOCYTOPENIA ....

37. PHAGOCYTOSIS ....

38. HEMOSTASIS ....

39. LYMPHANGIOMA ....

40. ATHEROSIS ....

41. IMMUNOGENIC ....

42. PHLEBOPLASTY ....

43. VENOSTASIS ....

44. NODULE ....

45. RETICULOCYTE ....

II. Make medical words from the following phrases. Indicate the primary stress by underlining the stressed letter(s). *Example:*

a substance that stimulates the production of red blood cells

erythrop__oi__etin
....

1. a blood cell

....

2. incision of a vein

....

3. abnormal enlargement of the heart

....

4. inflammation of an artery

....

5. inflammation of a blood vessel

    . . . .

6. deficiency of oxygen

    . . . .

7. increase in the number of eosinophils in the blood

    . . . .

8. production of granulocytes

    . . . .

9. causing blood vessels to expand

    . . . .

10. suture of the aorta

    . . . .

11. incision of a ventricle

    . . . .

12. pertaining to the heart and the aorta

    . . . .

13. pertaining to the vein (vena cava) and the atrium

    . . . .

14. within a vein

    . . . .

15. a type of white blood cell having an affinity for *neither* (NEUTR/O neither) an acid nor
    base stain

    . . . .

16. one who specializes in the study of blood and the treatment of its diseases

    . . . .

17. a disease affecting the aorta

    . . . .

18. instrument for cutting the atrium

....

19. incision of a valve

....

20. hardening of the arteries

....

21. excess of basophils in the blood

....

22. having oxygen

....

23. instrument for recording pulse and heartbeat

....

24. destruction of (red) blood cells

....

25. surgical repair of a valve

....

26. tendency to form blood clots

....

27. production of red blood cells

....

28. having an osmotic pressure less than that of another solution

....

29. abnormal enlargement of the spleen

....

30. inflammation of the tonsils

....

31. excision of a varicose vein

. . . .

32. excision of the thymus gland

. . . .

33. disease of the lymph gland(s)

. . . .

34. iron deficiency

. . . .

35. process by which microorganisms or blood cells are clumped together

. . . .

36. without a nucleus

. . . .

37. destruction of phagocytes

. . . .

38. breaking up of a clot

. . . .

39. production of white blood cells

. . . .

40. abnormal decrease in the amount of fibrinogen in the blood

. . . .

III. True or false: Circle T or F for each of the following statements. If the statement is false, provide the correct answer.

1. The parietal pericardium is that portion of the pericardial sac directly attached to the heart.

   T / F . . . .

2. Blood enters the heart through the two upper chambers called the atria.

   T / F . . . .

3. All arteries carry oxygenated blood. T / F ....

4. Blood leaving the right ventricle circulates throughout the body.

   T / F ....

5. Listening for sounds produced within the body such as the "lub-dup" sound of the heart is

   called palpation. T / F ....

IV. Match the following descriptions with their medical words.

1. contraction of the heart	a. bundle of His
2. the area of the heart muscle where the contractions of the heart begin	b. cardiac cycle
3. the area of the heart muscle that causes the ventricles to contract	c. cardiac output
	d. foramen ovale
4. the contractory muscle fibers that permeate the ventricular walls	e. sinoatrial node
	f. medulla
5. period in which the heart rests	g. placenta
6. centers stimulated by changes in blood pressure	h. systole
7. the term for the amount of blood pumped by the left ventricle per minute	i. pulse
	j. baroreceptors
8. the term for the time between one heartbeat and the next	k. hepatic portal system
9. a microscopic blood vessel that joins arteries and veins	l. arterioles
	m. diastole
10. venous blood from the stomach, intestines, pancreas, and spleen emptying into one large vein leading to the liver	n. capillary
11. the organ that connects the blood vessels of the mother with those of the fetus	o. atrioventrical node

12. an opening in the fetal heart through which blood entering the

fetus passes   ....

13. blood vessels that play a significant role in blood

pressure   ....

14. the "throbbing" of the arteries as blood is pumped through

them   ....

15. the portion of the brain controlling the diameter of the

blood vessels   ....

V.   Fill in the blank spaces for the following statements.

1. .... is the fluid portion of blood, and the remaining volume of blood is

composed of ...., which are ....,

...................., and ....

2. The pigment portion of red blood cells is called ....

3. Primitive blood cells are called .... or ....

....

4. .... cells, produced in the liver, spleen, and bone marrow, consume
particles of broken-down erythrocytes.

5. .... is a bile pigment formed from the remains of destroyed
erythrocytes.

6. Two major divisions of leukocytes are .... and ....

....

7. .... are leukocytes that stain easily with acid dyes.

8. .... is the chief function of leukocytes.

9. .... seal tears in blood vessels and release a substance that begins the
coagulation process.

10. .... is the series of reactions that occurs when a blood vessel is broken.

11. Excessive, violent bleeding is known as ...., and it can be controlled by

    applying pressure to certain areas of the body called ....

12. A substance that maintains the pH of the blood is called a blood ....

13. Lymph is filtered in the ....

14. A lymphatic structure, located in the thorax above the heart, that contributes to the

    development of immune response is the ....

15. The .... is a storage bank for blood and a place where old erythrocytes
    are destroyed.

VI. Multiple choice: Circle the correct letter.

1. The obstruction of electrical impulses moving from the atria to the ventricles is called
   (a) heart block
   (b) angina pectoris
   (c) myocardial infarction
   (d) cardiac arrest

2. Inflammation of the sac surrounding the heart is known as
   (a) myocarditis
   (b) endocarditis
   (c) pericarditis
   (d) carditis

3. A type of arrhythmia
   (a) AV block
   (b) cardiac tamponade
   (c) infarction
   (d) tachycardia

4. Necrosis of an area of heart tissue due to insufficient blood supply
   (a) coronary thrombosis
   (b) myocardial infarction
   (c) embolism
   (d) coronary occlusion

5. The medical term for high blood pressure
   (a) atherosclerosis
   (b) arteriosclerosis
   (c) stenosis
   (d) hypertension

6. The ballooning of a blood vessel
    (a) thrombophlebitis
    (b) aneurysm
    (c) atherosclerosis
    (d) vasoconstriction

7. Abnormal heart sound resulting from incompetent heart valves
    (a) flutter
    (b) murmur
    (c) fibrillation
    (d) defibrillation

8. Abnormal condition in which fatty plaques adhere to the walls of a blood vessel
    (a) arteriostenosis
    (b) atherosclerosis
    (c) arteriosclerosis
    (d) thrombosis

9. A congenital malformation in which the blood vessel that connects the pulmonary trunk
    with the aorta does not wither
    (a) patent foramen ovale
    (b) patent ductus arteriosus
    (c) ventricular septal defect
    (d) hypertrophy of the right ventricle

10. Increased blood cell formation in the bone marrow, which may lead to leukemia
    (a) hemophilia A
    (b) hemopoiesis
    (c) aplastic anemia
    (d) polycythemia vera

11. The type of anemia brought on by the absence of an intrinsic factor necessary for the
    absorption of vitamin B12
    (a) pernicious anemia
    (b) aplastic anemia
    (c) sickle cell anemia
    (d) iron-deficiency anemia

12. A viral infection characterized by enlarged lymph glands, sore throat, fever, and fatigue
    (a) infectious mononucleosis
    (b) leukemia
    (c) polycythemia vera
    (d) lymphoma

13. Abnormal enlarging and twisting of the leg veins
    (a) thrombophlebitis
    (b) atheromas
    (c) varicose veins
    (d) venous stasis

14. A type of anemia in which the erythrocytes change their shape at low oxygen levels
    (a) aplastic anemia
    (b) sickle cell anemia
    (c) thalassemia
    (d) pernicious anemia

15. Hereditary bleeding disease affecting only male offspring
    (a) Von Willebrand's syndrome
    (b) erythroblastosis fetalis
    (c) hemophilia
    (d) Hodgkin's disease

16. A form of cancer in which there is an uncontrolled increase of white blood cells
    (a) infectious mononucleosis
    (b) polycythemia
    (c) leukemia
    (d) aplastic anemia

ANSWERS TO EXERCISES

I.

1. small blood vessel from which capillaries connect arterioles and venules, met/arteriole
2. tumor developing from blood or lymph vessels, angi/oma
3. instrument for measuring the expansion of the chest, steth/o/meter
4. pathogenic organisms and their toxins in the blood, blood poison, septic/emia
5. tumor developing from plasma-forming cells in the bone marrow plasm/o/cyt/oma
6. retention of urea in the blood, ur/emia
7. pertaining to the pulse, sphygm/ic
8. instrument for studying blood vessels, angi/o/scope
9. originating in the heart, cardi/o/gen/ic
10. inflammation of an arteriole, arteriol/itis
11. x ray of the blood vessels, vas/o/graphy
12. pertaining to the nutrients carried in the blood, hem/o/troph/ic
13. deficiency of basophils in the blood, bas/o/cyt/o/penia
14. abnormal decrease in the number of granulocytes in the blood a/granul/o/cyt/osis
15. without oxygen, deficient in oxygen, an/ox/ia
16. narrowing of a blood vessel, angi/o/sten/osis
17. pertaining to/having blood vessels, vascul/ar
18. inflammation of a venule, venul/itis
19. located between ventricles, inter/ventricul/ar
20. pertaining to the nerves having muscular control over the blood vessel walls, vas/o/motor
21. stem cell from which all blood cells arise, hem/o/cyt/o/blast
22. within a blood or lymph vessel, intra/vascul/ar
23. increase in the number of neutrophils in the blood, neutr/o/phil/
24. death of a portion of arterial tissue, arteri/o/necr/osis
25. pertaining to the heart and lungs, cari/o/pulmon/ary
26. antibody that causes agglutination, agglutin/in

27. pertaining to the phagocytes of the reticuloendothelial system, reticul/o/endo/<u>thel</u>/ial
28. a chemical essential for clotting (factor II), pro/<u>thromb</u>/in
29. abnormal hardening of the spleen, splen/o/<u>kerat/</u>osis
30. abnormal heartbeat accompanied by a rapid heart rate, tachy/a/<u>rrhythm</u>/ia
31. inflammation of a vein followed by the development of a clot, thromb/o/<u>phleb/</u>itis
32. excision of an aneurysm, aneurysm/<u>ectomy</u>
33. serum having antibodies for a specific antigen, immune serum, anti/<u>ser</u>/um
34. a simple plasmic protein containing most of the body's antibodies, <u>gamma</u> <u>globul</u>/in
35. abnormal development of fibrous tissue in an artery, arteri/o/<u>fibr/</u>osis
36. an abnormal decrease in the number of clotting cells (platelets), thromb/o/cyt/o/<u>penia</u>
37. destruction of microscopic particles and bacteria by phagocytes, phag/o/cyt/<u>osis</u>
38. halting of bleeding or circulation, hem/o/<u>stasis</u>
39. tumor developing from lymph vessels, lymph/angi/<u>oma</u>
40. buildup of fatty plaques in arterial walls, ather/<u>osis</u>
41. producing immunity, immun/o/<u>gen</u>/ic
42. surgical repair of a damaged vein, <u>phleb</u>/o/plasty
43. halting of the flow of blood in a vein, <u>ven</u>/o/stasis
44. small node, <u>nod</u>/ule
45. immature red blood cell having a network of granules, re<u>ticul</u>/o/cyte

II.

1. he<u>mat</u>ocyte;   2. ven<u>ot</u>omy or phle<u>bot</u>omy;   3. cardiome<u>gal</u>y;   4. arter<u>it</u>is;
5. vascu<u>lit</u>is;   6. hyp<u>ox</u>ia;   7. eosino<u>phil</u>ia;   8. granulocytopoi<u>es</u>is;
9. vasodil<u>at</u>or;   10. aort<u>orr</u>haphy;   11. vent<u>ric</u>ulotomy;   12. aorto<u>cor</u>onary;
13. veno<u>atr</u>ial;   14. intra<u>ven</u>ous;   15. <u>neu</u>trophil;   16. hemot<u>ol</u>ogist;
17. aort<u>op</u>athy;   18. <u>atr</u>iotome;   19. val<u>vot</u>omy or valvul<u>ot</u>omy;
20. arterioscler<u>os</u>is;   21. basocyt<u>os</u>is;   22. <u>ox</u>ygenated;
23. sphygmo<u>car</u>diograph;   24. he<u>mol</u>ysis;   25. <u>val</u>vuloplasty;
26. thrombo<u>phil</u>ia;   27. erythropoi<u>es</u>is;   28. hypot<u>on</u>ic;   29. splenomegaly;
30. tonsil<u>lit</u>is;   31. vari<u>cot</u>omy;   32. thy<u>mec</u>tomy;   33. lymphaden<u>op</u>athy;
34. sidero<u>pen</u>ia;   35. agglutin<u>at</u>ion;   36. an<u>uc</u>leate;   37. phagocyt<u>ol</u>ysis;
38. throm<u>bol</u>ysis;   39. leukopoi<u>es</u>is;   40. fibrinogeno<u>pen</u>ia.

III.

1. F, visceral pericardium
2. T
3. F, only systemic arteries
4. F, goes to lungs (pulmonary circulation)
5. F, auscultation

IV.

1. h;   2. e;   3. o;   4. a;   5. m;   6. j;   7. c;   8. b;   9. n;
10. k;   11. g;   12. d;   13. l;   14. i;   15. f.

V.

1. plasma, formed elements, erythrocytes, leukocytes, thrombocytes (or platelets);

2. hemoglobin;   3. hemocytoblasts, stem cells;   4. reticuloendothelial;
5. bilirubin;   6. granulocytes, agranulocytes;   7. eosinophils;   8. phagocytosis;
9. platelets;   10. hemostasis;   11. hemorrhage, pressure points;   12. buffer;
13. lymph nodes;   14. thymus;   15. spleen.

VI.

1. (a);   2. (c);   3. (d);   4. (b);   5. (d);   6. (b);   7. (b);   8. (b);
9. (b);   10. (d);   11. (a);   12. (a);   13. (c);   14. (b);   15. (c);
16. (c).

12 The Respiratory System

COMBINING FORMS

	Meaning	Example
SPIR/O (spi'ro)	breathing	RESPIRATION (res-pir-ay'shun), process of taking oxygen and giving off carbon dioxide
PECTOR/O (pek'to-ro)	chest	PECTORAL (pek'to-ral), pertaining to the chest
NAS/O (nay'zo)	nose	ORONASAL (or-o-nay'zal), pertaining to the mouth and nose
RHIN/O (ry'no)	nose	RHINITIS (ry-ny'tis), inflammation of the nose, especially the mucous membrane
PHARYNG/O (far-in'go)	pharynx, the passageway from the nasal cavity to the larynx	PHARYNGOTOMY (far-in-got'o-me), incision of the pharynx
LARYNG/O (lar-in'go)	larynx, voice box	LARYNGOPHONY (lar-in-gof'o-ne), sounds heard during auscultation of the larynx
EPIGLOTT/O (ep-e-glot'to)	epiglottis	EPIGLOTTITIS (ep-e-glot-eye'tis), inflammation of the epiglottis
TRACHE/O (tray'ke-o)	trachea, windpipe	TRACHEOSTOMY (tray-ke-os'to-me), incision of the trachea for the insertion of a tube

	Meaning	*Example*
MEDIASTIN/O (me-de-as-tie'no)	mediastinum, a cavity located between two parts of an organ	MEDIASTINAL (me-de-as-tie'nal), pertaining to the mediastinum
BRONCH/O (bron'ko)	bronchus, bronchial tube	BRONCHOSTENOSIS (bron-ko-sten-o'sis), narrowing of a bronchial tube
BRONCHI/O (bron'ke-o)	bronchus, bronchial tube	BRONCHIOGENIC (bron-ke-o-jen'ik), originating in the bronchus
BRONCHIOL/O (bron-ke'o-lo)	bronchiole, small bronchus	BRONCHIOLAR (bron-ke'ol-ar), pertaining to a bronchiole
ALVEOL/O (al-vee'o-lo)	alveolus, a small hollow or cavity, an air cell of the lung	ALVEOLITIS (al-vee-o-ly'tis), inflammation of an alveolus
PULM/O (pul'mo)	lung	PULMOMETRY (pul-mom'e-tre), measurement of the air capacity of the lungs
PULMON/O (pul'mo-no)	lung	PULMONARY (pul'mo-na-re), pertaining to the lung
PNEUM/O (new'mo)	air, lung	PNEUMOCOCCI (new-mo-kok'eye), oval-shaped bacteria that cause pneumonia
PNEUMON/O (new-mon'o)	air, lung	PNEUMONIA (new-mon'ya), inflammation of the lungs
LOB/O (lo'bo)	lobe, a division of an organ	LOBAR (lo'bar), pertaining to a lobe
PLEUR/O (plur'o)	pleura, serous membrane covering the lungs and thoracic wall	PLEURAL (plur'al), pertaining to the pleura
MUC/O (mu'ko)	mucus, a thick fluid secreted by membranes	MUCOSAL (mu-ko'sal), pertaining to a mucous membrane
DIAPHRAGM/O (dy-a-frag'mo)	diaphragm, the wall separating the thoracic and abdominal cavities	DIAPHRAGMITIS (dy-a-frag-my'tis), inflammation of the diaphragm
DIAPHRAGMAT/O (dy-a-frag-mat'o)	diaphragm	DIAPHRAGMATIC (dy-a-frag-mat'ik), pertaining to the diaphragm
PHREN/O (fren'o)	diaphragm	PHRENIC (fren'ik), pertaining to the diaphragm

	Meaning	*Example*
PHRENIC/O (fren'ik-o)	phrenic nerve	PHRENICECTOMY (fren-i-kek'to-me), excision of the phrenic nerve
PTY/O (ty'o)	saliva	PTYSIS (ty'sis), spitting
PTYAL/O (ty'al-o)	saliva	PTYALOGRAPHY (ty-al-og'ra-fe), x ray of salivary glands and ducts
-PNEA (nee'a)	breathing	EUPNEA (youp-nee'a), normal breathing
-CAPNIA (kap'ne-a)	carbon dioxide	ACAPNIA (a-kap'ne-a), absence of carbon dioxide
ATEL/O (at'e-lo)	imperfect, defective	ATELECTASIS (at-e-lek'ta-sis), a birth defect in which the lungs of the newborn do not expand
MYC/O (my'ko)	fungus	MYCOPLASMAS (my-ko-plaz'maz), a strain of bacteria that causes pneumonia

ANATOMY OF THE RESPIRATORY SYSTEM

The taking in of oxygen by the body and the elimination of carbon dioxide are accomplished through *respiration*, more commonly called breathing. Through this process oxygen from the external environment enters the bloodstream and carbon dioxide leaves the bloodstream and enters the external environment. The procedure is called *external respiration*, which is performed in the *respiratory tract* (Figure 12-1). The exchange of gases between the cells and blood is called *internal respiration*.

Air enters the body through the *nose*, which consists of two cavities (called *nostrils* or *nares*) lined with the same type of mucous membrane that lines most of the respiratory system. *Cilia* (sil'e-a), hairlike projections, also cover the respiratory passageways and filter out dirt and dust. The nasal membrane secretes *mucus*, a thick, sticky substance, which protects the passageway by trapping entering particles. The *paranasal sinuses*, which drain into the nose, add to the mucus.

Next, the air passes through the *pharynx*. The pharynx begins behind the nasal cavities and through it air passes to the *trachea*, food to the *esophagus*. The pharynx can be divided into three parts: the *nasopharynx* behind the nasal cavities and where the nostrils and eustachian tubes open, the *oropharynx* behind the mouth whose opening (called *fauces* faw'sez) joins the pharynx, and the *laryngopharynx*, which is connected to the larynx and esophagus. All three pairs of tonsils are located in the first two portions of the pharynx.

After passing the *larynx*, the organ of voice, the air enters the trachea. The *trachea* or windpipe is composed of smooth muscle that is supported by C-shaped rings

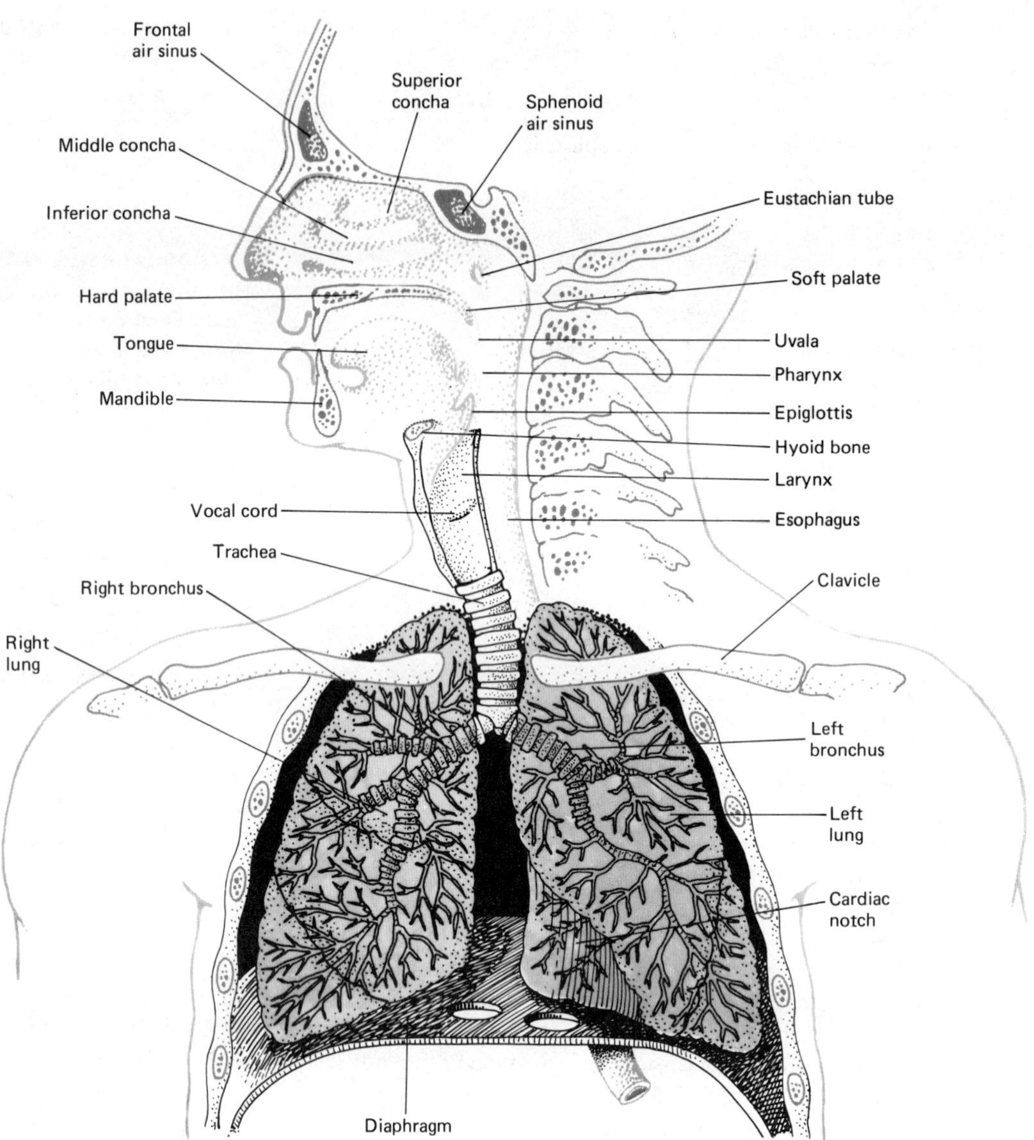

Figure 12-1 The respiratory tract and some associated structures.

of cartilage. The trachea descends into the *mediastinum*, a cavity located between the right and left lungs. About the fifth thoracic vertebra the trachea (Figure 12-2) branches off into the right and left *pulmonary bronchi*, which also branch off into *secondary bronchi* on entering the lungs at the *hilus* (hil'us), where blood and lymph vessels and nerves also enter the lungs. This process of *ramification* or branching off into smaller bronchi continues until microscopic bronchi made entirely of smooth muscle appear. These microscopic bronchi are called *bronchioles*. The numerous *air sacs* containing clusters of *alveoli* that are clumped around the ends of the bronchioles, much like grapes on a vine (Figure 12-3), are called *alveolar sacs*. They are attached to a bronchiole by an *alveolar duct*. The exchange of gases occurs in the alveoli, which are surrounded by capillary networks.

The *lungs* are two nearly cone-shaped lobes with the pointed end (called an *apex*) on top slightly above the level of the first rib. The base of each lung begins at the sternum and tapers off somewhere around the eighth rib. The *costodiaphragmatic sinus* is a space located below each lung to allow for greater expansion. A serous membrane, the *visceral pleura*, covers both lungs and separates them into lobes. (Lobes are obvious curved divisions of an organ.) The visceral pleura is continuous with the *parietal* (PARIET/O wall) *pleura* that lines the thoracic cavity. Both pleuras are separated by a space, the *pleural space*, where serous fluid keeps both membranes from

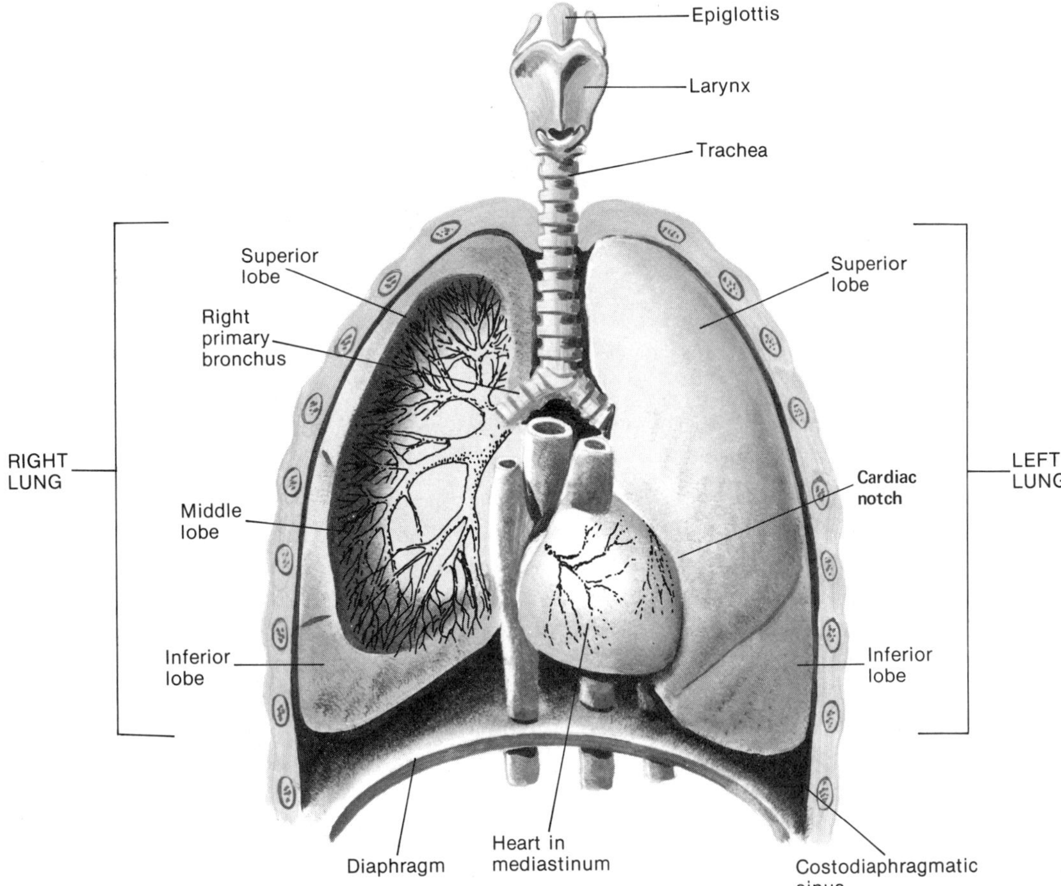

Figure 12-2 The lungs and related structures in place within the thorax. A portion of the right lung has been cut away to show the branching of the bronchial "tree."

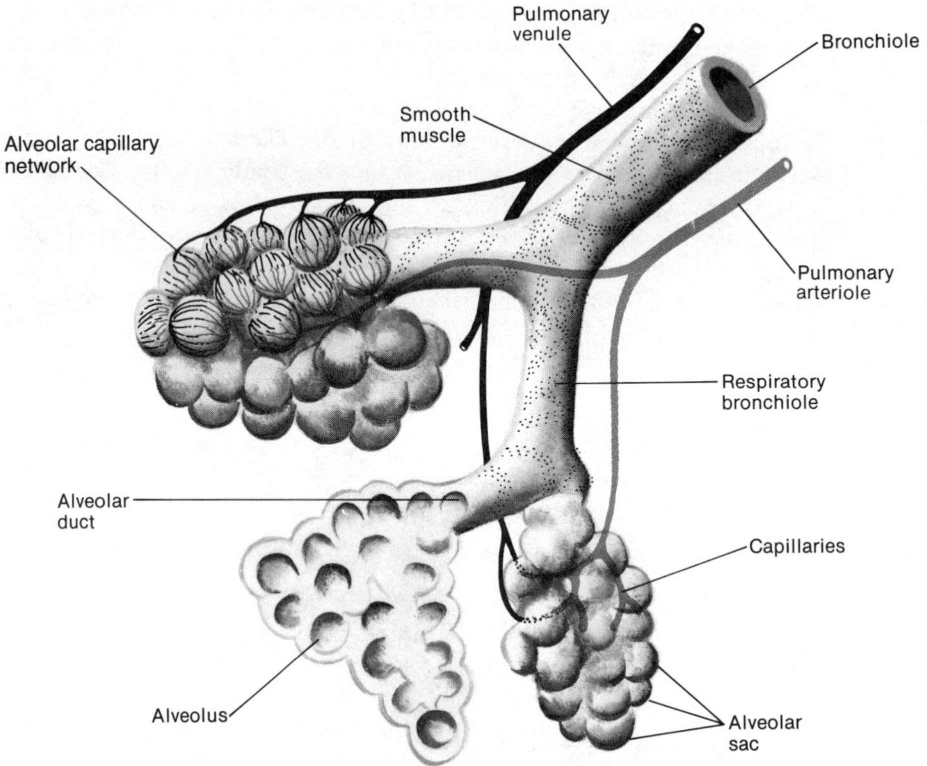

Figure 12-3   The structure of alveoli and the capillary network that surrounds them.

rubbing together during breathing. Each lobe can be further divided into *broncho-pulmonary segments* that contain their own blood and air supply.

Using a stethoscope, one can hear inhaled or exhaled air making a sharp, high-pitched sound called a *bronchial sound* as it passes through the trachea and bronchi. Inhaled air also makes a murmur called a *vesicular murmur*. When the thoracic walls are tapped (called *percussion*), a hollow sound is normal. Abnormal breath sounds are called *adventitious sounds*. Adventitious sounds can be divided into two groups: rales and wheezes. *Rales* (also called crackles) are sharp bubbling sounds. *Wheezes* are harsh, high pitched whistling sounds. Abnormal breath sounds may indicate chronic obstructive pulmonary disease or diseases such as asthma or atelectasis.

BREATHING

Breathing—taking air in (inspiration) and expelling air (expiration)—is accomplished through up and downward movements of the *diaphragm*, a muscular wall separating the thoracic and abdominal cavities. Because the thorax is a closed cavity, when the diaphragm moves downward, intrathoracic pressure becomes lower than atmospheric pressure, thus creating a vacuum in the lungs. As a result, outside air is under a greater pressure, which causes it to fill the lungs. When the diaphragm moves upward, greater than atmospheric pressure is created, forcing the air to leave the lungs. This *respiratory cycle*, inspiration-respiration, occurs about 16 to 18 times every minute without any physical activity. The internal and external intercostal muscles also contribute to respiration by raising and lowering the ribs, resulting in the expansion and contraction of the chest. The entire breathing mechanism is an involuntary reflex controlled by the respiratory centers of the medulla and pons of the brainstem, which are extremely sensitive to the level of carbon dioxide in the blood.

PULMONARY FUNCTION TESTS

Pulmonary function tests are used to detect any problems or abnormalities in lung function. They are especially useful in assessing the degree or stage of a *chronic obstructive pulmonary disease*, such as emphysema. The following tests represent the major types of pulmonary function tests.

Spirometry
A spirometer is a bell-shaped device that is placed in water, but air is able to pass into and out of it. By measuring the passage of air into and out of the spirometer, lung volume, capacity, and flow can be determined.

Nitrogen-washout technique
The patient breathes a 100% oxygen, which he then exhales into a closed unit. In this way, the nitrogen content of the lungs is collected in the unit, measured, and the *functional residual capacity* (FRC) of the lungs determined.

Helium-dilution technique
A measured amount of helium is circulated in a closed container. After the entrapped air has been exhausted, the remaining concentration of helium is determined. This test is used to determine the FRC of the lungs.

Carbon monoxide test
The patient inhales a measured amount of carbon monoxide, which diffuses into the blood and combines with the hemoglobin. In this way, the degree and rate of gas exchange can be determined.

Arterial blood gases
Carbon dioxide levels in the blood are used to determine the degree and rate of gas exchange.

Plethysmography (plee-thiz-mog'ra-fe)
A unit, the plethysmograph (a pressure chamber), is used to measure air pressure and the volume of all gases found in the lungs.

Chest x ray
Chest x rays are used to visualize the increase and decrease in lung size and the movement of the diaphragm.

VOCAL MECHANISM

The *larynx* or voice box (Figure 12-4) is made up of four sections of cartilage—two arytenoid (ar-i-tey'noid, ladle-shaped) cartilages, a cricoid (kre'koid, ring-shaped) cartilage, and the thyroid cartilage, also called the Adam's apple. Sound is caused by the tensing of the *vocal folds*, which causes the *glottis*, the space between the two vocal folds, to close. In addition to vocalization, the larynx is part of the mechanism that enables us to cough, swallow, and expectorate (expel mucus from the throat). The *epiglottis* is attached to the thyroid cartilage and prevents food from entering the respiratory tract.

CLINICAL AND PATHOLOGICAL CONDITIONS

Abnormal breathing
Breathing that deviates from normal respiration (*eupnea*) may be symptomatic of a disease or illness (e.g., emphysema). Some examples of abnormal breathing are

> *Dyspnea:* difficult or labored breathing.
>
> *Hypernea:* deep breathing.
>
> *Tachypnea:* rapid succession of short breaths.
>
> *Polypnea:* extremely rapid breathing accompanied by *hyperventilation* (very deep breathing).
>
> *Cheyne-Stokes* (kay'n* sto'ks): hypernea followed by the cessation of breathing (apnea).

Disruptions of the acid-base balance of the blood

Respiratory acidosis. Carbon dioxide is not adequately removed by the lungs; this results in an increased level of carbonic acid. Hypoventilation brought on by impaired alveolar function (in such conditions as pneumonia and emphysema; also

---

*Also pronounced chain'ee.

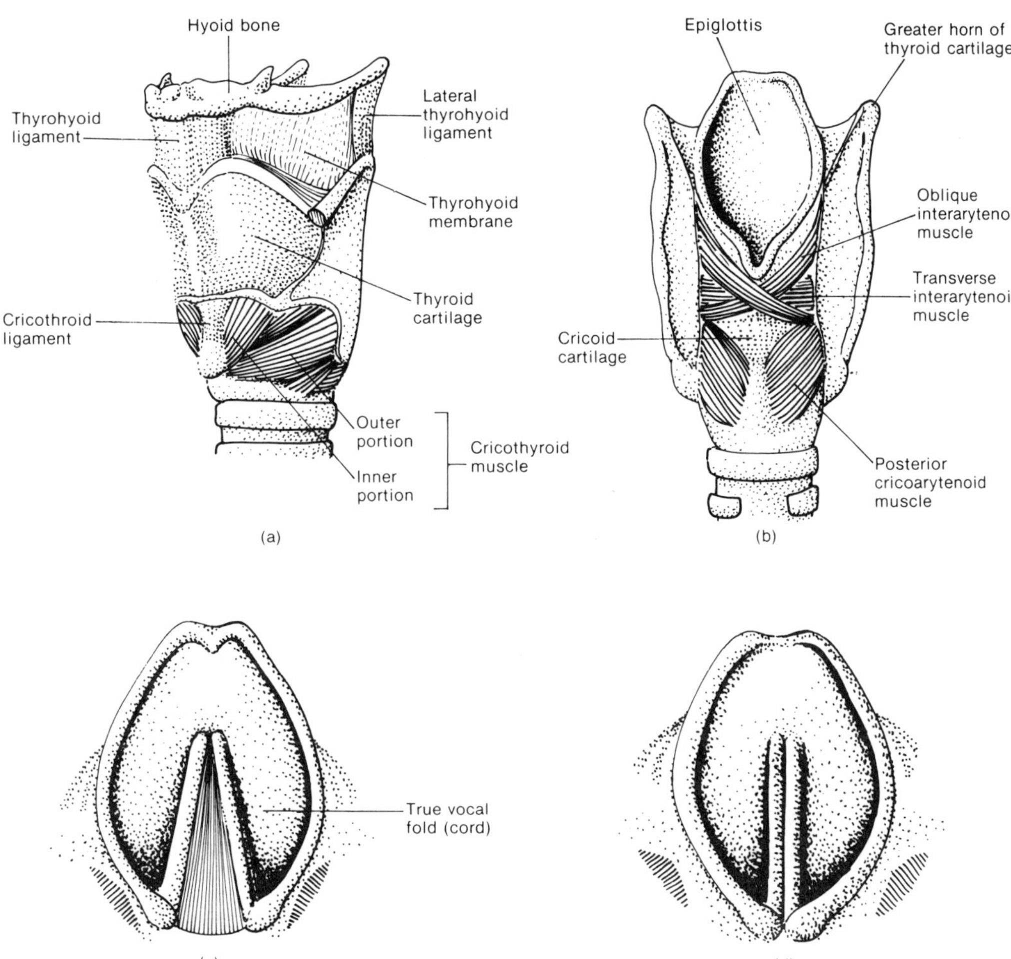

Figure 12-4 The larynx: (a) anterolateral view; (b) posterior view; (c) true vocal folds open, or abducted; (d) true vocal folds closed, or adducted.

after abdominal surgery or as a result of certain medications) is the major cause of respiratory acidosis.

Respiratory alkalosis. An imbalance in the acid-base levels produces a higher concentration of base. Hyperventilation, which produces a decrease in the level of carbon dioxide (hypocapnia), is the cause of respiratory alkalosis.

Coughing

Coughing occurs when the mucosal nerves of the respiratory tract are irritated. Not all coughing is a sign of disease; a cough, however, may indicate a respiratory disease.

Sometimes coughing produces secretions called *sputum* (spew'tum). *Hemoptysis* is bloody sputum. *Whooping cough* (*pertussis*) is an infectious disease characterized by a *paroxysmal* (par-ok-siz'mal, PAROXYSM/O sudden, sharp recurrence of the symptoms of a disease) whooping type of cough. There are usually three stages: (a) catarrhal (katar'al)—symptoms of a common cold, (b) paroxysmal—frequent outbursts of the whooping cough, and (c) decline—coughing is less frequent and finally ceases.

Hyaline (hy'a-lin) membrane disease

Hyaline membrane disease, also called *respiratory distress syndrome* of the newborn, occurs in a newborn baby shortly after birth. Instead of lubricating fluid, thick hyaline membranes cover the alveoli, preventing the normal diffusion of gases. The baby dies from *asphyxiation* (as-fik-se-ay'shun), a lack of oxygen and a buildup of carbon dioxide.

Atelectasis (at-e-lek'ta-sis)

This is usually a neonatal condition in which the lungs are collapsed due to either blockage or failure to expand properly. In older persons atelectasis results from fluid or air filling the plural cavity.

Pneumothorax

Air enters the pleural cavity from a wound and the lungs collapse.

Diphtheria

An infectious disease of the upper respiratory tract, diphtheria is produced by the *Corynebacterium diphtheriae* (kor-i-ne-bak-tee're-um dif-thee're- eye).This bacterium, which is infected with a virus, produces a potent toxin that causes the development of a false membrane in the pharynx. Eventually, the toxin is picked up by the blood and toxemia results. Myocardial necrosis and damage to the peripheral nervous system resulting in paralysis may develop if the condition is not treated; treatment is with diphtheria antitoxin.

Pneumonia

The lungs are inflamed, and as the bronchi and alveoli become fluid filled, breathing is difficult. Pneumonia is caused by bacteria or viruses and may affect both lungs, a single lung, or a portion of a lung (lobar pneumonia). Affected areas appear white on an x ray. "Walking pneumonia", which is characterized by a general feeling of fatigue and coughing, is caused by bacteria called *mycoplasmas*.

Pulmonary Abscesses

An *abscess* is an area of inflammed tissue containing pus. Pulmonary abscesses may result from pneumonia or may be induced by introducing bacteria into the lungs by accidentally breathing in food or other substances. Frequently pulmonary abscesses must be drained surgically.

Tuberculosis (TUBERCUL/O tubercle)

This is a highly infectious disease of the lungs characterized by the formation of *tubercles* (swollen areas, protrusions) on the lung. There are two forms of tuberculosis: primary and secondary. In *primary tuberculosis* the individual inhales the *bacilli* (ba-sil'lie) from an infected person. The body's immune response is activated and the bacilli are encapsulated. Surrounding tissue becomes fibrous and calcified. *Secondary tuberculosis* is a reactivation of the bacilli enclosed in the tubercles. The inflammation can spread to other parts of the body.

Asthma

Asthma is an allergic response caused by inhaling antigens, such as pollen. The bronchioles constrict and mucus plugs the airways, giving rise to a wheezing sound. Treatment is usually in the form of an *antihistamine* (HISTI/O tissue), which counters the allergic reaction of the tissues.

Pneumoconioses (nu-mo-ko-ne-o'sez, CONI/O dust)

These are lung diseases caused by the inhalation of airborne particles. *Silicosis* (SILIC/O flint, rock dust) causes fibrosis of the lungs as a result of the continuous inhaling of fine dust particles. *Asbestosis* is caused by the inhaling of asbestos particles. Until recently asbestos was used as a fireproofing material; however, it has now been linked to cancer. *Anthracosis* (an-thra-ko'sis, ANTHRAC/O coal) is an inflammation caused by the inhaling of coal dust. Gases (e.g., chlorine and ammonia) can also irritate the lungs. Inflammation of the lungs caused by an irritant gas is called *chemical pneumonitis*.

Pulmonary emphysema (em-fi-see'ma, EMPHYSEM/O inflation)

The lung tissues swell and lose their elasticity. Breathing becomes difficult and is accompanied by a heavy cough. Carbon dioxide builds up in the blood (called *respiratory acidosis*) and failure of the right side of the heart (*cor pulmonale*) may result.

Pleurisy

Pleurisy is an inflammation of the pleura. Fluid collects in the pleural cavity (*hydrothorax*). *Empyema* (em-py-ee'ma) is the collection of pus in the pleural cavity. Fluid is removed from the pleural cavity by *aspiration* (as-pi-ray'shun, to withdraw through suction).

Cancers of the respiratory tract

Cancers can occur in any part of the respiratory tract. The lips, mouth, pharynx, larynx, and lungs are common sites of cancer in smokers.

Laryngeal carcinoma. It is especially common among cigarette smokers. A hoarse or raspy voice is a sign of laryngeal cancer. A *laryngectomy* is performed to remove the cancerous larynx.

Lung cancer.   This form of cancer may develop in the trachea, bronchi, or air sacs; however, it often develops in the mucosal lining of a primary or secondary bronchus—hence the name *bronchiogenic carcinoma.* There are three characteristics of lung cancer: (a) tumorous growth within the lung, (b) the spread (metastasis) of the cancer to other areas of the body, especially the lymph nodes, liver, brain, bone, and adrenal glands, and (c) stimulation of adrenal glands. A large number of lung cancers are squamous cell or epidermoid carcinomas originating in the bronchial mucosa. Cancer developing from an *oat cell* (shaped like an oat seed) is another histologic type of lung carcinoma.

EXERCISES

I. Give the meaning for each of the following medical words. Divide each word into base(s), prefix, and suffix; underline the letter(s) that has the primary stress. *Example:*

NASOPHARYNGEAL   pertaining to the nose and pharynx   nas/o/pharyng/eal

1. ENDORHINITIS

2. PHARYNGEMPHRAXIS (-EMPHRAXIS obstruction)

3. MEDIASTINOPERICARDITIS

4. PNEUMOMELANOSIS

5. BRONCHIOLECTASIS

6. PLEUROPNEUMONIA

7. DIAPHRAGMATOCELE

8. APNEA

9. PTYALITH

10. HYPERCAPNIA

11. SPIROMETER

12. EXPECTORANT ....

13. RHINOMYCOSIS ....

14. LARYNGOTRACHEITIS ....

15. TRACHEOPYOSIS ....

16. PULMOAORTIC ....

17. PNEUMOGRAM ....

18. DIAPHRAGMODYNIA ....

19. PHRENOPLEGIA ....

20. MYCOSIS ....

21. PARANASAL ....

22. PHARYNGOLARYNGITIS ....

23. TRACHEOTOME ....

24. BRONCHORRAPHY ....

25. PNEUMOHYDROTHORAX ....

II. Make medical words from the following phrases. Indicate the primary stress by underlining the stressed letter(s). *Example:*

inflammation of a bronchus

bron<u>chi</u>tis
....

1. (watery) discharge from the nose

....

2. pertaining to the pharynx

....

3. the process of inhaling

....

4. the excision (of all or part) of a lung

    . . . .

5. the inflammation of a bronchiole

    . . . .

6. the attachment of a displaced lung to the chest wall

    . . . .

7. having or pertaining to small lobes

    . . . .

8. a mucous membrane

    . . . .

9. inflammation of the pleura

    . . . .

10. spitting up blood

    . . . .

11. labored breathing

    . . . .

12. an abnormal decrease in the level of carbon dioxide

    . . . .

13. the elimination of mucus from the throat or lung

    . . . .

14. a narrowing of the larynx

    . . . .

15. pertaining to the epiglottis

    . . . .

16. inflammation of mediastinal tissue

    . . . .

17. pertaining to the bronchi and lungs

....

18. pertaining to the air cells of the lungs

....

19. hernia of the pleura

....

20. excision of the larynx

....

III. Trace the path of air through the respiratory system.

trachea	**1.**	....
primary bronchi	**2.**	....
alveoli	**3.**	....
nose	**4.**	....
secondary bronchi	**5.**	....
capillaries	**6.**	....
larynx	**7.**	....
bronchioles	**8.**	....
pharynx	**9.**	....

IV. Match the following descriptions with their medical words.

1. the exchange of gases between the external environment

and the respiratory tract ....   a. hilus

2. the cellular exchange of gases with the blood ....   b. parietal pleura

3. the hairs that line the respiratory tract ....   c. larynx

4. the windpipe ....   d. epiglottis

5. the voicebox ....   e. diaphragm

6. a cavity located between the two parts of an

   organ ....   f. cilia

7. the site where the bronchi enter the lungs ....   g. vocal folds

8. clustered around the air sacs ....   h. external respiration

9. the "reserve" space below each lung ....   i. alveoli

10. membrane covering both lungs ....   j. internal respiration

11. membrane attached to the thoracic cavity ....   k. bronchopulmonary segments

12. divisions of the lungs ....

13. the wall separating the thoracic and abdominal   l. trachea

   cavities ....   m. costodiaphragmatic sinus

14. Adam's apple ....   n. thyroid cartilage

15. air passes through them to produce sound ....   o. mediastinum

16. guards the glottis ....   p. visceral pleura

      V.   Multiple choice: Circle the correct letter.

1. Labored breathing
   (a) hyperpnea
   (b) dyspnea
   (c) eupnea
   (d) hypopnea

2. Hyperpnea followed by apnea
   (a) tachypnea
   (b) polypnea
   (c) Cheyne–Stokes
   (d) hyperventilation

3. An infectious disease that produces a paroxysmal whooping type of cough
   (a) hemoptysis
   (b) pertussis
   (c) asphyxia
   (d) atelectasis

4. A respiratory disease affecting the newborn in which the alveoli are covered with a thick membrane
    (a) atelectasis
    (b) pneumothorax
    (c) lobar pneumonia
    (d) hyaline membrane disease

5. Collapse of the lungs
    (a) atelectasis
    (b) hyaline membrane disease
    (c) pneumothorax
    (d) pneumohydrothorax

6. An infectious disease of the lungs in which the bacteria become encapsulated
    (a) pneumonia
    (b) pulmonary abscess
    (c) tuberculosis
    (d) mycoplasmas

7. An example of a pneumoconiosis
    (a) silicosis
    (b) secondary tuberculosis
    (c) mycoplasmas
    (d) abscesses

8. A condition in which lung tissues swell and lose their elasticity
    (a) pleurisy
    (b) anthracosis
    (c) emphysema
    (d) acidosis

9. Inflammation of the serous membrane covering the lungs and thoracic cavity
    (a) pneumonia
    (b) pleurisy
    (c) emphysema
    (d) pneumoconiosis

10. Process of removing fluid from the pleural cavity
    (a) aspiration
    (b) percussion
    (c) hydrothorax
    (d) palpation

ANSWERS TO EXERCISES

I.

1. inflammation of the mucosa of the nose, endo/rhin/itis
2. obstruction of the pharynx, pharyng/emphraxis

3. inflammation of the tissue of the mediastinum and the pericardium, mediastin/o/peri/card/itis
4. abnormal blackening of a lung as a result of inhaling a substance such as coal dust, pneum/o/melan/osis
5. stretching of the bronchioles, bronchiol/ectasis
6. pneumonia, including pleurisy, pleur/o/pneumon/ia
7. hernia of the diaphragm, diaphragmat/o/cele
8. cessation of breathing, a/pnea
9. calculus originating in a salivary gland, pty/a/lith
10. excess of carbon dioxide, hyper/capnia
11. an instrument for measuring the air capacity of the lungs, spir/o/meter
12. a substance that aids in the elimination of mucus from the throat or lungs, ex/pector/ant
13. a fungus infection of the mucous membrane of the nose, rhin/o/myc/osis
14. inflammation of the larynx and trachea, laryng/o/trache/itis
15. suppurative inflammation of the trachea, trache/o/py/osis
16. pertaining to the lungs and the aorta, pulm/o/aort/ic
17. x ray of an area of the body that has been injected with air, pneum/o/gram
18. pain in the diaphragm, diaphragm/odynia
19. paralysis of the diaphragm, phren/o/plegia
20. any disease caused by a fungus, myc/osis
21. located near the nose, para/nas/al
22. inflammation of the pharynx and larynx, pharyng/o/laryng/itis
23. an instrument for cutting the trachea, trache/o/tome
24. the suturing of a bronchus, bronch/o/rraphy
25. air and fluid in the pleural cavity, pneum/o/hydr/o/thorax

II.

1. rhinorrhea;   2. pharyngeal;   3. inspiration;   4. pulmonectomy;
5. bronchiolitis;   6. pneumonopexy;   7. lobular;   8. mucosa;   9. pleuritis;
10. hemoptysis;   11. dyspnea;   12. hypocapnia;   13. expectoration;
14. laryngostenosis;   15. epiglottal;   16. mediastinitis;
17. bronchopulmonary;   18. alveolar;   19. pleurocele;   20. laryngectomy.

III.

1. nose;   2. pharynx;   3. larynx;   4. trachea;   5. primary bronchi;
6. secondary bronchi;   7. bronchioles;   8. alveoli;   9. capillaries.

IV.

1. h;   2. j;   3. f;   4. l;   5. c;   6. o;   7. a;   8. i;   9. m;
10. p;   11. b;   12. k;   13. e;   14. n;   15. g;   16. d.

V.

1. (b);   2. (c);   3. (b);   4. (d);   5. (a);   6. (c);   7. (a);   8. (c);
9. (b);   10. (a).

13 The Digestive System

COMBINING FORMS

	Meaning	*Example*
OR/O (or'o)	mouth	ORAL (or'al), pertaining to the mouth
STOMAT/O (sto'ma-to)	mouth	STOMATOPATHY (sto-ma-top'a-thee), any disease of the mouth
LABI/O (lay'be-o)	lip	LABIAL (lay'be-al), pertaining to the lip(s)
CHEIL/O (ky'lo)	lip	CHEILOSTOMATO-PLASTY (ky-lo-sto-mat'o-plas-te), surgical reconstruction of the lips and mouth
BUCC/O (buk'o)	cheek	BUCCAL (buk'al), pertaining to the cheeks
DENT/I (den'ti)	tooth, teeth	DENTALGIA (den-tal'je-a), toothache
ODONT/O (o-don'to)	tooth, teeth	PERIODONTAL (per-e-o-don'tal), pertaining to the structures surrounding a tooth
LINGU/O (ling'wo)	tongue	SUBLINGUAL (sub-ling'wal), under the tongue
GLOSS/O (glos'o)	tongue	GLOSSITIS (glos-eye'tis), inflammation of the tongue
ADEN/O (ad'e-no)	gland	ADENOID (ad'e-noid), resembling a gland, adenoid, the pharyngeal tonsils

	Meaning	Example
SALIV/A (sa-ly'va)	saliva	SALIVATION (sal-i-vay'shun), secretion of saliva
SIAL/O (sy'a-lo)	saliva	SIALOANGITIS (sy-a-lo-an-jy'tis), inflammation of a salivary duct(s)
SIALADEN/O (sy-al-ad'e-no)	salivary gland	SIALADENITIS (sy-al-ad-e-ny'tis), inflammation of a salivary gland
PHARYNG/O (far-in'go)	pharynx	PHARYNGOLARYNGITIS (far-in-go-lar-in-jy'tis), inflammation of the pharynx and larynx
ESOPHAG/O (ee-sof'a-go)	esophagus	ESOPHAGEAL (ee-sof-a-jee'al), pertaining to the esophagus
SPHINCTER/O (sfink'ter-o)	sphincter, valvelike muscle ring	SPHINCTERITIS (sfink-ter-eye'tis), inflammation of a sphincter
GASTR/O (gas'tro)	stomach	GASTRIC (gas'trik), pertaining to the stomach
PYLOR/O (py-lor'o)	pylorus, the opening of the stomach that empties into the duodenum	PYLOROSPASM (py-lor'o-spazm), spasmodic closure of the pylor opening
CELI/O (se'le-o)	abdomen	CELIOTOMY (se-le-ot'o-me), incision of the abdomen
LAPAR/O (lap'ar-o)	abdominal wall	LAPAROTOMY (lap-ar-ot' o-me), incision of the abdominal wall
ENTER/O (en'ter-o)	small intestine	PARENTERAL (par-en'ter-al), outside of the intestines
DUODEN/O (du-o-dee'no)	duodenum	DUODENOSTOMY (du-od-e-nos'to-me), surgical formation of an opening of the duodenum through the abdominal wall
JEJUN/O (jey-ju'no)	jejunum	JEJUNITIS (jey-ju-ny'tis), inflammation of the jejunum
ILE/O (il'ee-o)	ileum	ILEAL (il'ee-al), pertaining to the ileum
COL/O (ko'lo)	colon	COLITIS (ko-ly'tis), inflammation of the colon

	Meaning	*Example*
CEC/O (see′ko)	cecum	CECAL (see′kal), pertaining to the cecum
APPENDIC/O (a-pen′de-ko)	appendix	APPENDICITIS (a-pen-de-sy′tis), inflammation of the appendix
APPEND/O (a-pen′do)	appendix	APPENDECTOMY (a-pen-dek′to-me), excision of the appendix
SIGMOID/O (sig′moi-do)	sigmoid colon	SIGMOIDOPEXY (sig-moi′do-pek-se), fixation of the sigmoid colon to the abdominal wall
RECT/O (rek′to)	rectum	RECTAL (rek′tal), pertaining to the rectum
AN/O (ay′no)	anus	ANAL (ay′nal), pertaining to the anus
PROCT/O (prok′to)	anus and rectum	PROCTALGIA (prok-tal′je-a), pain of the anus and rectum
HEPAT/O (he-pat′o)	liver	HEPATITIS (hep-a-tie′tis), inflammation of the liver
CHOLECYST/O (ko-lee-sis′to)	gallbladder	CHOLECYSTOTOMY (ko-lee-sis-tot′o-me), incision of the gallbladder
BIL/I (bi′le)	bile	BILIRUBIN (bil-i-rou′bin), bile pigment—a product of the breaking down of hemoglobin
CHOL/E (ko′le)	bile	CHOLEMIA (ko-lee′me-a), presence of bile or bile pigment in the blood
CHOLEDOCH/O (ko-lee-do′ko)	common bile duct	CHOLEDOCHOLITHOTOMY (ko-lee-do-ko-lith-ot′o-me), removal of a gallstone from the common bile duct
PANCREAT/O (pan-kree-at′o)	pancreas	PANCREATIC (pan-kree-at′ik), pertaining to the pancreas
PERITONE/O (per-e-toe-nee′o)	peritoneum, the serous membrane of the abdominal wall and viscera	INTRAPERITONEAL (in-tra-per-e-to-nee′al), inside the peritoneal cavity
MESENTER/O (mez-en′ter-o)	mesentery	MESENTERITIS (mez-en-ter-eye′tis), inflammation of the mesentery

	Meaning	*Example*
OMENT/O (o-men′to)	omentum	OMENTORRHAPHY (o-men-tor′ra-fe), suture of the omentum
-ASE (ays)	enzyme	PROTEASE (pro′tee-ays), enzyme that breaks down protein
SUCC/O (sou′ko)	juice, secretion	SUCCAGOGUE (sou′ka-gog), a substance that stimulates glandular secretion
PEPT/I (pep′ti)	digestion	PEPTIC (pep′tik), pertaining to digestion
PEPS/I (pep′si)	digestion	DYSPEPSIA (dis-pep′se-a), indigestion
CHLORHYDR/O (klor-hy′dro)	hydrochloric acid	ACHLORHYDRIA (a-klor-hy′dre-a), absence of hydrochloric acid
GLUC/O (glou′ko)	sugar	GLUCATONIA (glou-ka-toe′ne-a), reduction of blood sugar, insulin shock
GLYC/O (gly′ko)	sugar	GLYCEMIA (gly-see′me-a), presence of sugar in the blood
SACCHAR/O (sak′a-ro)	sugar	POLYSACCHARIDE (pol-e-sak′a-rid), a complex carbohydrate group containing more than two molecules of sugar
AMYL/O (am′i-lo)	starch	AMYLOID (am′i-loid), resembling starch
LIP/O (lip′o)	fat	LIPEMIA (li-pee′me-a), (excess of) fat in the blood
STEAT/O (stee′a-toe)	fat	STEATOLYSIS (stee-a-tol′i-sis), breakdown (emulsification) of fats
FEC/A (fee′ka)	feces, stool	FECAL (fee′kal), pertaining to feces
-LITHIASIS (li-thy′a-sis)	production of calculi (stones)	CHOLELITHIASIS (ko′lee-li-thy′ a-sis), gallstones
OREX/I (o-reks′e)	appetite	ANOREXIA (an-o-reks′e-a), lack of appetite
-HELCOSIS (hel-ko′sis)	formation of ulcers	GASTROHELCOSIS (gas-tro-hel-ko′sis), formation of a stomach ulcer

	Meaning	*Example*
HERNI/O (her'ne-o)	hernia	HERNIORRHAPHY (her-ne-or'a-fe), repair (by suturing) of a hernia
ICTER/O (ik'ter-o)	jaundice	ICTEROHEPATITIS (ik-ter-o-hep-a-ty'tis), inflammation of the liver accompanied by jaundice
POLYP/O (pol'i-po)	polyp	POLYPOSIS (pol-i-po'sis), condition in which polyps are present

DENTAL TERMS

GNATH/O (na'tho)	jaw	GNATHITIS (nath-eye'tis), inflammation of the jaw
MENT/O (men'to)	chin	LABIOMENTAL (lay-be-o-men'tal), pertaining to the lips and chin
GINGIV/O (jin'je-vo)	gums	GINGIVITIS (jin-je-vie'tis) inflammation of the gums
DENTIN/O (den'tin-o)	dentin	DENTINOMA (den-tin-o'ma), tumor developing from dentin
CEMENT/O (see-men'to)	cementum	CEMENTOBLAST (see-men'to-blast), a cementum-forming cell
ALVEOL/O (al-vee'o-lo)	hollow, socket of a tooth	ALVEOLITIS (al-vee-o-ly'tis), inflammation of the socket of a tooth
OCCLUS/O (o-klou'zo)	a closing, alignment of the teeth when the jaws are closed	MALOCCLUSION (mal-o-klou'shun), poor alignment of the teeth
PROSTH/O (pros'tho)	artificial, the replacement of real body parts with artificial ones	PROSTHODONTIST (pros-tho-don'tist), a dentist who specializes in making and fitting false teeth
ORTH/O (or-tho)	straight	ORTHODONTICS (or-tho-don'tiks), area of dentistry that deals with correcting teeth that are irregularly set
PY/O (py'o)	pus	PYORRHEA (py-o-ree'a), discharge of pus

ANATOMY OF THE DIGESTIVE SYSTEM

Two main functions are performed by the digestive system: food is broken down both physically and chemically in the process called *digestion* and through the process of *absorption* the digested foods leave the digestive tract and are distributed to the cells throughout the body by way of the circulatory system. The utilization of these digested substances by the body cells is called *metabolism*.

The structures of the digestive system (Figure 13-1), also called the *alimentary* (al-e-men′tar-e, ALIMENT/O nourish) *tract*, are the mouth, pharynx, esophagus, stomach, small intestines, large intestines, rectum, and anus. Several other structures, called accessory structures, contribute to digestion; they are the salivary glands, the liver, and the pancreas.

The *mouth* or *buccal cavity* is formed by the cheeks, hard and soft palates, the tongue muscles, and the lips. This enclosed space is called the *oral cavity*. When food enters the mouth (*ingestion*), it undergoes the first form of reductions: *mastication* (mas-ti-kay′shun) or chewing. In this process, the cheek muscles cause the teeth to move against one another so that the food is torn apart, cut, and ground. Besides containing taste receptors, the tongue aligns the food so that it can be chewed and swallowed.

As the food is being reduced mechanically by the action of the teeth, the *salivary glands* produce *saliva*, a mucous substance, which moistens and lubricates the food to prepare it for swallowing; and through the action of *ptyalin*, a salivary *amylase*, the saliva begins the process of chemically breaking down the food into simpler compounds. There are three salivary glands. The largest is called the *parotid* because it is located in front of the ear. The *sublingual* is located under the tongue, and the *submandibular* is located beneath the base of the tongue under the jawbone. When the food is sufficiently reduced and properly lubricated, it takes on a ball-like shape called a *bolus* (bo′lus, BOL/O mass, lump).

Deglutition (dee-glou-tish′un), more commonly called swallowing, is performed by the action of the tongue against the hard palate. The food mass descends into the *oropharyngeal canal*, where it is prevented from entering the larynx by the pharyngeal muscles, which cause the epiglottis to cover the larynx. As it proceeds to the stomach, the food mass is carried along the *esophagus* by a series of muscle contractions called *peristalses* (per-e-stal′sez), which are waves of alternating muscle contraction and relaxation. When the food arrives at the entrance to the stomach, it passes through a sphincterlike valve called the *cardiac sphincter valve*.

The *stomach* (Figure 13-2), which both stores food and continues the chemical and physical reduction begun in the mouth, looks like a J-shaped bag. The portion of the stomach that protrudes above the gastroensophageal junction is called the *fundus* (fun′dus, FUND/O base). The cardiac region is the point where the esophagus and stomach join. The distal end of the stomach is called the *pylorus*. The *pyloric sphincter valve* (a sphincter is a ring of muscle) allows the partially digested food to enter the small intestine. The *lesser curvature* and the *greater curvature* constitute the right and left borders of the stomach. Like the other digestive structures, the stomach is lined

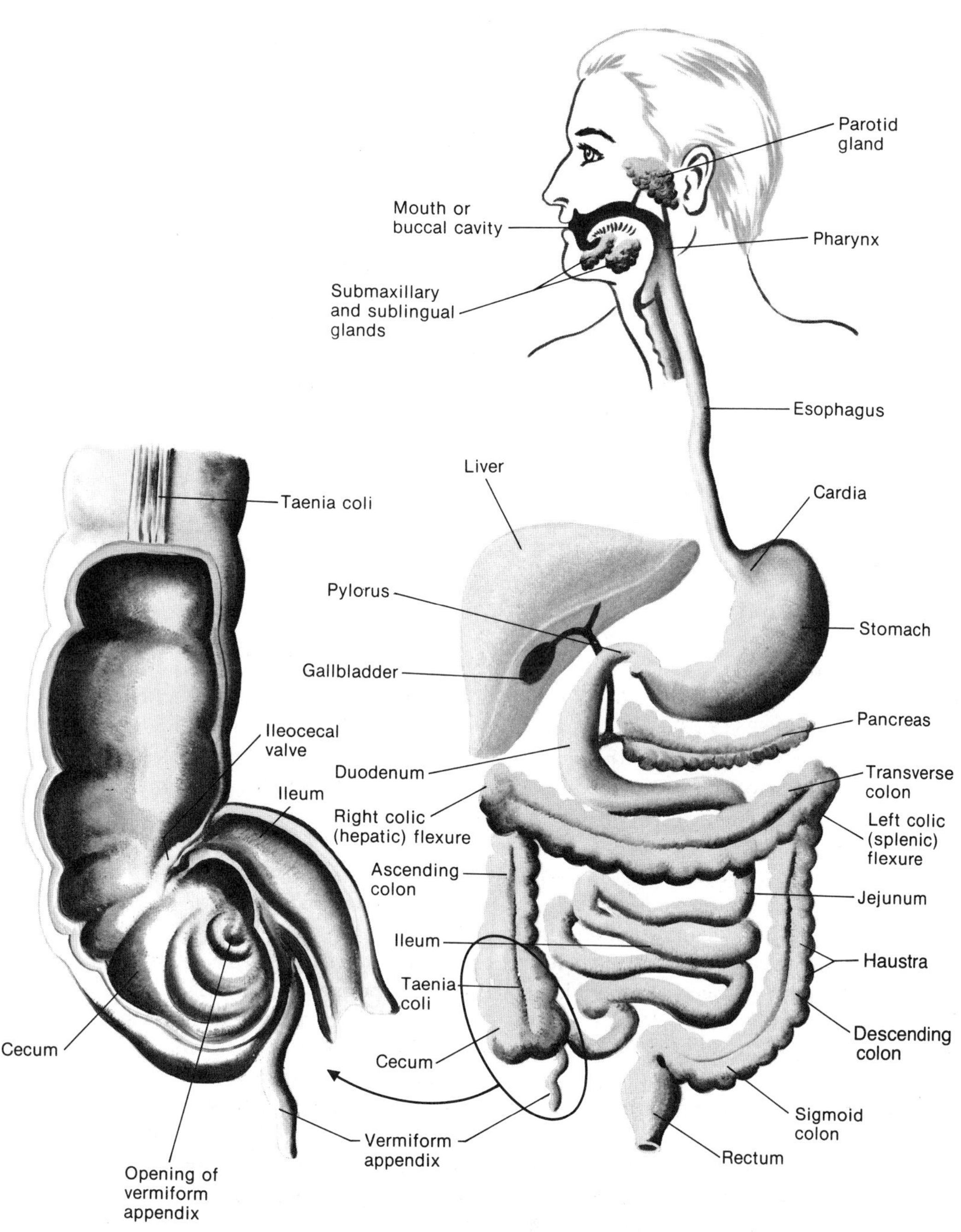

Figure 13-1 The digestive system.

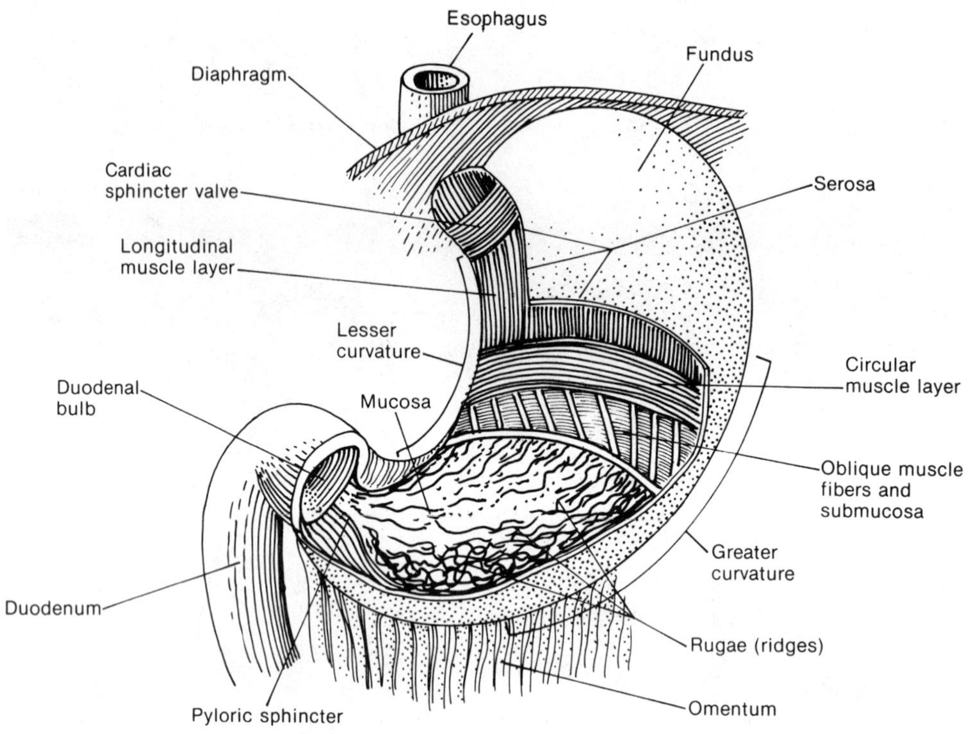

Figure 13-2 Structure of the stomach.

with mucus-producing glands. The mucous lining itself appears as a series of folds or wrinkles called *rugae* (ru′guy, RUG/O wrinkle). Mucin, pepsinogen, and hydrochloric acid are all produced by the mucous lining. *Intrinsic factor*, which is necessary for the absorption of vitamin B_{12}, is also produced by the mucous lining. The roughly digested food, called *chyme* (ky′m), leaves the lower part of the stomach and enters the *duodenum*, the first portion of the *enteron* or small intestine.

The inner surface of the small intestines (except for the last half of the ileum) is formed into numerous circular folds (*plicae circulares*, pli′ki sir-ku-lar′ez) that protrude into the intestinal *lumen* (lou′men), the space or hollow of the intestines. On the surfaces of these circular folds are countless fingerlike protrusions called *villi*. The absorption of digested food takes place through the capillaries and lacteals (lak′te-als, lymph vessels of the intestines) of the villi. Although the duodenum is a mere 12 inches in comparison with the 8 feet of the *jejunum* and 12 feet of the *ileum* (the other two portions of the small intestine), an amazing number of processes occur here. Waves of peristaltic movements rigorously churn the chyme, further reducing it in preparation for the next process. It is in the descending portion of the duodenum that the secretions from the liver, gallbladder, and pancreas are mixed with the chyme.

The *liver*, the largest organ in the body, performs two important digestive functions: the secretion of *bile* and the absorption of *glucose* from the blood carrying the newly absorbed nutrients. In addition, the liver performs several other important functions.

242

1. The synthesis of fibrinogen and prothrombin and many other substances (e.g., heparin).
2. The storage of glucose in the form of glycogen (*glycogenesis*) and the production of glucose from substances other than carbohydrates (*gluconeogenesis*).
3. Regulation of blood sugar.
4. Initial metabolism of proteins, carbohydrates, and lipids.
5. Filtration of the blood through the *hepatic sinusoids* to remove harmful organisms.

The hepatic function most directly related to digestion is the secretion of *bile*, a greenish fluid that emulsifies the *lipids* or fat globules by further reducing them. When bile is released from the liver, it travels through the *hepatic duct* (Figure 13-3) where it is concentrated by the action of the *gallbladder*, the repository for extra bile. Next, it passes through the *common bile duct*. Meanwhile, secretions (proteases, amylases, lipases) from the *pancreas* further break down food substances. The secretions of the liver, gallbladder, and pancreas enter the duodenum. When the chyme enters the *jejunum*, the second part of the small intestine, absorption of the digested food occurs.

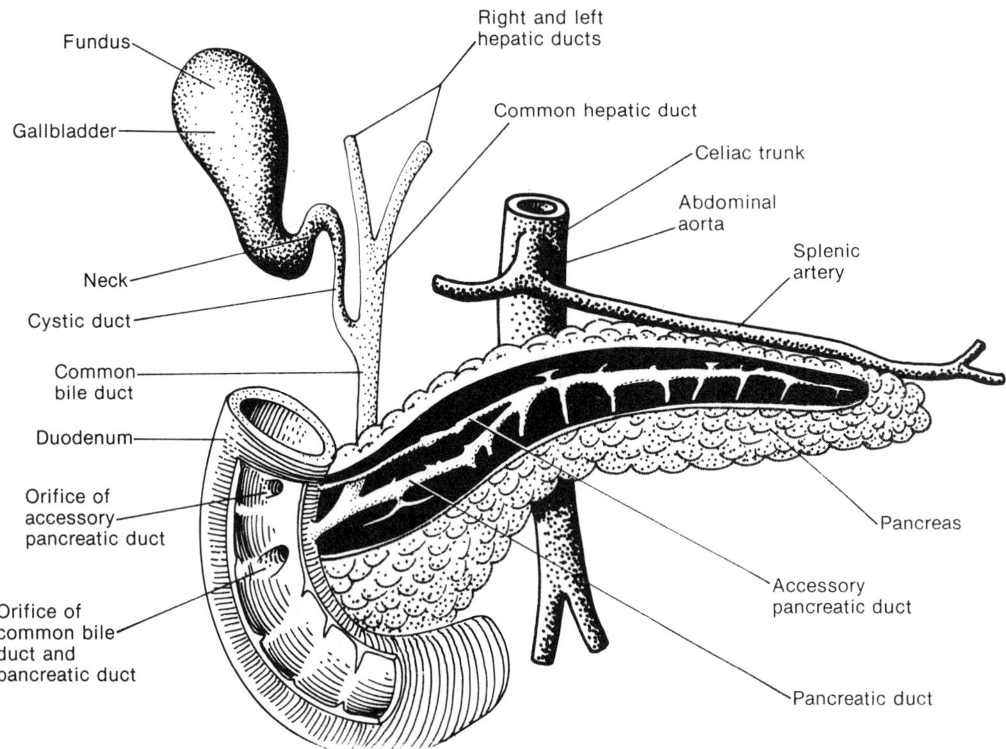

Figure 13-3   The gallbladder and pancreas and their systems of ducts. Both empty into the duodenum, often by a common orifice.

The *colon* or large intestine is about 6 feet long and 2½ inches in diameter. Except for the rectum, the entire colon is lined with little sacs called *haustra* (haw'stra). The first portion of the colon, the *cecum*, is a pouch that is situated below the place where the large and small intestines join (*ileocecal junction*). At the tip of the cecum, the *appendix*, called a *vermiform* (VERM/O worm) structure because it resembles a worm, is located. As the byproducts of digestion make their way through the *ascending*, *transverse*, and *descending* portions of the colon, water and essential body salts are reabsorbed. Vitamin K and the vitamin B-complex are manufactured in the colon by the bacterial *flora* (flor'a, microorganisms adapted to a certain environment). *Feces*, the waste material of digestion, are formed in the colon. Until evacuated from the body, feces are stored in the *sigmoid colon*. From here the wastes pass through the *rectum* and out through the *anus*.

THE PERITONEUM

The abdominopelvic cavity and the visceral organs are lined by double layers of a serous membrane called the *peritoneum*. The peritoneum covering the visceral organs is called the *visceral* peritoneum, and the peritoneum lining the abdominopelvic cavity is called the *parietal peritoneum*. When the folds of peritoneum adhere to one another, they form *mesenteries*, *omenta*, and *ligaments* (not true ligaments). A mesentery joins a viseral organ to the abdominal wall. An omentum attaches visceral organs to one another. A ligament is a thick portion of peritoneum that supports an organ or connects it to another organ.

THE TEETH

Teeth are the structures used for chewing. An adult has 32 teeth, 8 in each half jaw: 2 incisors (in-sy'sors, CIS/O cut), 1 canine (tearing teeth CAN/O dog), 2 premolars or bicuspids (MOL/O grind, CUSPID/O point), and 3 molars. In the adult the teeth are permanent; a child, however, has only 20 teeth that are called *deciduous* (de-sid'ou-us, DECIDU/O falling) teeth. The deciduous teeth begin to appear at the age of six months and have fallen out by the age of 13.

A tooth (Figure 13-4) can be divided into *crown, neck,* and *root.* The portion of the tooth above the gum is covered with a hard substance called *enamel* that develops from *ameloblasts* (a-mel'o-blasts, AMEL/O enamel), specialized epithelial cells. The root of the tooth is held firmly in the gum by a bonelike substance called *cementum.* The *pulp* (PULP/O) or connective tissue inside the tooth contains nerves, blood vessels, and lymphatics. *Odontoblasts*, cells lining the pulp cavity, produce *dentin*, the bulk of the body of the tooth.

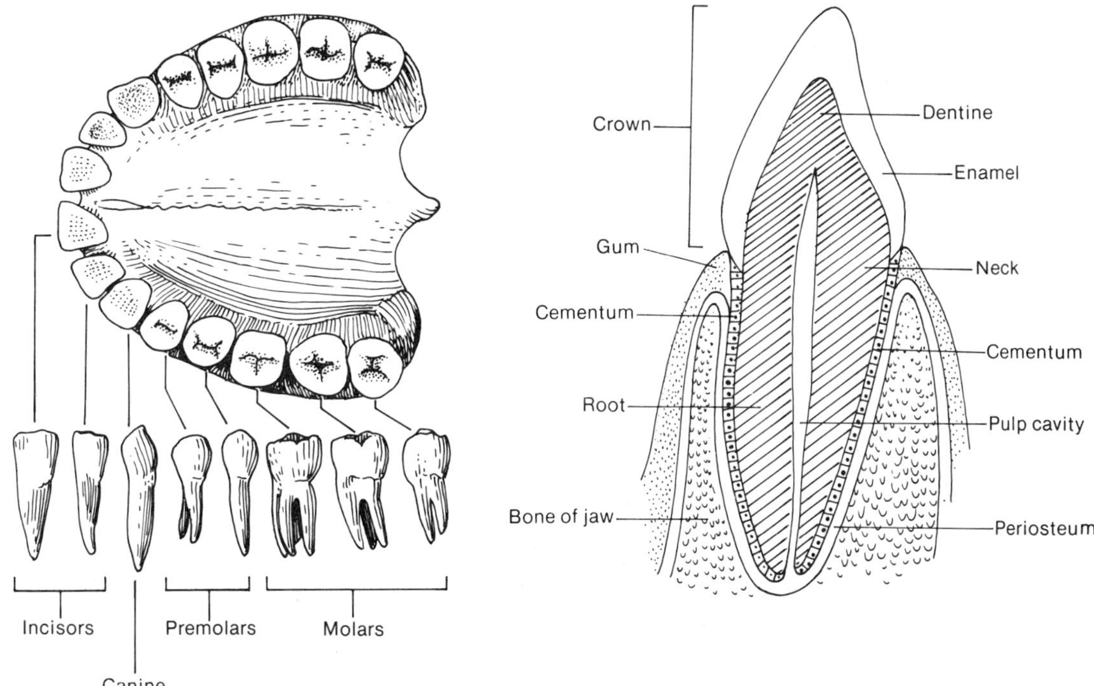

Figure 13-4 The teeth: left, permanent teeth of upper jaw; right, longitudinal section of a tooth.

CLINICAL AND PATHOLOGICAL CONDITIONS

Oral Cavity

Dental caries (ka'rez)

Patches of microorganisms and debris called plaque accumulate on the surface of teeth. The tooth enamel is destroyed by the lactic acid released by the bacteria, which then enter the tooth, causing caries (decay).

Cold Sore

A virus, *herpes simplex*, inflames a portion of the mucous membrane lining the mouth, which forms a blister called a cold sore.

Aphtha (af'tha)

Tiny ulcers develop on the mucous membrane of the mouth as a result of a general inflammation of the mouth (stomatitis).

Leukoplakia (lu-ko-play'ke-a)

White patches form on the mucus membranes of the mouth, which become dry and inflamed. The patches may become malignant if the irritation continues.

Mumps

The mumps virus infects the salivary glands (sialadenitis), especially the parotid, causing the area to become swollen and painful. After about a week the swelling subsides; in some cases, however, complications may develop. A common complication is the inflammation of the testicles in the male and the inflammation of the breasts and fallopian tubes in the female.

Gastrointestinal Tract

Hernia

A hernia is the protrusion of an organ or part of it through the wall of the cavity in which it is normally contained. For example, a *hiatal* (hy-ay'tal) *hernia* occurs when the stomach protrudes upward through the diaphragm. A hernia becomes *incarcerated* when it is trapped so that the blood supply of the organ is obstructed and tissue begins to die (*necrosis*). Two other types of obstruction are related to hernias. A *volvulus* (vol'vou-lus) is a condition in which the bowel becomes entangled as the result of twisting itself. Volvulus is frequently caused by a prolapsed mesentery. When one portion of an intestine *invaginates* (falls into) another portion of intestine, the obstruction is termed an *intussusception* (in-tu-su-sep'shun). Vovulus occurs chiefly in older persons, intussusception in children.

Diverticulosis (di-ver-tik-you-loo'sis)

Diverticula are pouches that form on the wall of an intestine or organ as a result of the degeneration of the structure's wall. Feces can become lodged in the diverticula of the colon, causing diverticulitis.

Peptic ulcer

An *ulcer* is a localized destruction of a mucous membrane, resulting in a open sore. Peptic ulcers are caused by the destruction of mucosa by peptic acid. Most peptic ulcers occur in the distal portion of the stomach or in the first part of the duodenum. Severe hemorrhaging, especially of a duodenal ulcer, is the most common complication of an ulcer. An ulcerated duodenum can be bypassed by performing a *gastrojejunostomy* in which the stomach and jejunum are anastomized. To correct the oversecretion of hydrochloric acid in the stomach, the vagus nerves can be cut (*vagotomy*) or a portion of the stomach can be removed (*gastrectomy*). Frequently vagotomy and *pyloroplasty* (widening of the pylorus) are performed to reduce the conditions that cause ulcers.

Gastrointestinal cancer

Gastrointestinal cancer is a leader in cancer-caused deaths. If detected early, the tumor can be removed (e.g., gastrectomy); gastric cancer, however, frequently metastasizes to the liver. The colon and rectum are also common sites of cancerous growth. *Melena* (mel'e-na) or bloody stools are a frequent indication of gastrointestinal cancer. *Polyps* (pol'ips), tumors on long stalks, are common in the rectum and often become malignant.

Liver, Gallbladder, Pancreas

Hepatitis

Hepatitis is an acute inflammation of the liver, usually resulting from a viral infection. *Infectious hepatitis* (A virus) is caused by the ingestion of contaminated food or water. In *serum hepatitis* (B virus) the virus is transmitted by needles, blood transfusions, and so on. *Alcoholic hepatitis* is the result of prolonged and excessive drinking of alcoholic beverages and frequently leads to cirrhosis of the liver.

Cirrhosis (si-ro'sis, CIRRH/O orange)

Cirrhosis is a chronic liver disease in which the liver cells attempt to regenerate. The liver becomes scarred with fibrous and nodular growths. As a result, the circulation of blood through the liver is hindered. *Jaundice* (jawn'dis), a yellowing of the skin, develops due to a buildup of the bile pigment, bilirubin, in the blood (*bilirubinemia*).

Neoplasms (abnormal new tissue) of the liver

Adenomas (benign tumors) of the hepatic blood vessels is the chief benign liver neoplasm. Adenomas may also develop from hepatocytes. Malignant growths metastasizing to the liver from other areas of the body are the most common type of cancer in the liver. Cancer originating in the liver, *hepatocarcinoma*, is frequently associated with cirrhosis that extends over a long period.

Gallstones

Stones (also called *calculi* or *concretions*) can form in the gallbladder or bile ducts. They are formations of cholesterol, bilirubin, and minerals and protein. Jaundice is frequently an indication that the bile duct is blocked.

Peritoneum

Ascites (a-see'teez)

An excessive amount of fluid accumulates in the peritoneal cavity. Ascites is frequently a complication of cirrhosis in which the portal veins and lymphatics become obstructed in the cirrhotic liver.

EXERCISES

I. Give the meaning for each of the following medical words. Divide each word into base(s), prefix, and suffix; underline the letter(s) that has the primary stress. *Example:*

GASTRITIS   inflammation of the stomach   gastr/itis

1. PYLOROSTENOSIS

2. DUODENAL

3. SIALOGOGUE (-gogue, a substance that stimulates the production of secretion)

4. CHEILOSCHISIS

5. ODONTOCLASIS (-clasis, a break, fracture)

6. ILEOCOLOSTOMY

7. APPENDICOLITHIASIS

8. ORONASAL

9. STOMATOSIS

10. GLOSSOTOMY

11. ADENOMA

12. ESOPHAGECTASIA

13. GASTROENTEROPTOSIS

14. LAPARORRHAPHY

15. RETOCLYSIS

16. STOMATITIS

17. DENTOALVEOLITIS

18. PHARYNGEMPHRAXIS ....

19. GASTRODUODENOSTOMY ....

20. CELIOMYOSITIS ....

21. ENTERECTOMY ....

22. RETORRHAPHY ....

23. PYLOROMYOTOMY ....

24. ODONTOBLAST ....

25. OROLINGUAL ....

26. RETROPERITONEAL ....

27. OREXIGENIC ....

28. GNATHODYNAMOMETER ....

29. PANCREATHELCOSIS ....

30. CHOLECYSTOKININ ....

31. SUCCORRHEA ....

32. LIPASE ....

33. CHOLANGIOCARCINOMA ....

34. ICTEROGENIC ....

35. ORTHODONTIST ....

36. GLYCOGENOLYSIS ....

37. MESENTERIC ....

38. CHOLEPOIESIS ....

39. PROCTITIS ....

40.   HEPATOMEGALY ....

41.   PEPSIN ....

42.   HYPOGLYCEMIA ....

43.   DEFECATION ....

44.   PROSTHESIS ....

45.   STEATOMA ....

II.   Make medical words from the following phrases. Indicate the primary stress by underlining the stressed letter(s). *Example:*

process of x–raying the gallbladder

   cholecystography
....

1.   constriction (narrowing) of a salivary gland

....

2.   anastomosis of the esophagus and stomach

....

3.   excision of the appendix

....

4.   inflammation of the tissue surrounding a gland

....

5.   inflammation of the ileum

....

6.   excision of a sphincter

....

7.   examination of the duodenum

....

8.   formation of an opening into the stomach through the abdominal wall

....

9. pertaining to the abdomen

. . . .

10. prolapse of the colon

. . . .

11. hemorrhage from the mouth

. . . .

12. pertaining to the tongue

. . . .

13. area of dentistry concerned with correcting poorly aligned teeth

. . . .

14. inflammation of the glands of the small intestine

. . . .

15. disorder of the small intestine

. . . .

16. incision of the jejunum

. . . .

17. pertaining to the ileum and cecum

. . . .

18. instrument for examining the sigmoid colon

. . . .

19. pertaining to the lips, tongue, and pharynx

. . . .

20. pertaining to the teeth and the cheeks

. . . .

21. inflammation of the lips

. . . .

22. pertaining to the pharynx

   ....

23. inflammation of the stomach glands

   ....

24. surgical formation of an opening into the colon (through the abdominal wall)

   ....

25. prolapse of the cecum

   ....

26. presence of bilirubin in the blood

   ....

27. surgical repair of an ulcer

   ....

28. inflammation of the pancreas

   ....

29. presence of sugar in the urine

   ....

30. enzyme that breaks down starch

   ....

31. incision of the omentum

   ....

32. surgery to correct a hernia

   ....

33. formation of dentin

   ....

34. inflammation of the peritoneum

   ....

35. formation of calculi in the liver

. . . .

36. pertaining to the anus and rectum

. . . .

37. substance that stimulates the secretion of bile

. . . .

38. an instrument for removing polyps

. . . .

39. one who specializes in the treatment of the diseases of the anus and rectum

. . . .

40. inflammation of the common bile duct

. . . .

III.   Match the following descriptions with their medical words.

1. synonym for oral cavity	a.	pylorus
2. chewing	b.	villi
3. a salivary gland	c.	appendix
4. a salivary secretion that breaks down starch	d.	mesentery
5. food after it has been reduced by chewing	e.	bolus
6. swallowing	f.	cardiac
7. carries the food to the stomach	g.	parotid
8. wave of muscle contraction that moves food	h.	insulin
9. the area of the stomach where the esophagus and stomach meet	i.	rugae
10. the opening in the distal end of the stomach	j.	omentum

11. a ring of muscle that closes an orifice by contracting   ....   k. buccal

12. the folds in the lining of the stomach   ....   l. esophagus

13. a mixture of partially digested food and gastric juices   ....   m. sphincter

14. the space inside an intestine or any tubelike structure   ....   n. mastication

15. fingerlike projections   ....   o. gallbladder

16. a function of the liver   ....   p. peritoneum

17. a substance that emulsifies fats   ....   q. deglutition

18. a respository for extra bile   ....   r. cecum

19. a secretion of the pancreas   ....   s. ptyalin

20. the blind portion of the colon   ....   t. lumen

21. a wormlike structure   ....   u. bile

22. waste products of digestion   ....   v. peristalsis

23. a serous membrane lining the abdominal cavity and visceral

     organs   ....   w. glycogenesis

                                                                                x. chyme

24. attaches visceral organs to one another   ....

                                                                                y. feces

25. attaches a visceral organ to the abdominal wall   ....

         IV.   List the order in which food passes through the digestive system.

     1. ....   a. jejunum

     2. ....   b. descending colon

     3. ....   c. rectum

     4. ....   d. esophagus

     5. ....   e. pyloric orifice

     6. ....   f. ileocecal junction

7. ....   g. oral cavity

8. ....   h. ascending colon

9. ....   i. anus

10. ....   j. stomach

11. ....   k. pharynx

12. ....   l. sigmoid colon

13. ....   m. ileum

14. ....   n. cardiac sphincter valve

15. ....   o. transverse colon

16. ....   p. duodenum

V. Fill in the blank spaces for each of the following statements.

1. An adult has .... teeth that are called permanent teeth; a child has only 20 teeth

   that are called .... teeth.

2. .... cut food, ... teeth tear food, and ....

   grind it.

3. .... which develops from cells called .... covers the portion

   of the tooth above the gum.

4. A tooth is held firmly in its socket by a bonelike substance called ....

5. Odontoblasts produce ...., which fills up most of the tooth.

6. The tooth's nerve and blood vessels are contained in the ....

VI. Multiple choice: Circle the correct letter.

1. A virus, herpes simplex, causes a blister to erupt on the mucous membrane lining of the
   mouth.
   (a) aphtha
   (b) cold sore
   (c) leukoplakia
   (d) mumps

2. Inflamed patches of mucous membrane that can become malignant
   (a) caries
   (b) aphtha
   (c) cold sores
   (d) leukoplakia

3. The invagination of one portion of intestine into another
   (a) volvulus
   (b) hernia
   (c) intussusception
   (d) diverticulosis

4. Pouches that form on the intestinal wall.
   (a) volvulus
   (b) diverticula
   (c) intussusception
   (d) incarcerated hernia

5. Bloody stools
   (a) melena
   (b) polyp
   (c) ulcer
   (d) diverticula

6. A form of liver disease caused by a blood transfusion with contaminated blood
   (a) infectious hepatitis
   (b) serum hepatitis
   (c) cirrhosis
   (d) jaundice

7. Scarred condition of the liver that results in impeded circulation of blood
   (a) cirrhosis
   (b) infectious hepatitis
   (c) jaundice
   (d) bilirubinema

8. The development of new but abnormal tissue
   (a) adenoma
   (b) carcinoma
   (c) neoplasm
   (d) sarcoma

9. The buildup of excessive fluid in the peritoneal cavity
   (a) aphtha
   (b) ascites
   (c) cirrhosis
   (d) diverticulosis

ANSWERS TO EXERCISES

I.

1. narrowing of the pyloric opening, pylor/o/sten/osis
2. pertaining to the duodenum, duoden/al
3. substance that stimulates salivation, sial/o/gogue
4. harelip, cheil/o/schisis
5. breaking of a tooth, odont/o/clasis
6. anastomosis between the ileum and colon, ile/o/col/ostomy
7. formation of stones in the appendix, appendic/o/lithiasis
8. pertaining to the nose and mouth, or/o/nas/al
9. any mouth disease, stomat/osis
10. incision of the tongue, gloss/o/tomy
11. a tumor developing from glandular tissue, aden/oma
12. stretching of the exophagus, esophag/ectasia
13. prolapse of the stomach and intestines, gastr/o/enter/o/ptosis
14. suture of the abdominal wall, lapar/o/rrhaphy
15. irrigation of the rectum, rect/o/clysis
16. inflammation of the mouth, stomat/itis
17. purulent inflammation of the tooth socket accompanied by a loosening of the tooth, dent/o/alveol/itis
18. obstruction of the pharynx, pharyng/emphraxis
19. anastomosis between the stomach and duodenum, gastr/o/duoden/ostomy
20. inflammation of the adbominal muscles, celi/o/myos/itis
21. excision of a portion of the small intestine, enter/ectomy
22. suture of the rectum (to the anus), rect/o/rrhaphy
23. incision of the pyloric muscle (sphincter), pylor/o/my/o/tomy
24. a cell that forms dentin, odont/o/blast
25. pertaining to the mouth and tongue, or/o/lingu/al
26. behind the peritoneum, retro/peritone/al
27. stimulating the appetite, orex/i/gen/ic
28. instrument for measuring the force exerted by the closing of the jaw, gnath/o/dynam/o/meter
29. ulceration of the pancreas, pancreat/helcosis
30. a substance that stimulates gallbladder contractions, cholecyst/o/kin/in
31. abnormal flow of glandular secretion, succ/o/rrhea
32. an enzyme that breaks down fat, lip/ase
33. cancer in the bile ducts (of the liver), cholangio/o/carcin/oma
34. producing jaundice, icter/o/gen/ic
35. a dentist who specializes in correcting irregularly aligned or placed teeth, orth/odont/ist
36. conversion of glycogen to glucose, glyc/o/gen/o/lysis
37. pertaining to the mesentery, mesenter/ic
38. formation of bile, chole/poiesis
39. inflammation of the rectum and anus, proct/itis
40. enlargement of the liver, hepat/o/megaly

41. digestive secretion that breaks down protein, peps/in
42. decrease in the level of blood sugar, hypo/glyc/emia
43. process of eliminating feces, de/fec/a/tion
44. process of replacing a body part with an artificial part, prosthe/sis
45. tumor composed of fatty tissue, steat/oma

II.

1. sialostenosis;   **2.** esophagogastrostomy;   **3.** appendectomy;   **4.** periadenitis;
5. ileitis;   **6.** sphincterectomy;   **7.** duodenoscopy;
8. celigastrostomy or laparograstrostomy;   **9.** abdominal or celiac;   **10.** coloptosia;
11. stomatorrhagia;   **12.** glossopharyngeal;   **13.** orthodontics;
14. enteradenitis;   **15.** dysentery;   **16.** jejunotomy;   **17.** ileocecal;
18. sigmoidoscope;   **19.** labioglossopharyngeal;   **20.** dentibuccal;
21. cheilitis;   **22.** pharyngeal;   **23.** gastradenitis;   **24.** colostomy;
25. cecoptosis;   **26.** bilirubinemia;   **27.** helcoplasty;   **28.** pancreatitis;
29. glycosuria;   **30.** amylase;   **31.** omentotomy;   **32.** herniotomy;
33. dentinogenesis;   **34.** peritonitis;   **35.** hepatolithiasis;   **36.** anorectal;
37. cholagogue;   **38.** polypotome;   **39.** proctologist;   **40.** choledochitis.

III.

1. k;   **2.** n;   **3.** g;   **4.** s;   **5.** e;   **6.** q;   **7.** l;   **8.** v;
9. f;   **10.** a;   **11.** m;   **12.** i;   **13.** x;   **14.** t;   **15.** b;   **16.** w;
17. u;   **18.** o;   **19.** h;   **20.** r;   **21.** c;   **22.** y;   **23.** p;   **24.** j;
25. d.

IV.

1. g;   **2.** k;   **3.** d;   **4.** n;   **5.** j;   **6.** e;   **7.** p;   **8.** a;   **9.** m;
10. f;   **11.** h;   **12.** o;   **13.** b;   **14.** l;   **15.** c;   **16.** i.

V.

1. 32, deciduous;   **2.** incisors, canine, molars;   **3.** enamel, ameloblasts;
4. cementum;   **5.** dentin;   **6.** pulp.

VI.

1. (b);   **2.** (d);   **3.** (c);   **4.** (b);   **5.** (a);   **6.** (b);   **7.** (a);
8. (c);   **9.** (b).

14 The Urinary System

COMBINING FORMS

	Meaning	Example
REN/O (ree'no)	kidney	RENAL (ree'nal), pertaining to the kidney
NEPHR/O (nef'ro)	kidney	NEPHROMEGALY (nef-ro-meg'a-le), enlargement of the kidney
PYEL/O (py'e-lo)	renal pelvis	PYELOLITHOTOMY (py-e-lo-lith-ot'o-me), incision to remove a calculus from the renal pelvis
GLOMERUL/O (glo-mer'ou-lo)	a cluster, glomerulus	GLOMERULITIS (glo-mer-ou-ly'tis), inflammation of the renal glomeruli
TUBUL/O (tou'bu-lo)	small tube, tubule	TUBULAR (tou'bu-lar), pertaining to or having tubules
PAPILL/O (pa-pil'o)	a small nipplelike projection	PAPILLOMA (pa-pi-lo'ma), a tumor with nipplelike projections
URETER/O (you-ree'ter-o)	ureter	URETEROLITH (you-ree'ter-o-lith), calculus in the ureter
VESIC/O (ves'i-ko)	bladder	VESICOTOMY (ves-i-kot'o-me), incision of the bladder
CYST/O (sis'to)	sac, bladder	CYSTITIS (sis-ty'tis), inflammation of the bladder

	Meaning	*Example*
URETHR/O (you-ree'thro)	urethra	URETHROPEXY (you-reeth'ro-pek-se), surgical fastening of the urethra
UR/O (your'o)	urine, urinary tract	DIURETIC (dy-you-ret'ik), substance that increases the output of urine
HYDR/O (hy'dro)	water	HYDRONEPHROSIS (hy-dro-nef-ro'sis), accumulation of water in the kidney resulting from an obstruction
LITH/O (lith'o)	stone, calculus	LITHONEPHROTOMY (lith-o-ne-frot'o-me), incision of the kidney to remove a calculus
STAPHYL/O (staf'il-o)	bunch	STAPHYLOCOCCUS (staf-il-o-kok'us), bacteria arranged in bunches
COCC/O (kok'o)	spherical bacteria	MICROCOCCUS (my-kro-kok'us), a genus of spherical bacteria
RETRO- (ret'ro)	backward, behind	RETROPERITONEAL (re-tro-per-e-to-nee'al), situated behind the peritoneum
-EMPHRAXIS (em-frak'sis)	obstruction blockage	NEPHREMPHRAXIS (nef-rem-frak'sis), renal obstruction
-CLASIS (kla'sis)	breaking	HEMOCLASIS (he-mok'la-sis), destruction of red blood cells
-CLAST (klast')	instrument to break	OSTEOCLAST (os'tee-o-klast), instrument for breaking a bone.
-TRIPSY (trip'se)	rubbing crushing	LITHOTRIPSY (lith'o-trip-se), crushing of a calculus

ANATOMY OF THE URINARY SYSTEM

The body eliminates a major portion of its metabolic wastes through the urinary system. Although the lungs, skin, and digestive system also eliminate body wastes, it is through the *kidney* that *nitrogenous byproducts* resulting from protein metabolism are eliminated from the blood. Such substances as water and salts that are in excess of the amount necessary for proper body function are also excreted through the urinary system.

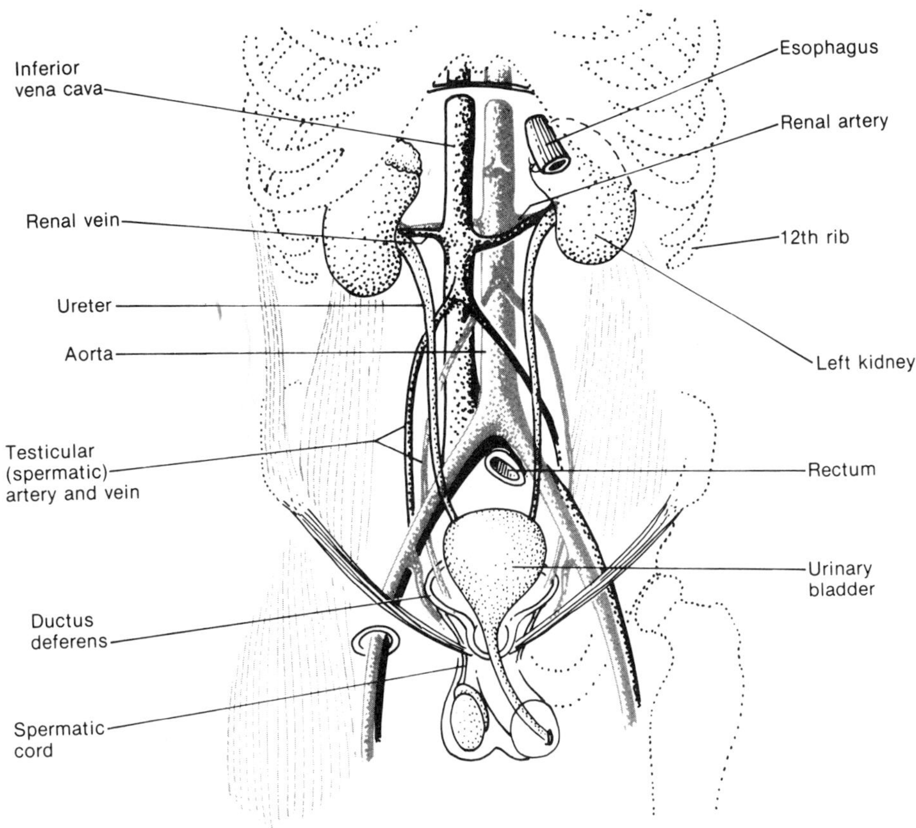

Figure 14-1   Organs of the urinary system and related structures.

The structures of the urinary system are the kidneys, ureters, urinary bladder, and the urethra (Figure 14-1).

The *kidneys* are red, bean-shaped structures weighing about one-half pound each and are located in the upper posterior portion of the abdomen. Because they are not covered by the peritoneum, they are called *retroperitoneal.* The renal artery and vein, the lymph vessels, and the ureter all enter the kidney at the *hilus,* the indented portion of the kidney. Internally the kidney (Figure 14-2) has two major portions: an outer, granulated area called the *cortex* and an inner, striated area called the *medulla.* The functional unit of the kidney is the *nephron.* Millions of nephrons make up the cortex, and they collect wastes by filtering the blood. The nephrons send *tubules* to the medullary area. In the medulla, *calyces* (ka'le-sez, CALYC/O cup), which are extensions of the renal pelvis, collect urine from the *papillary ducts* of the nephrons. The calyces then empty their contents into the *renal pelvis,* the portion of the ureter within the kidney.

The *ureters* (Figure 14-3), one for each kidney, are tubes a little over a quarter of an inch in diameter. They convey the urine from the kidneys through the abdomen to the bladder located in the pelvic region. The ureters enter the bladder posteriorly at the

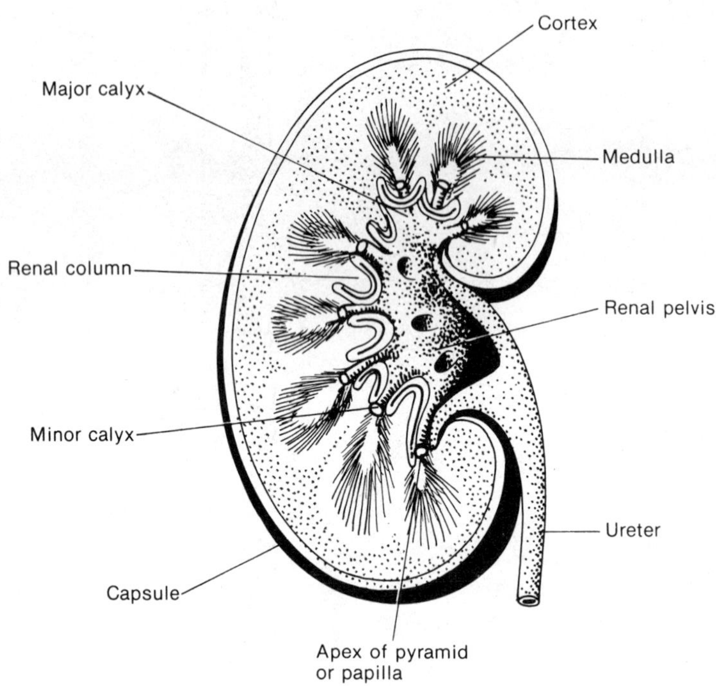

Figure 14-2   Frontal section of the kidney showing major anatomical details.

urinary trigone, a triangle formed by the entrance of the ureters and the exit of the urethra.

The urinary *bladder* (Figure 14-3) is located behind the pubic symphysis and acts as a reservoir for the urine. The bladder has three heavy muscle layers that enable it to contract and expand in expelling urine. *Micturition* (mik-tou-ri′shun) or urination is accomplished through the contraction of this structure.

THE MECHANISM OF MICTURITION

With the increase of urine in the renal pelvis there is a corresponding increase in pressure, which produces a series of peristaltic muscle contractions. When these contractions reach the ureters, they cause the urine to move to the bladder. In the bladder the urine accumulates, causing the bladder to relax to the point at which the micturition reflex is stimulated. The muscles of the bladder then contract while the internal sphincter relaxes. Finally, the external sphincter is voluntarily relaxed to allow the urine to be eliminated from the body.

The *urethra* begins at the lower portion of the bladder and conveys urine to the outside of the body. In the female the urethra is less than 2 inches long and opens above the vaginal orifice. In the male, however, the urethra is nearly 8 inches long and serves

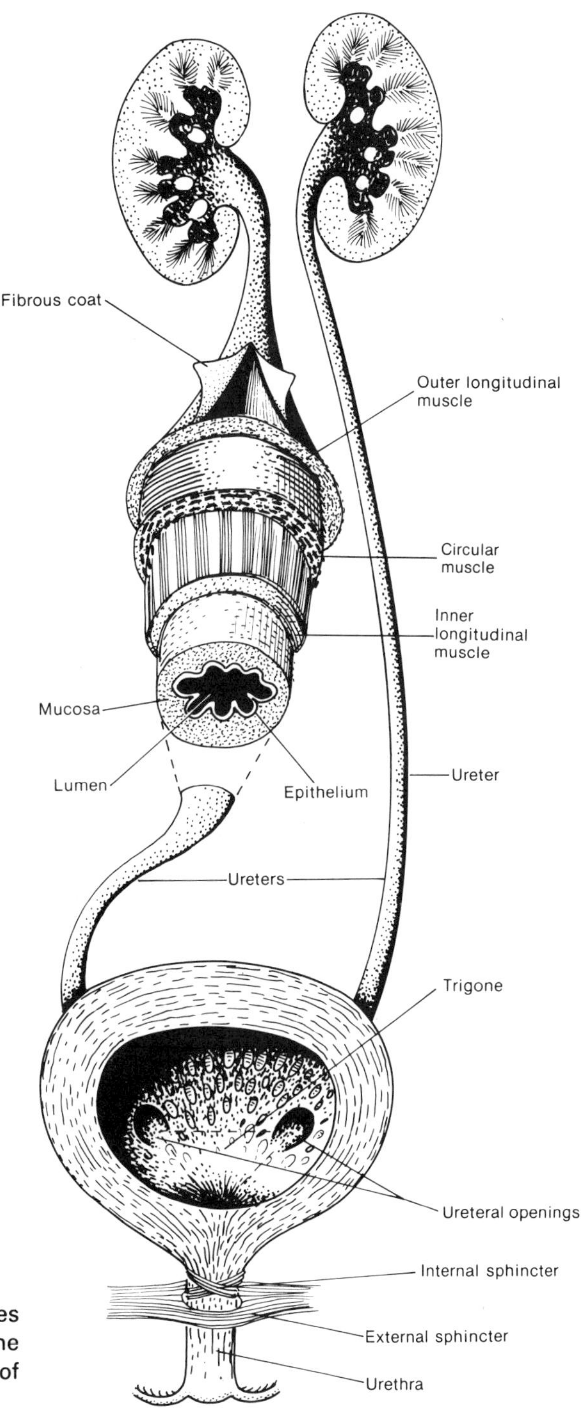

Figure 14-3 Sphincter valves of the urethra, trigone of the bladder, and layers of the wall of the ureter.

both the urinary and reproductive systems. In the male the urethra can be divided into three portions: the *prostatic urethra*, which passes through the prostate gland, the *membranous urethra*, which passes through the floor of the pelvis, and the *cavernous urethra*, which passes through the penis.

THE FORMATION OF URINE

The entire blood volume passes through the kidney about every five minutes. The *renal corpuscle*, which is the filtration unit of a nephron, consists of a clump of capillaries, called the *glomerulus*, enclosed in a hollow chamber known as *Bowman's capsule* (Figure 14-4). The osmotic pressure of the blood causes certain substances to diffuse through the capillary walls into the capsule. Next, these substances, now called *glomerular filtrate*, move from the capsule wall into the tubular system of the nephron. *Urea* and *uric acid* are formed as the glomerular filtrate passes through the tubules. In addition, much of the water and essential substances are reabsorbed as they move through the tubules.

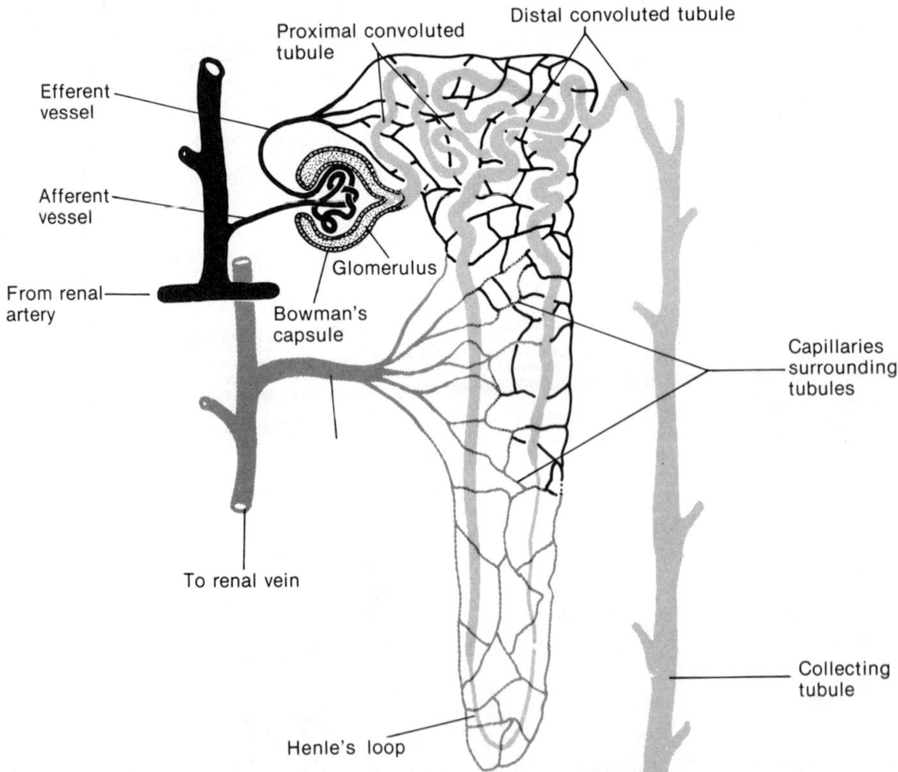

Figure 14-4 Diagrammatic drawing of a nephron, the functional unit of the kidney.

Table 14-1   The Normal Constituents of Urine

Constituent	*Weight (grams per 24 hr)*
Water	500–2500*
Urea	25.0
Sodium chloride	9.0
Potassium chloride	2.5
Sulfuric acid	2.0
Phosphoric acid	1.7
Creatinine	1.0
Ammonia	0.7
Uric acid	0.6
Calcium	0.2
Magnesium	0.2

*Since 1 cc of water weighs 1 g, the weight of water in urine is determined by simply measuring its volume.

Urine (see Table 14-1) is a yellowish fluid, slightly acidic, and close to the specific gravity of water. Water is the major component of urine, and such solids as urea, uric acid, ammonia, sodium, and potassium chloride make up the remaining 5%. Glycose and protein are completely reabsorbed (by the process called *pinocytosis*, pee-no-sy-toe'sis, PIN/O drink); so they do not normally appear in the urine. Hormones are normally excreted in the urine.

The substances in the table below occur abnormally in the urine.

Substance	*Condition*
Proteins, such as albumin and globulin	Proteinuria
Carbohydrates in the form of glucose	Glycosuria
Ketone bodies (acetone and beta-hydroxy-butyric acid) are present in the urine as a result of the catabolism of fatty acids	Ketonuria (frequently a sign of diabetes mellitus)
Blood	Hematuria
Pus	Pyuria
Urinary casts*	Proteinuria, Kidney disease

*A *cast* is a particle shaped like the structure where it has developed; casts vary in composition: fat, blood, pus, etc.

CLINICAL AND PATHOLOGICAL CONDITIONS

There are five symptoms of urinary disease:

1. Blood in the urine (hematuria)
2. Accumulation of fluid in body tissues (edema)

3. Pain located near the urinary organs
4. Enlargement of one or both kidneys (nephromegaly)
5. Anemia

Renal failure

Nitrogenous wastes that are not sufficiently removed from the blood will produce *azotemia* (az-o-tee′me-a, AZOT/O nitrogen), also called *uremia*. As a result of uremia, other body systems, especially the cardiovascular and muscular, become affected. Shock caused by low blood pressure (e.g., as a result of surgery), severe hemorrhaging, infection, or external injury are the causes of *acute renal failure*. Many of the nephrons die (called *tubular necrosis*) and urine output decreases or ceases. Within two weeks the tubular cells regenerate and urine excretion increases. In *chronic renal failure* there is no cellular regeneration; so the kidneys shrink and die. The only treatment for chronic renal failure is *hemodialysis* or renal transplantation. In hemodialysis the patient's blood is sent via a special tube through which toxic substances pass into the surrounding solution.

Acute glomerulonephritis

The glomeruli become inflamed, usually following an infection in another area of the body. Hypertension, hematuria, and edema occur. Glomerulonephritis is caused by the circulation of immune complexes (antigen–antibody) in the blood. These complexes become entrapped in the glomeruli. *Chronic glomerulonephritis* sometimes develops from acute glomerulonephritis but more commonly develops from other diseases (e.g., systemic lupus erythematosis). The glomeruli become thick, and the tubules wither. The kidneys become scarred and atrophy.

Cystitis

The urinary bladder becomes inflamed as a result of a bacterial infection (e.g., *staphylococcus*). Frequent urination, burning urine (dysuria), and sometimes hematuria are the symptoms of cystitis. Antibiotics are an effective treatment.

Pyelonephritis

In *acute pyelonephritis* the kidney and renal pelvis become inflamed as a result of a bacterial infection. The patient is weak, chilled, feverish, and experiences pain in the flank above the kidneys. Renal function may be hindered and numerous leukocyte casts are present in the urine. An infected kidney is swollen and its surface is covered with abscesses. In *chronic pyelonephritis* the tubules are destroyed and fibrous tissue develops. The kidney shrinks and uremia occurs.

Urinary tract stones

Calculi or stones are generally formed in the kidneys from a mixture of proteins, calcium, and other substances. They may pass from the kidney to any part of the urinary tract. Sometimes they can be easily passed in the urine; frequently, however, they must be removed surgically or with a cystoscope.

Urinary tract obstruction

The urinary tract can be obstructed at any point by calculi, prostatic enlargement in the male, blood vessels, and so on. An obstruction causes a portion of the tract to become distended by the accumulation of urine. *Hydroureter* is the distension of a ureter as a result of a blockage. *Hydronephrosis* is the swelling of a kidney with urine as a result of an obstruction.

Neoplasms of the urinary tract

Nephroblastoma or *Wilms' tumor* is a malignant renal tumor that occurs in children. It can metastasize to the liver, lungs, and lymph nodes.

Renal carcinomas are malignant tumors of the kidneys that occur in adults. These solid mass tumors can be surgically removed before they metastasize. Sometimes they develop in the renal pelvis or ureters where they form projections that obstruct the flow of urine.

Urinary bladder carcinomas develop from the epithelial lining of the urinary tract and are usually *papillomas*, tumors that send out branches into a space or cavity. Bladder cancer develops most frequently in male smokers and those who are exposed to certain chemicals (*carcinogenic agents*).

EXERCISES

I. Give the meaning for each medical word. Divide each word into base(s), prefix, and suffix; underline the letter(s) that has the primary stress. *Example:*

CYSTOSCOPY examination of the bladder with a cystoscope cyst/o/scopy

1. CYSTOGRAPHY

2. UROBILINOGEN

3. DIURESIS

4. STAPHYLOTOXIN

5. URETHREMPHRAXIS

6. URETEROURETEROSTOMY

7. UROGRAM

8. ENURESIS

9. NOCTURIA (NOCT/O night)

10. HYDROPYONEPHROSIS ....

11. COCCI ....

12. CYSTOLITHIASIS ....

13. URETHRALGIA ....

14. URETEROSPASM ....

15. NEPHROLITHIASIS ....

16. NEPHRITIS ....

17. GLOMERULAR ....

18. URETERONEOCYSTOSTOMY (NE/O new) ....

19. RENOGASTRIC ....

20. PYELONEPHRITIS ....

21. NEPHROPHYDROSIS ....

22. PAPILLOCARCINOMA ....

23. URETEROSTENOSIS ....

24. RENOPATHY ....

25. INTRATUBULAR ....

    II. Make medical words from the following phrases. Indicate the primary stress by underlining the stressed letter(s). *Example:*

the presence of blood in the urine

    hemat<u>u</u>ria
....

1. inflammation of the urethra

....

2. painful, burning urine

....

3. instrument used for crushing a stone

. . . .

4. the branch of medicine that deals with the urinary tract

. . . .

5. irrigation of a bladder

. . . .

6. presence of clusters of spherical bacteria in the blood

. . . .

7. incision of the bladder to remove a calculus

. . . .

8. decreased excretion of urine

. . . .

9. anastomosis of the bladder and kidney

. . . .

10. cessation of urine excretion

. . . .

11. surgical formation of an opening into the renal pelvis

. . . .

12. inflammation of the glomeruli of the kidney

. . . .

13. excision of a papilla(e)

. . . .

14. suppurative infection of a ureter

. . . .

15. hardening of a kidney

. . . .

III. Match the medical words with their descriptions.

1. the major body waste excreted by the urinary

    tract ....   a. medulla

2. location of the kidneys in the abdomen ....   b. micturition

3. site where nerves, blood and lymph vessels, and ureter enter

                                                                             c. proteinuria
    the kidney ....

                                                                             d. calyces
4. the outer, granulated area of the kidney ....

                                                                             e. nitrogenous
                                                                                 byproducts
5. the inner, striated area of the kidney ....

                                                                             f. glomerular filtrate
6. the functional unit of the kidney ....

7. they collect urine from the papillary ducts of the nephron   g. glycosuria

    tubules ....   h. hilus

8. tube connecting the kidney with the bladder ....   i. retroperitoneal

9. the reservoir for urine ....   j. ureter

10. urination ....   k. glomerulus

11. from here urine is expelled from the body ....   l. cortex

12. cluster of capillaries ....   m. bladder

13. passes through the tubular system of the

                                                                             n. urethra
    nephron ....

                                                                             o. nephron

14. appearance of albumin and globulin in the urine ....

15. sugar in the urine ....

IV. Multiple choice: Circle the correct letter.

1. Particles formed like the structure where they have developed
    (a) clasts
    (b) casts
    (c) hematuria
    (d) pyuria

2. Accumulation of fluid in tissues
   (a) adenoma
   (b) anemia
   (c) hematuria
   (d) edema

3. Accumulation of nitrogenous wastes in the blood
   (a) azotemia
   (b) hematuria
   (c) ketonuria
   (d) pinocytosis

4. The kidneys become injured and both tubular necrosis and anuria result; however, within a few weeks the tubular cells regenerate and urine excretion increases.
   (a) hemodialysis
   (b) acute renal failure
   (c) chronic renal failure
   (d) cystitis

5. Infection of the capillary clusters of the kidney
   (a) cystitis
   (b) chronic renal failure
   (c) acute glomerulonephritis
   (d) hydronephrosis

6. An inflammation in which the kidney becomes swollen and abscessed
   (a) cystitis
   (b) hydronephrosis
   (c) acute pyelonephritis
   (d) hydroureter

7. A malignant tumor that occurs chiefly in children
   (a) nephroblastoma
   (b) papillomas
   (c) renal carcinoma
   (d) bladder carcinoma

8. A tumor that branches out into a space or cavity
   (a) neoplasms
   (b) carcinomas
   (c) papillomas
   (d) sarcomas

ANSWERS TO EXERCISES

I.

1. x ray of the bladder using a dye, cyst/o/graphy
2. the substance that produces urobilin, the yellow coloring of urine, ur/o/bil/in/o/gen
3. increased excretion of urine, di/ur/esis

4. poisonous waste produced by staphlococci, staphyl/o/<u>tox</u>/in
5. obstruction of the urethra, urethr/em<u>phra</u>xis
6. anastomosis between the two ureters, ureter/o/ureter/<u>os</u>tomy
7. x ray of the urinary tract, <u>ur</u>/o/gram
8. involuntary urination, en/<u>ur</u>/esis
9. excessive urination during the night, noct/<u>ur</u>/ia
10. accumulation of urine and pus in the renal pelvis as a result of an obstruction, hydr/o/py/o/ne<u>phr</u>/osis
11. spherical bacteria, plural form, <u>cocc</u>/i
12. calculi in the bladder, cyst/o/li<u>thi</u>asis
13. pain in the urethra, urethr/<u>algia</u>
14. spasm of the ureter, u<u>re</u>ter/o/spasm
15. calculi in the kidney, nephr/o/li<u>thi</u>asis
16. inflammation of a kidney, ne<u>phr</u>/itis
17. pertaining to a glomerulus, glo<u>mer</u>ul/ar
18. surgical formation of a new connection between a ureter and the bladder, ureter/o/ne/o/cyst/<u>ostomy</u>
19. pertaining to the kidneys and stomach, ren/o/<u>gastr</u>/ic
20. inflammation of a kidney and renal pelvis, pyel/o/ne<u>phr</u>/itis
21. accumulation of urine in the kidneys as a result of an obstruction, nephr/o/<u>hydr</u>/osis
22. a malignant tumor containing papillae, papill/o/carcin/oma
23. narrowing of a ureter, ureter/o/<u>sten</u>/osis
24. any kidney disease, ren/o/pathy
25. within a tubule, intra/<u>tubul</u>/ar

II.

1. ure<u>thr</u>itis;   2. dysu<u>ria</u>;   3. <u>lith</u>oclast;   4. u<u>rol</u>ogy;   5. vesi<u>coc</u>lysis;
6. staphylo<u>he</u>mia;   7. lithocys<u>tot</u>omy;   8. oliguria;   9. nephrocystanasto<u>mos</u>is;
10. anu<u>ria</u>;   11. pye<u>los</u>tomy;   12. glomerulone<u>phr</u>itis;   13. papil<u>lec</u>tomy;
14. ureteropy<u>os</u>is;   15. nephroscler<u>os</u>is.

III.

1. e;   2. i;   3. h;   4. l;   5. a;   6. o;   7. d;   8. j;   9. m;
10. b;   11. n;   12. k;   13. f;   14. c;   15. g.

IV.

1. (b);   2. (d);   3. (a);   4. (b);   5. (c);   6. (c);   7. (a);   8. (c).

15 The Reproductive Systems

COMBINING FORMS

	Meaning	Example
MALE REPRODUCTIVE SYSTEM		
TEST/O (tes'to)	testis, testicle	TESTOSTERONE (tes-tos'ter-own), male sex hormone
ORCHI/O (or'ke-o)	testis, testicle	ORCHIOCELE (or'ke-o-seel), hernia of the testis
ORCHID/O (or'ke-do)	testis, testicle	ORCHIDOPEXY (or'kid-o-pek-se), attaching an undescended testis to the scrotum
ANDR/O (an'dro)	male, masculine	ANDROGEN (an'dro-jen), hormone that produces male characteristics
EPIDIDYM/O (ep-e-did'e-mo)	epididymis	EPIDIDYMOVASOSTOMY (ep-e-did-e-mo-vas-os'to-me), anastomosis between the epididymis and the vas deferens
SCROT/O (skro'to)	scrotum	SCROTAL (skro'tal), pertaining to the scrotum
VAS/O (vas'o)	vessel, vas deferens	VASECTOMY (vas-ek'to-me), cutting of the vas deferens to produce sterility
VESICUL/O (ve-sik'you-lo)	small vessel, seminal vesicles	VESICULOGRAM (ve-sik'you-lo-gram), an x ray of the seminal vesicles

	Meaning	*Example*
PROSTAT/O (pros'ta-to)	prostate gland	PROSTATECTOMY (pros-ta-tek'to-me), excision of all or part of the prostate gland
BULB/O (bul'bo)	bulb	BULBOURETHRAL (bul-bo-you-ree'thral), pertaining to the bulbourethral glands
PEN/O (pee'no)	penis	PENILE (pee'nyl), pertaining to the penis
PHALL/O (fal'o)	penis	PHALLIC (fal'ik), pertaining to the penis
BALAN/O (bal'a-no)	glans (head) penis	BALANITIS (bal-a-ny'tis), inflammation of the glans penis
GENIT/O (jen'i-to)	reproductive organs (male or female), genitals	GENITAL (jen'i-tal), pertaining to the reproductive organs
GON/O (gon'o)	reproductive organs (male or female), genitals	GONORRHEA (gon-o-ree'a), a venereal disease causing a purulent mucous discharge from the penis or vagina
GONAD/O (go-na'do)	male or female sex gland, gonad	GONADOTROPHIC (go-na-do-trof'ik), nourishing or stimulating the gonads
SPERM/O (sper'mo)	spermatozoa, semen (sperm: spermatozoa and spermatic fluid)	SPERMICIDE (sper'mi-syd), substance that destroys spermatozoa
SPERMAT/O (sper'ma-to)	spermatozoa, semen	SPERMATOCYTE (sper-mat'o-syt), a diploid cell that divides into spermatids, which, in turn, divide into spermatozoa
SEMIN/O (sem'i-no)	semen, a mixture of glandular secretions and spermatozoa	SEMINIFEROUS (sem-in-if'er-us), transporting semen
ZO/O (zo'o)	animal life	SPERMATOZOON (sper-mat-o-zo'on), a fully developed male sex cell
GAMET/O (ga-me'to)	a fully developed reproductive cell (spermatozoon and ovum), a gamete	GAMETOGENESIS (ga-me-to-jen'e-sis), production of gametes

	Meaning	*Example*
FEMALE REPRODUCTIVE SYSTEM		
OV/O (o'vo)	egg, ovum	OVULATION (ov-you-lay'shun), release of a mature ovum from the ovary
OO/O (o'o-o)	egg, ovum	OOPHORITIS (o-of'o-ry'tis, ou-fo-ry'tis), inflammation of an ovary
OVARI/O (o-var'e-o)	ovary	OVARITIS (o-va-ry'tis), inflammation of an ovary
OOPHOR/O (o-of'or-o)	ovary	OOPHORRHAPHY (o-of-or'a-fe), suture of an ovary to the pelvic wall
SALPING/O (sal-ping'o)	tube, fallopian (uterine) tube	SALPINGOPEXY (sal-ping'o-pek-se), fixation of a displaced fallopian tube
UTER/O (you'ter-o)	uterus, womb	UTERITIS (you-ter-eye'tis), inflammation of the uterus
HYSTER/O (his'ter-o)	uterus, womb	HYSTERECTOMY (his-ter-ek'toe-me), excision of the uterus
METR/O (mee'tro)	uterus, womb	METROCYTOSIS (mee-tro-sis-toe'sis), formation of cysts in the uterus
CERVIC/O (ser'vi-ko)	neck, the cervix	CERVICECTOMY (ser-vi-sek'to-me), excision of the cervix
VAGIN/O (va-jy'no)	vagina	INTRAVAGINAL (in-tra-va-jy'nal), within the vagina
COLP/O (kol'po)	vagina	MYOCOLPITIS (my-o-kol-py'tis), inflammation of the muscle tissue of the vagina
VULV/O (vul'vo)	vulva	VULVITIS (vul-vy'tis), inflammation of the vulva
EPISI/O (e-pez'e-o)	vulva	EPISIOTOMY (e-pez-e-ot'o-me), incision of the peritoneal portion of the vulva

	Meaning	*Example*
PERINE/O (per-e-nee′o)	perineum (male or female)	PERINEOTOMY (per-e-nee-ot′o-me), incision of the perineum
MEN/O (men′o)	menses, menstruation	MENORRHAGIA (men-o-ra′je-a), excessive menstrual flow
GYNEC/O (gy′ne-ko)	woman, female	GYNECOLOGIST (gy-ne-kol′o-jist), one who specializes in the diseases of the female reproductive organs

PREGNANCY AND BIRTH

EMBRY/O (em′bre-o)	embryo	EMBRYONIC (em-bre-on′ik), pertaining to an embryo
CHORI/O (ko′re-o)	chorion	CHORIONIC (ko-re-on′ik), pertaining to the chorion
AMNI/O (am′ne-o)	amnion	AMNIORRHEXIS (am-ne-o-rek′sis), rupture of the amniotic sac
GRAVID/O (gra′vi-do)	pregnant	PRIMIGRAVIDA (pre-me-grav′i-da), a woman who is pregnant for the first time
CYES/O (sy-ee′so)	pregnancy	OVARIOCYESIS (o-vay-re-o-sy-ee′sis), ectopic pregnancy occurring in the ovary
TOC/O (to′ko)	birth, labor	EMBRYOTOCIA (em-bre-o-to′she-a), abortion
PAR(T)/O (par′(t)o)	give birth	POSTPARTUM (post-par′tum), after childbirth
UMBILIC/O (um-bil′i-ko)	navel	UMBILICAL (um-bil′i-kal), pertaining to the navel
OMPHAL/O (om′fal-o)	navel	OMPHALOTOMY (om-fal-ot′o-me), cutting of the umbilical cord at birth
MAMM/O (mam′o)	breast	MAMMOGRAPHY (mam-og′ra-fe), process of making a breast x ray to detect cancer
MAST/O (mas′to)	breast	MASTECTOMY (mas-tek′to-me), removal of the breast(s)

	Meaning	*Example*
PSEUD/O (sou'do)	false	PSEUDOHERMAPHRO-DITE (sou-do-her-maf'ro-dyt), an individual who has the sex glands of one sex and the genitals of the other
CRYPT/O (crip'to)	hidden	CRYPTORCHIDISM (kript-or'kid-izm), undescended testicles
-PLASIA (play'ze-a)	formation, development	HYPERPLASIA (hy-per-play'ze-a), abnormal increase in the size of an organ due to an increase in the number of cells

Reproduction is the process whereby living organisms produce offspring. In human beings the reproductive systems of the male and female produce *sperm* and *ova*, and the newly formed organism is housed in the female until it is sufficiently developed to enter the external environment.

THE MALE REPRODUCTIVE SYSTEM

The primary sex organs of the male are the *testes* (Figure 15-1). Here the production of sperm (*spermatogenesis*) takes place. A testis has an oval shape and is divided by septa into several compartments. Each compartment contains one or several coiled *seminiferous tubules*. Germinal epithelium lines these tubules and in this lining sperm cells are produced. *Spermatozoa*, mature sperm cells, leave the testis by way of the *efferent ductules* and are stored in the *epididymis*, a coiled tube of about 20 feet attached to the superior portion of the testis. In addition to producing sperm; the testes also produce *testosterone*, the male sex hormone (called an *androgen*).

Gametogenesis is the production of sperm and egg cells. In the male this process is called *spermatogenesis*. With the exception of mature reproductive cells all body cells are *diploid*: they have the full number of chromosomes (46). The chromosomes contain the genetic material that is the basis of all hereditary characteristics. *Gametes*, however, are *haploid* cells, which means that they have only 23 chromosomes. Thus when a sperm penetrates an ovum, a cell containing 46 chromosomes is formed. The process by which gametes undergo a reduction in the number of chromosomes is called *miosis* (my-o'sis, MI/O less, also spelled meiosis). In the male diploid spermatocytes undergo two miotic divisions, resulting in the production of four primitive spermatozoa called *spermatids*, each having 23 chromosomes. The mature spermatozoon has a *head*, a *neck*, and a *tail* called a *flagellum* (fla-jel'um, FLAGELL/O whip).

Because spermatozoa cannot tolerate the body's internal temperature, they are enclosed in the *scrotum*, which is suspended from the body. Within the scrotum the testes are divided by a septum and externally by the *median raphe* (ray'fee), a seam that

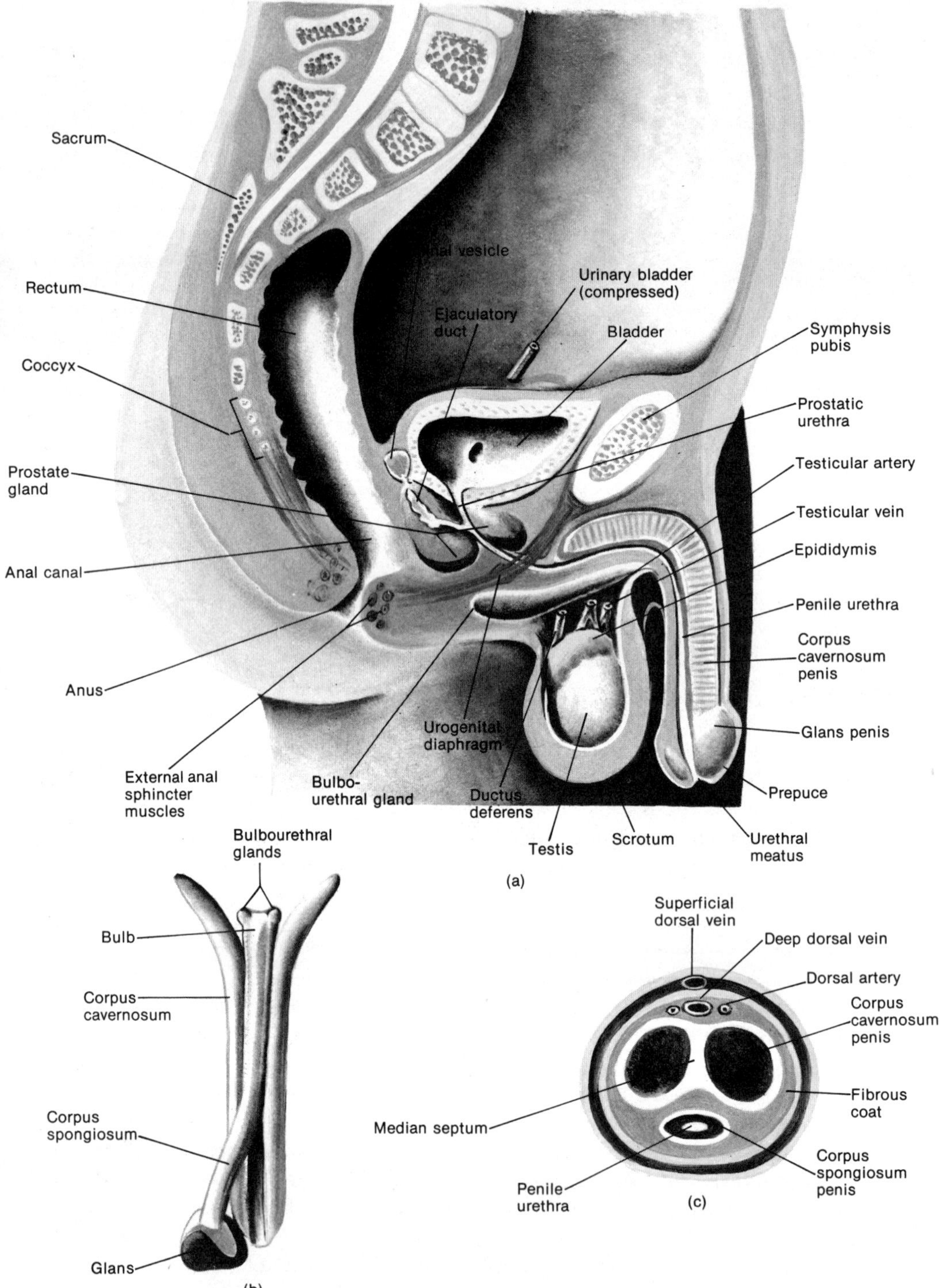

Figure 15-1 The male reproductive system: (a) sagittal section through the pelvis; (b) structure of the penis; (c) cross-section through the penis.

runs from the perineum to the penis. The *dartos* (dar'tos), the muscular tissue of the scrotum, allows the testes to move toward or away from the body, depending on the external temperature.

From the *epididymis*, the storage areas located on the top of each testis, sperm moves along the *vas deferens* (one for each testis) and enters the body along the *spermatic cord*, a structure that supports the testes and contains the blood and lymph vessels and nerves. Before each vas deferens enters the prostate, it connects with the ejaculatory duct of a *seminal vesicle*, which contributes to the seminal fluid. Inside the prostate, both structures empty into the urethra. The *prostate gland* is a walnut-shaped structure that secretes an alkaline fluid that is added to the semen and helps to neutralize any acidity caused by urine. Before the urethra enters the penis, two pea-shaped glands, the *bulbourethral* or *Cowper's glands*, add to the seminal fluid and produce a lubricant that is secreted during sexual arousal.

The *penis* is the male *copulatory* (kop'you-la-to-re, COPUL/O a joining) *organ*. It is made up of three masses of erectile tissue called cavernous tissue because they contain numerous hollow spaces. Blood fills these hollow spaces to produce an erection. The urethra passes through the bottom layer of cavernous tissue. The *glans* (glanz') or head of the penis is covered by a fold of skin called the *prepuce* (pree'pus). *Preputial* (pree-pou'shal, also called Tyson's glands) *glands* secrete a thick, cheeselike substance called *smegma* (smeg'ma). *Circumcision* is the removal of the prepuce. *Ejaculation* is the reflex by which the semen is expelled from the genital tract. The vas deferens, seminal vesicles, and prostate contract, expelling the semen.

THE FEMALE REPRODUCTIVE SYSTEM

The *ovaries* are the primary sex organs of the female and the equivalent of the male testes (Figure 15-2). Each ovary is attached laterally to the uterus by an ovarian ligament. Like the testes, the ovaries not only produce female gametes, the *ova*, but also produce the female hormones *estrogen* (ESTR/O, sexual desire), and *progesterone*. A thin cortex makes up the outer portion of an ovary, and the inner portion or medulla contains the *follicles*—hollow, round vesicles where the ova develop. Ova are formed from *primary oocytes*, each of which divides into two cells: an ovum and a polar body that quickly breaks down.

Ovulation occurs in cycles of about 28 days. The follicle containing an ovum surfaces from the ovary and enters one of the uterine tubes. The *uterine tubes* (also called oviducts or fallopian tubes), one on each side of the uterus, are actually continuations of the uterus. The structures of the uterine tubes are the isthmus (is'mus), an narrow end opening to the uterus; the *infundibulum* (in-fun-di'bou-lum), the funnel-shaped end; and the *ostium* (os'te-um), the opening of the infundibulum. One of the fingerlike projections of the ostium is attached to the ovary and provides a way for the ovum to enter the uterus. Occasionally an egg that does not enter the uterine tube is fertilized, resulting in an *ectopic* (ek-top'ik, EC-, out and TOP/O place) pregnancy.

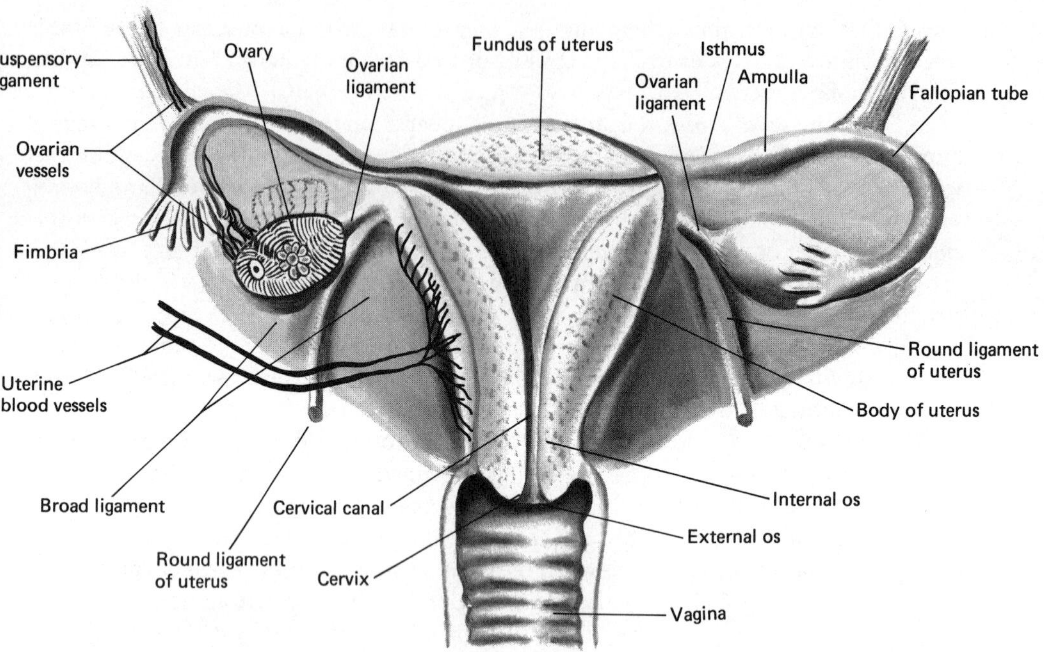

Figure 15-2   Details of the uterus, ovary, and associated structures.

Menstruation (men-strou-ay′shun) is the periodic discharge of fluid from the uterus that occurs regularly unless an egg is fertilized. The entire menstrual cycle has four stages.

1. Menstrual stage: period of bleeding lasting about four to five days during which the uterine lining is shed.
2. Proliferative or follicular stage: eight to fourteen days; restoration of the uterine lining, maturation of another follicle, release of an ovum around the fourteenth day.
3. Secretory stage: ten to fourteen days; secretion of progesterone by the corpus luteum of the ruptured follicle, preparation of uterus to receive a fertilized egg.
4. Premenstrual stage: a few days before menstruation; breakdown of tissue.

The *uterus* or womb is a pear-shaped structure in which the fertilized egg is implanted and the fetus is housed until birth. It has a wide upper portion (its fundus), a body, and a long neck called the *cervix*. The uterine cavity is lined with epithelial tissue called *endometrium*. It has very thick muscular walls that are stretched during pregnancy.

The last internal structure of the female reproductive system is the *vagina*. The vagina is a tubular organ that receives the penis during intercourse and serves as a passageway for the menstrual flow and childbirth.

Externally the vagina is covered by the *vulva*, the external structure of the female genitals. The vulva consists of the labia majora (la'be-a may-jor'a), the labia minora, the clitoris, the vestibule of the vagina, and the vestibular bulbs. The *labia majora* and *minora* are two sets of protective folds of skin. The *clitoris* is a small structure composed of erectile tissue and is the female counterpart of the male penis. The vagina is bounded on either side by the labia minora, which form a *vestibule*. Two mucus-secreting glands, *Bartholin's glands*, are located on either side of the vagina orifice, which is covered by a membrane, the *hymen*. The hymen may or may not be present before the first intercourse but is lost after that.

GESTATION (jes-tay'shun)

When the pronuclei (called *pro*nuclei because they are haploid) of the sperm and ovum unite, a *zygote* (zy'goat) is formed. This fertilized egg or zygote immediately begins to divide. The cells do not entirely separate but form a *cleavage*. The result is a ball of cells called a *morula* (mor'ou-la). At the same time a developing cavity, the *blastocele*, forms a *blastocyst*, which consists of an inner cell mass, the future embryo, and an outer layer, the *trophoblast* or primitive placenta. By the second week the blastocyst attaches itself to the uterine wall by fixing *chorionic villi* from the chorion membrane into the uterine wall (Figure 15-3). Meanwhile, a fluid-filled membrane, the *amnion*, also develops. Next, two cell layers develop in the embryo, the ectoderm and

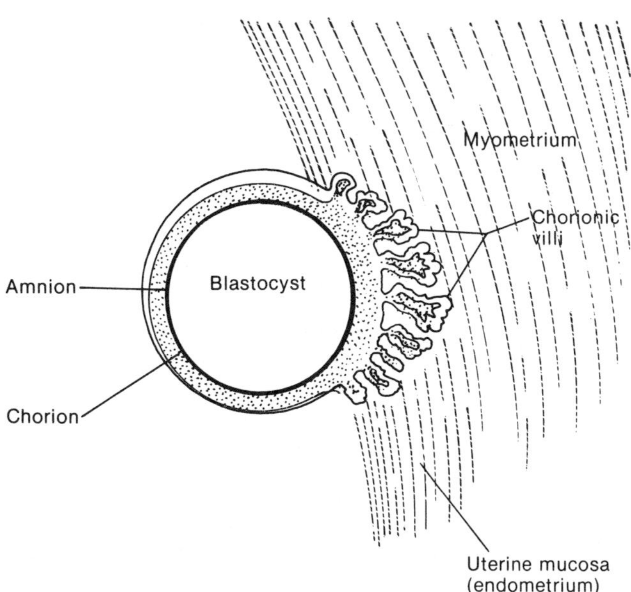

Figure 15-3 Early implantation.

endoderm. Finally, a middle layer, the mesoderm, develops. These three cell layers are called the *primary germ layers*, and they begin to form specialized tissues (*histogenesis*) that will become body organs and structures. At this time the embryo begins to form body shapes (*morphogenesis*, MORPH/O shape). As tissue differentiation proceeds, the cells of the ectoderm, mesoderm, and endoderm produce the linings of all systems.

Extraembryonic structures—the yolk sac, amnion, chorion, and allantois (see Figure 15-4)—sustain and protect the fetus. Blood vessels develop in the *yolk sac* and in the early stages provide the embryo with nourishment. For protection, the embryo is enclosed in a fluid-filled sac, the *amnion*. The *chorion* gives rise to much of the *placenta*, which is the organ of communication between the mother's blood vessels and the fetus'. The umbilical vein and arteries develop from the *allantois* (a-lan'toe-is). The fetal stage of pregnancy lasts from the third month to birth. During this period the body structures develop and growth of the fetus continues.

CHILDBIRTH

Parturition (par-tou-rish'un) is the expulsion of the fully developed fetus from the uterus. There are three stages lasting several hours.

First stage. The progesterone level is decreased and the uterus begins to contract, pushing the fetus downward and causing the cervix to dilate.

Second stage. Labor pains become more frequent and severe. Finally, the infant is expelled head first. Sometimes an *episiotomy* is performed to prevent the infant from tearing through the perineum.

Third stage. Ten to thirty minutes after the birth the *placenta* ("afterbirth") is expelled.

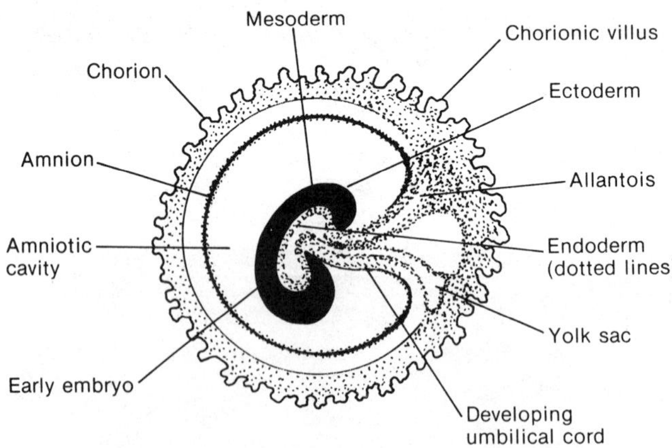

Figure 15-4 Extraembryonic structures.

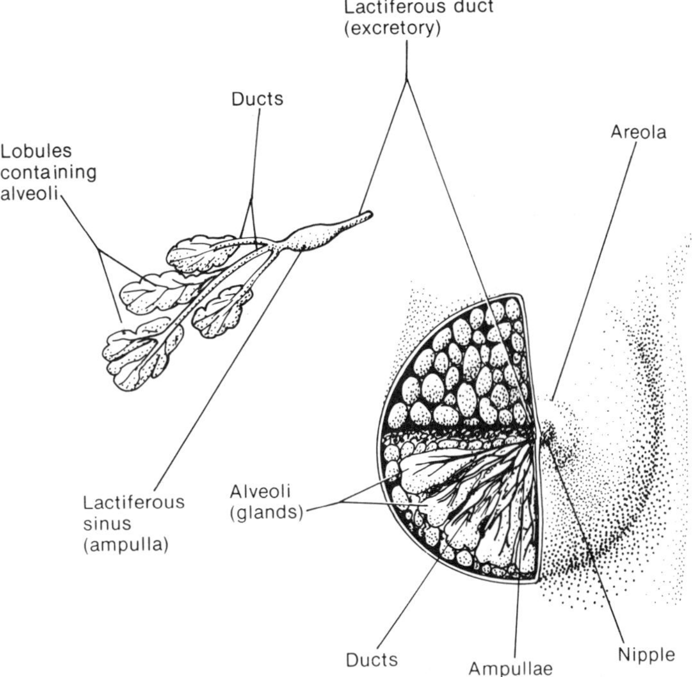

Figure 15-5 The mammary gland.

THE MAMMARY GLANDS

The *mammary glands* or breasts (Figure 15-5) are modified apocrine sweat glands. At puberty they become more fully developed in females than in males or children. The center of each gland has a *nipple* surrounded by a pink area called the *areola* (a-ree-o'la), which becomes brown permanently after pregnancy. Each nipple has about 10 to 15 ducts called *lactiferous ducts* (LACT/O, milk). Each duct is connected to a lobe of glandular tissue. The lobes divide into smaller lobes, which in turn divide into small sacs called *alveoli*. Here the milk-producing cells are located and begin to produce milk soon after childbirth. *Lactation*, the production of milk, is preceded by the secretion of a watery fluid called *colostrum* (ko-los'trum). This "first milk" provides the infant with essential proteins and immunological substances.

CLINICAL AND PATHOLOGICAL CONDITIONS

Infertility

Infertility is the inability of the male to produce sperm that can fertilize the ovum; in the female it is the inability to conceive. Several factors may lead to infertility. Congenital defects, irregular development, and disease are the major causes of infertility. A low sperm count is a common cause of infertility in the male.

Syphilis (sif'i-lis)
Syphilis is an infectious venereal (VENERE/O, love, sexual intercourse) disease that is communicated by direct contact with infected areas. There are three stages.

Primary syphilis. A *chancre* (shang'ker, a hard ulcer) develops on the skin, especially the genetalia. The sore contains infectious microorganisms called *spirochetes* (spe'ro-kets).

Secondary syphilis. About a month after the primary stage a body rash develops and quickly disappears.

Tertiary syphilis. Ten to twenty years later the cardiovascular and nervous systems become affected. In the former, arterial fibrosis and aneurysm of the aorta may develop; in the latter, meningitis and the destruction of the spinal cord and cerebral cortex.

Penicillin is effective in treating the first two stages; there is no cure for the last stage.

Gonorrhea
This highly contagious venereal disease causes an acute inflammation of the urethra. In men dysuria and a purulent discharge develop. In chronic conditions the prostate may become inflamed. In females dysuria and suppuration occur but may not be as pronounced as in the male. Inflammation of the cervix may lead to inflammation of the pelvic reproductive organs (*pelvic inflammatory disease*). Sterility can result from abscesses and stenosis of the reproductive organs. Penicillin is the most common form of treatment.

Congenital defects of the reproductive organs (*Gonadal Dysgenesis*)
Since the fetus is neither male nor female, abnormal development of the sex organs can occur. Gonadal malformations fall into two categories.

1. Infertility with differentiation in genital development
   (a) Extra X chromosome (called Klinefelter's syndrome). The breasts become enlarged and the testes are atrophic. Mental retardation is also common.
   (b) X chromosome lacking (called Turner's syndrome). The sex organs do not develop (gonadal agenesis). Skin and skeletal abnormalities are common.

2. Infertility accompanied by a lack of sexual differentiation
   (a) Hermaphroditism (her-maf'ro-dyt-izm). The individual possesses the primary sex organs of both sexes.
   (b) Pseudohermaphroditism. The individual has the sex glands of one sex and the genitalia of the other.

Conditions of the Male Reproductive Organs

Hypospadia (hy-po-spay'de-a)
This is a congenital defect in which the urethra opens on the underside of the penis.

Cryptorchidism

The testes do not descend into the scrotum. Frequently the testes will descend within the first year. A *cryptorchidectomy* is performed to place the testes in the scrotum.

Balanitis

This inflammation of the glans penis usually spreads to the foreskin and is accompanied by a discharge of pus.

Phimosis (fy-mo'sis)

The foreskin tightens over the glans and cannot be easily pushed back. This situation frequently leads to balanitis. Circumcision is performed to remove the foreskin.

Hydrocele

Fluid accumulates in the scrotum, causing a swelling.

Varicocele (var'i-ko-seal)

The veins of the spermatic cord become enlarged, causing a mild ache. Large varicoceles may require surgery.

Prostatic hyperplasia

Declining testosterone levels in older men, together with the adrenal production of estrogen, cause the prostate to enlarge, resulting in an obstructed urethra. Nocturia and urinary tract infection are signs of prostatomegaly. The obstructing prostate tissue can be surgically removed by *curettage* (kou-re-tohz'), a scraping or cutting of tissue.

Prostatic carcinoma

Cancer of the prostate is one of the most common causes of cancer in elderly men. The symptoms are those for prostatic hyperplasia. A tumor in the prostate can frequently be palpated through the rectum. Prostatectomy, sometimes accompanied by orchidectomy, is the usual treatment for prostatic carcinoma.

Testicular carcinoma

Carcinoma of the testicles is rather rare and usually occurs during the period when the individual is most sexually active. Swelling of the testicle and abdominal pain are signs of testicular carcinoma. Testicular cancers metastasize early to the lungs and bones.

Conditions of the Female Reproductive Organs

Vulvovaginitis

This is an infection of the vulva and vagina characterized by the discharge of white pus (leukorrhea) and itching. The infection is caused by such microorganisms as fungi or protozoa. Treatment is with penicillin, sulfa applications, and vaginal suppositories.

Endocervicitis

This is a viral (herpes) inflammation of the lining of the cervix. Painful erruptions develop along with a mucous discharge. These lesions have been linked to cervical cancer.

Pelvic inflammatory disease

This is a general term for an infection of any of the pelvic reproductive organs. Two examples are *salpingitis* and *endometritis*. Penicillin is the usual form of treatment.

Placental tumors

These are tumors that develop from placental tissue. A *hydatidiform* (hy-da-tid'i-form) *mole* is a benign tumor. A *choriocarcinoma* is a malignant tumor whose cause is unknown. It sometimes develops from the hydatidiform mole. Both tumors develop from the chorionic membrane.

Vaginal neoplasms

Cervicovaginal adenocarcinoma can develop in young women as a result of *stilbestrol* (stil-bes'trol) being given to their mothers during pregnancy to prevent abortion. Vaginal squamous cell carcinoma sometimes occurs in elderly women.

Uterine neoplasms

Leiomyoma is a benign fibroid tumor of smooth muscle that develops from the smooth muscle of the uterus. Leiomyomas can cause hemorrhaging and can put pressure on the pelvic organs. A partial or complete hysterectomy frequently accompanies the removal of this tumor.

Polyps are benign tumors that can develop in the endocervical canal and the endometrium. Spotting (discharge of blood) is sometimes caused by polyps.

Cervical carcinoma

Although the cause of cervical carcinoma is unknown, it has been linked to the herpes II simplex virus. Spotting is frequently a sign of cervical carcinoma. The cancer has four stages.

Stage I. The tumor has not spread from the cervix. This is usually preceded by another stage: *carcinoma in situ*, merely a malignant lesion of the cervical mucosa.

Stage II. The surrounding tissues are affected.

Stage III. The cancer begins to invade the pelvis.

Stage IV. Cancer spreads to the rectum and urinary bladder.

Endometrial cancer

Adenocarcinoma of the uterine wall might result from excessive estrogen. It usually affects women past menopause. Treatment is by the implantation of radiation *seeds*, followed by a hysterectomy. Like cervical carcinomas, endometrial cancers metastasize to surrounding tissues and organs.

Ovarian cancer

Papillary cystadenocarcinoma is the most common malignant tumor of the ovaries. It is a fluid-filled tumor. *Solid adenocarcinoma* is a solid mass tumor. Both malignancies can be *bilateral*, occurring in both ovaries, which makes the prognosis worse. *Teratomas* are benign tumors that develop from the primary germ layers (ectoderm, mesoderm, and endoderm).

Diseases of the Breasts

Diseases of the breasts normally produce masses that may or may not be malignant.

Nonmalignant breast masses

1. *Fibroadenoma.* This is a benign tumor composed of fibrous and glandular tissue. It chiefly occurs in women under 35.

2. *Breast tissue dysplasia.* Dysplasia is the abnormal growth of tissue. There are three types of breast dyplasia.
   (a) *Fibrosis* arises from fibroblasts.
   (b) *Cystic disease* produces cysts from the glandular ducts and is considered precancerous.
   (c) *Adenosis* produces a tough lesion and the glands become compressed.

Carcinoma of the breast

Breast cancer is a major form of cancer in women. It occurs in one out of every 12 women and is found most often in families where it has previously occurred. The most common sign of breast cancer is a lump on the breast. Swelling of the surrounding lymph nodes, discharge from a nipple, or a retracted nipple may also point to cancer. Most breast cancers arise in the ducts, and it takes about five years for the cancerous cells to reach the stage where they can be felt with the fingers. By this time the cancer has usually spread to surrounding tissue and lymph nodes.

When the lump is surgically removed, a pathologist examines it. He cuts a portion of the lump and freezes it in a special unit called a *cryostat* (kry′o-stat, CRY/O cold). He then prepares a thin section of it for examination under the microscope. If the biopsy indicates that the tumor is malignant, a *mastectomy* is performed. In a *simple mastectomy* only the tumor, breast tissue, and overlying skin are removed. When a *radical mastectomy* is performed, the surrounding muscles (pectoris major and minor) and tissue containing lymph nodes are removed in addition to the preceding structures.

As a result of a radical mastectomy, the arm becomes swollen (lymphedema) and difficult to move and must be exercised regularly. Also, the tumor may reappear in the scar tissue or in the axillary area. If the tumor has already metastasized, other organs of the body will develop malignancies. Brain tumors in women are usually caused by metastasized breast cancer.

EXERCISES

I. Give the meaning for each of the following medical words. Divide each word into base(s), prefix, and suffix; underline the letter(s) that has the primary stress. *Example:*

TESTICULAR   pertaining to the testes   testicul/ar

1. ORCHIORRAPHY ....

2. VASOLIGATION (LIG/O tie) ....

3. PROSTATOVESICULITIS ....

4. SEMINAL ....

5. OVIDUCT ....

6. OOPHOROCYSTOSIS ....

7. OOCYTE ....

8. TESTES ....

9. SCROTECTOMY ....

10. VESICULITIS ....

11. BALANORRHEA ....

12. PHALLITIS ....

13. GONADOPATHY ....

14. SPERMATOGENESIS ....

15. SALPINGO-OOPHORECTOMY ....

16. OVULATORY ....

17. EPIDIDYMOTOMY ....

18. BULBAR ....

19. PROSTATOMEGALY ....

20. GENITALIA ....

21. HYPOGONADISM ....

22. SPERMOLYTIC ....

23. ASPERMIA ....

24. OVARIORRHEXIS ....

25. ANDROID ....

26. ORCHIDECTOMY ....

27. OVARIOCENTESIS ....

28. PANHYSTEROCOLPECTOMY (PAN- all, entire) ....

29. DYSMENORRHEA ....

30. EMBRYOTROPH ....

31. TOCOPHOBIA ....

32. VARICOMPHALUS ....

33. MAMMOPLASTY ....

34. DYSPLASIA ....

35. METROFIBROMA ....

36. COLPOPERINEORRHAPHY ....

37. PERINEOCELE ....

38. GRAVIDITY ....

39. BIPAROUS ....

40. UTERINE ....

41. EPISIORRHAPHY ....

42. CHORIOCARCINOMA ....

43. OMPHALOPHLEBITIS ....

44. CRYPTORCHIDECTOMY ....

45. ENDOMETRIOSIS ....

46. VAGINAL ....

47. GYNECOMASTIA ....

48. CYESEDEMA ....

49. AMNIOTIC ....

50. HYSTEROPTOSIS ....

II. Make medical words from the following phrases. Indicate the primary stress by underlining the stressed letter(s). *Example:*

excision of a portion of the seminal vesicles

vesicul_ect_omy
....

1. pertaining to the prostate gland

....

2. a hormone that stimulates the gonads

....

3. pus in a uterine tube

....

4. production of ova

....

5. presence of semen in the urine

. . . .

6. study of animal life

. . . .

7. inflammation of the epididymis

. . . .

8. sperm duct

. . . .

9. fixation of a displaced ovary

. . . .

10. formation of an opening into an occluded fallopian tube

. . . .

11. excision of the vas deferens and seminal vesicles

. . . .

12. hernia in the scrotum

. . . .

13. pertaining to the glans penis and prepuce

. . . .

14. inflammation of the bulbourethral portion of the urethra

. . . .

15. inflammation of the prostate gland

. . . .

16. overdevelopment of the genitals (resulting from glandular disturbance)

. . . .

17. to convey semen into the vagina

. . . .

18.   pertaining to gametes

....

19.   absence of a testis (or both testes)

....

20.   a seminal vesicle

....

21.   excision of an ovary

....

22.   inflammation of the cervical lining

....

23.   excision of the uterus

....

24.   pertaining to the vulva and vagina

....

25.   pregnancy in a uterine tube

....

26.   pertaining to the breasts

....

27.   a woman who has given birth to her first child

....

28.   instrument for cutting the uterus

....

29.   inflammation of the cervix

....

30.   absence of menstruation

....

31. inflammation of the vagina

. . . .

32. normal childbirth

. . . .

33. puncture of the amniotic sac to remove fluid

. . . .

34. inflammation of a breast

. . . .

35. tumor of the muscular tissue of the uterus

. . . .

36. stricture of the vagina

. . . .

37. suture of the perineum

. . . .

38. pertaining to the uterine lining

. . . .

39. before pregnancy

. . . .

40. pregnancy in an ovary

. . . .

III. Match the following descriptions with their medical words.

1. male primary sex organs . . . .   a. prepuce

2. structure that stores sperm . . . .   b. uterus

3. an androgen . . . .   c. gametogenesis

4. production of sperm and ova . . . .   d. Bartholin's glands

5. sac that encloses the testes ....   e. Cowper's glands

6. transports sperm into pelvic area ....   f. fallopian

7. a walnut-shaped gland that adds to seminal fluid ....   g. menstruation

8. another name for the bulbourethral glands ....   h. vulva

9. fold of skin covering the glans penis ....   i. testes

10. female primary sex organs ....   j. prostate

11. female sex hormones ....   k. epididymis

12. another name for the uterine tubes ....   l. ectopic

13. describes a pregnancy occurring outside its normal

place ....   m. vas deferens

n. endometrium

14. periodic discharge of fluid from the uterus ....

o. testosterone

15. the fertilized egg is implanted here ....

p. ovaries

16. uterine lining ....

q. estrogen
progesterone

17. external portion of the female genitals ....

18. glands located on either side of the vaginal   r. scrotum

opening ....

       IV. Match the following descriptions with their medical words.

1. result of the union of a spermatozoon and an

ovum ....   a. allantois

2. specialized division of cells following   b. colostrum

fertilization ....

3. formation of the fertilized egg into a ball of   c. trophoblast

d. parturition

cells ....

e. fetus

4. primitive placenta ....

5. means of attaching the blastocyst to the uterine

wall ....

6. formation of body shapes ....

7. source of the umbilical vein and arteries ....

8. term for the unborn child from the third month until

birth ....

9. childbirth ....

10. pink ring around the nipple ....

11. watery fluid known as "first milk" ....

12. production of milk ....

f. zygote

g. lactation

h. morphogenesis

i. morula

j. areola

k. cleavage

l. chorionic villi

V. Multiple choice: Circle the correct letter.

1. A venereal disease that is characterized by the development of a chancre on the genitals
   (a) gonorrhea
   (b) vaginitis
   (c) syphilis
   (d) cervicitis

2. A gonadal malformation characterized by enlarged breasts, atrophic testes, and frequently mental retardation
   (a) hermaphroditism
   (b) Klinefelter's syndrome
   (c) Turner's syndrome
   (d) pseudohermaphroditism

3. A condition in which the urethra opens on the underside of the penis
   (a) hypospadia
   (b) balanitis
   (c) cryptorchidism
   (d) Turner's syndrome

4. Abnormal tightness of the foreskin of the penis
   (a) cryptorchidism
   (b) balanitis
   (c) hydrocele
   (d) phimosis

5. A congenital malformation in which the testes do not descend into the scrotum
   (a) hypospadia
   (b) cryptorchidism
   (c) phimosis
   (d) hydrocele

6. Accumulation of fluid in the scrotum
   (a) variocele
   (b) hyperplasia
   (c) hydrocele
   (d) hypospadia

7. Inflammation of the cervical lining
   (a) cervicitis
   (b) vulvovaginitis
   (c) pelvic inflammatory disease
   (d) endocervicitis

8. A highly malignant tumor developing from placental tissue
   (a) choriocarcinoma
   (b) hydatidiform mole
   (c) leiomyoma
   (d) polyps

9. An example of a pelvic inflammatory disease
   (a) vulvovaginitis
   (b) endometritis
   (c) hydatidiform mole
   (d) leukorrhea

10. A uterine neoplasm
    (a) squamous cell carcinoma
    (b) cervical adenocarcinoma
    (c) leiomyoma
    (d) teratomas

11. Benign ovarian tumors
    (a) papillary cystadenocarcinomas
    (b) endometrial carcinomas
    (c) teratomas
    (d) fibroadenomas

12. A form of breast tissue dyplasia
    (a) fibrosis
    (b) fibroadenoma
    (c) adenocarcinoma
    (d) leiomyoma

ANSWERS TO EXERCISES

I.

1. attaching an undescended testis (or testes) to the scrotum, orchi/o/rrhaphy
2. tying of the vas deferens, vas/o/lig/a/tion
3. inflammation of the prostate and seminal vesicles, prostat/o/vesicul/itis
4. pertaining to semen, semin/al
5. a fallopian tube, ov/i/duct
6. formation of an ovarian cyst, oophar/o/cyst/osis
7. a diploid egg cell that gives rise to a mature ovum, o/o/cyte
8. the testes, plural form of testis, test/es
9. excision of a portion of the scrotum, scrot/ectomy
10. inflammation of the seminal vesicles, vesicul/itis
11. purulent discharge from the glans penis, balan/o/rrhea
12. inflammation of the penis, phall/itis
13. any disease of the sex glands, gonad/o/pathy
14. production of spermatozoa, spermat/o/gen/esis
15. excision of a uterine tube and an ovary, salping/o/-oophor/ectomy
16. pertaining to ovulation, ov/u/latory
17. incision of the epididymis, epididym/o/tomy
18. bulb-shapped, bulb/ar
19. enlargement of the prostate gland, prostat/o/megaly
20. the genitals, genit/al/ia
21. decrease in the secretion of the sex glands, hypo/gonad/ism
22. destroying sperm, sperm/o/ly/tic
23. without ejaculate or the inability to ejaculate, a/sperm/ia
24. rupture of an ovary, ovari/o/rrhexis
25. manlike, andr/oid
26. removal of a testis, orchid/ectomy
27. surgical puncture of an ovary, ovari/o/centesis
28. removal of the entire uterus and vagina, pan/hyster/o/colp/ectomy
29. painful menstruation, dys/men/o/rrhea
30. substance that nourishes the embryo, embry/o/troph
31. extreme fear of childbirth, toc/o/phob/ia
32. varicose veins located in the navel, varic/omphal/us
33. plastic surgery of the breast, mamm/o/plasty
34. abnormal tissue development, dys/plasia
35. fibrous tumor of the uterus, metr/o/fibr/oma
36. suture of the perineal tears of the vagina, colp/o/perine/o/rrhaphy
37. hernia of the perineum, perine/o/cele
38. pregnancy, gravid/ity
39. giving birth to twins, bi/par/ous
40. pertaining to the uterus, uter/ine
41. suture of the perineal portion of the vulva, episi/o/rrhaphy
42. cancer developing from the chorion, chori/o/carcin/oma
43. inflammation of the umbilical veins, omphal/o/phleb/itis

44. operation to correct undescended testes, crypt/orchid/ectomy
45. abnormal condition in which endometrial tissue forms in the pelvis or abdomen, endo/metri/osis
46. pertaining to the vagina, vagin/al
47. abnormal condition in which the male possesses feminine breasts, gynec/o/mast/ia
48. swelling caused by pregnancy, cyes/edema
49. pertaining to the amnion, amni/o/tic
50. prolapse of the uterus, hyster/o/ptosis

II.

1. prostatic;   **2.** gonadotrophin;   **3.** pyosalpinx;   **4.** oogenesis;
5. spermaturia;   **6.** zoology;   **7.** epididymitis;   **8.** spermiduct;
9. oophoropexy;   **10.** salpingostomy;   **11.** vasovesiculectomy;   **12.** scrotocele;
13. balanopreputial;   **14.** bulbitis;   **15.** prostatitis;   **16.** hypergenitalism;
17. inseminate;   **18.** gametic;   **19.** anorchism;   **20.** spermatocyst;
21. oophorectomy;   **22.** endocervicitis;   **23.** hysterectomy;   **24.** vulvovaginal;
25. salpingocyesis;   **26.** mammary;   **27.** primipara;   **28.** uterotome;
29. cervicitis;   **30.** amenorrhea;   **31.** vaginitis;   **32.** eutocia;
33. amniocentesis;   **34.** mastitis;   **35.** hystermyoma;   **36.** colpostenosis;
37. perineorrhaphy;   **38.** endometrial;   **39.** pregravidic;   **40.** ovariocyesis.

III.

1. i;   **2.** k;   **3.** o;   **4.** c;   **5.** r;   **6.** m;   **7.** j;   **8.** e;   **9.** a;
10. p;   **11.** q;   **12.** f;   **13.** l;   **14.** g;   **15.** b;   **16.** n;
17. h;   **18.** d.

IV.

1. f;   **2.** k;   **3.** i;   **4.** c;   **5.** l;   **6.** h;   **7.** a;   **8.** e;   **9.** d;
10. j;   **11.** b;   **12.** g.

V.

1. (c);   **2.** (b);   **3.** (a);   **4.** (d);   **5.** (b);   **6.** (c);   **7.** (d);   **8.** (a);
9. (b);   **10.** (c);   **11.** (c);   **12.** (a).

16 The Endocrine System

COMBINING FORMS

	Meaning	Example
STER/O (ster'o)	solid	CHOLESTEROL (ko-les'ter-ol), a fatlike substance common in animal tissue and found in bile. It is used to manufacture several steroid hormones.
COLL/O (ko'lo)	glue	COLLOID (kol'oyd), a gluelike substance
-PHYSIS (fis'is)	growth	HYPOPHYSIS (hy-pof'i-sis), grown under the brain, the pituitary gland
SOMAT/O (so'ma-to)	body	SOMATOTROPIN (so-ma-toe-trop'in), body growth stimulating hormone
-TROPIN (trop'in)	a substance that stimulates or activates, hormone	ADRENOCORTICOTROPIN (ad-ree-no-kor-te-ko-trop'in), a hormone that stimulates the cortex of the adrenal gland
THYROID/O (thy'royd-o)	thyroid gland	THYROIDITIS (thy-royd-eye'tis), inflammation of the thyroid
THYR/O (thy'ro)	thyroid gland	THYROCELE (thy'ro-seel), enlargement of the thyroid, goiter
PARATHYROID/O (par-a-thy'royd-o)	parathyroid glands	PARATHYROIDOTROPIN (par-a-thy-ro-tro'pin), a hormone that stimulates the parathyroid glands
ADREN/O (ad-ree'no)	adrenal glands	ADRENAL (ad-ree'nal), pertaining to the adrenal glands
CALC/I (kal'se)	calcium	CALCIPENIA (kal-se-pee'ne-a), deficiency of calcium
NATR/I (na'tre)	sodium	HYPONATREMIA (hy-po-na-tree'me-a), decrease of sodium in the blood

	Meaning	*Example*
KAL/I (kay'le)	potassium	KALIEMIA (kay-le-ee'me-a), potassium in the blood
PINEAL/O (pin-ee'al-o)	pineal body	PINEALECTOMY (pin-ee-al-ek'to-me), excision of the pineal body
ACR/O (ak'ro)	top, extremity	ACROMEGALY (ak-ro-meg'a-le), enlargement of the bones of the extremities
CAC/O (ka'ko)	bad	CACHEXIA (ka-keks'e-a), state of poor health
DIPS/O (dip'so)	thirst	POLYDIPSIA (pol-e-dip'se-a), excessive thirst
CHROM/O (kro'mo)	color	CHROMAFFIN (kro-maf'in), cells that stain dark brown with chromic acid

The *endocrine system* (Figure 16-1) is a group of glands that regulate body functions. These glands are the hypophysis (pituitary), thyroid, parathyroids, adrenals, and gonads. Like the nervous system, the endocrine system initiates, maintains, and checks the biochemical reactions occurring in the body cells. Because the endocrine glands are ductless, they secrete their substances directly into the blood. *Hormones* (HORMON/O activate) are the secretions of these glands. Hormones are made from proteins, amines, and steroids. Nervous and chemical stimuli activate the secretion of hormones. Endocrine tissues are, in fact, controlled by the autonomic nervous system. Also, the level of various substances in the blood chemically induces the secretion of certain hormones (e.g., insulin).

Some hormones act on all cells. Thyroxine, for example, causes cells to grow. Other hormones act only on specific cells called *target cells*. For instance, gonadotrophin, stimulates the development of only the gonads. As its name indicates, a hormone activates a substance on the cellular membrane, which, in turn, causes the biochemical reaction. When its job is completed, the hormone is metabolized.

Endocrine disorders result from excessive glandular secretion (hyperfunction) or a decrease in secretion (hypofunction). *Hyperplasia*, the excessive growth of tissue—here glandular tissue—causes hyperfunction. Glandular *atrophy* produces hypofunction. The level of hormonal secretion can be determined by analyzing the hormone concentration in the blood and urine. The process by which blood and urine are analyzed to determine their hormone concentration is called *radioimmunoassay* (ray-de-o-im-you-no-as'ay).

THE PITUITARY GLAND

The *pituitary*, also called the *hypophysis*, is located in the sphenoid bone at the base of the brain. It has two lobes. The *adenohypophysis* is the anterior lobe and the

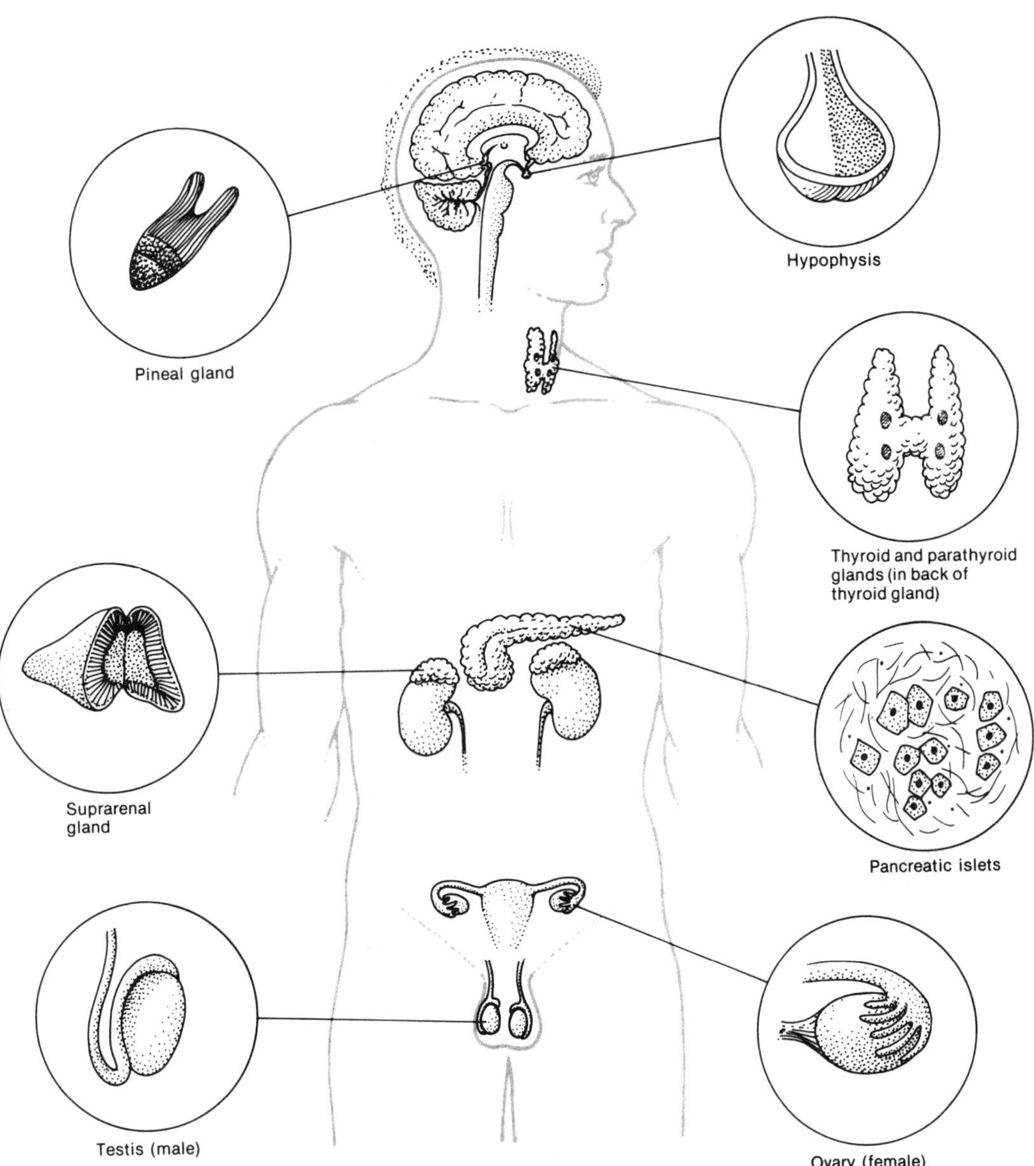

Figure 16-1   The endocrine glands and their locations in the body.

neurohypophysis the posterior lobe. The adenohypophysis consists of glandular tissue and secretes several hormones called *tropic* because they stimulate specific target tissues. The hormones of the adenohypophysis are as follows.

Somatotropin (SOMAT/O, body).   This hormone, known as the growth hormone (GH), is responsible for the growth of the body, especially the bones and muscles. Acidophils are the cells that secrete somatotropin.

Adrenocorticotropic hormone (ACTH) *or adrenocorticotropin.*   This hormone activates the cortex of the adrenal gland and causes it to produce adrenal cortical hormones. The secretion of adrenocorticotropin is regulated by the *hypothalamus*, which manufactures a corticotropin-releasing factor (CRF).

Thyrotropin or thyroid-stimulating hormone (TSH).   The development of the thyroid gland and its ability to secrete its own hormones are controlled by this hormone.

Follicle-stimulating hormone (FSH).   This is a *gonadotropin* that controls the growth of the ovarian follicles and the seminiferous tubules. It also controls the level of androgens and estrogens in the blood.

Luteinizing hormone (LH).   In the female this hormone activates the development of the ovarian follicles and the corpus luteum. It also brings about ovulation. In the male the interstitial cell-stimulating hormone (ISCH) stimulates the secretion of testosterone in the testes.

Lactogenic hormone, prolactin.   This hormone stimulates the production of milk and causes the breasts to enlarge during pregnancy.

Melanocyte-stimulating hormone (MSH).   This hormone stimulates the development of the skin pigment *melanin.* Of the above hormones, somatotropin and lactogenic hormones are produced by *acidophils*, cells that color well with an acid stain. The others are produced with *basophils*. All the hormones secreted by the hypophysis are regulated by the *hypothalamus*, which secretes a specific substance to stimulate the release of each hypophysic hormone. For example, a somatotropin-releasing factor (SRF) controls the secretion of somatotropin.

The neurohypophysis is the posterior lobe of the hypophysis and is composed of nervous tissue. It secretes two hormones that are stored in it but are produced by the hypothalamus.

Oxytocin.   This hormone causes uterine contractions during childbirth and activates the muscles of the mammary glands.

Antidiuretic hormone (ADH, vasopressin).   This substance stimulates the tubules of the kidneys to reabsorb water.

THE THYROID GLAND

The *thyroid gland* is located in front of the trachea. It is a two-lobed gland with each lobe lying on the sides of the trachea and connected by a neck called an isthmus. The thyroid is made up of little pockets or alveoli. These pockets contain a thick fluid called *colloid* that contains the thyroid hormones. TSH from the pituitary causes the colloidal substance *thyroglobin* to break down so that the thyroid hormones can be released into the blood. The two major hormones released by the thyroid are *thyroxin* and *triiodothyronine*, which control the rate of metabolism and are essential for normal growth.

THE PARATHYROID GLANDS

The *parathyroid glands* lie deep within the posterior portion of each thyroid lobe. They are composed of reticular connective tissue and have two types of cells. The *principal cells* secrete parathormone (PTH), which regulates the metabolism of calcium and phosphorus and their levels in the blood. This function is not controlled by the hypophysis but is determined by the level of calcium in the blood. The purpose of the *oxyphils*, the second type of cell, is not known.

THE ADRENAL GLANDS

The *adrenal glands*, also called *suprarenal glands*, are connected to the top of each kidney by connective tissue. The *adrenal medulla* contains *chromaffin cells*, cells that stain a dark brown with chromic acid and, under the control of the hypothalamus and autonomic nervous system, produce two important hormones: *epinephrine* (also called *adrenalin*) and *norepinephrine*. Both hormones are called *sympathicomimetic* because they act in a manner that is similar to the sympathetic division of the ANS. Epinephrine causes peripheral arteriole constriction, increased blood pressure, rapid heart rate, dilated bronchial tubes, dilated pupils, the halting of intestinal movements, and the conversion of glycogen into glucose. Norepinephrine, which is also produced in the postganglionic sympathetic nerves endings, constricts peripheral blood vessels and causes blood pressure to rise. Both hormones are also called *catecholamines* (kat-e-kol-am'eens), which are amino acids that imitate the sympathetic division of the ANS.

The *adrenal cortex* produces several hormones that are essential for life. These hormones are called *corticosteroids* or *corticoids* and they are grouped into three types: *glucocorticoids, mineralocorticoids,* and *sex hormones.* The glucocorticoids (e.g., cortisone and hydrocortisone) permit the conversion of glucose into glycogen in the liver. The mineralocorticoids promote water and electrolyte (acids, bases, and salts) balance, and the sex hormones are produced in only very small quantities. *Aldosterone*, an important mineralocorticoid that regulates sodium, chloride, and potassium metabolism, is controlled by a substance called *renin* that is produced in the kidneys.

THE PANCREAS

In addition to digestive enzymes, the *pancreas* also produces two important endocrine secretions: *insulin* and *glucagon.* The *isles of Langerhans* are groups of cells in the endocrine tissue that are responsible for hormonal secretions. The beta cells produce insulin, which lowers the blood glucose level by causing glucose to pass from the blood into the cells and by converting glucose into glycogen. The alpha cells produce glucagon (also called hyperglycemic-glycogenolytic factor, HCG), which promotes the conversion of glycogen to glucose when the level of blood sugar falls too low.

THE GONADS

The *gonads* or sex glands produce male or female hormones. The chief *androgen* (male sex hormone) is *testosterone*. Testosterone is produced in the interstitial cells of the testes called the *cells of Leydig*. All secondary sex characteristics—pubic hair, axillary hair, beard, masculine appearance, and sex drive—are the result of testosterone. The female sex hormones can be divided into two groups: *estrogens* and *progesterone*. The estrogens give the female her secondary sex characteristics and regulate the menstrual cycle. Progesterone prepares the uterine lining for pregnancy. The origin of the female hormones may be the follicular cells.

OTHER HORMONE-PRODUCING ORGANS

Several other organs produce endocrine secretions, but generally they are not included in the group of endocrine glands. Here is a table of the organs and their secretions.

Organ	Secretion	Function
Stomach	Gastrin	Stimulates gastric glands to secrete gastric enzymes and hydrochloric acid
Intestine	Secretin	Promotes the production of bile and pancreatic enzymes
	Pancreozymin	Activates pancreas
	Cholecystokinin	Regulates bile secretion
	Enterogasterone	Influences the secretion of the gastric glands
Kidneys	Renin	Regulates the secretion of aldosterone by the adrenal cortex
	Angiotensin	Influences vasoconstriction
Pineal body	Melatonin	Influences menstrual cycle
	Serotonin	Influences brain functions
	Adrenoglomerultropin	Stimulates the production of aldosterone
Placenta	Chorionic gonadotropin	Preserves the corpus luteum, which produces estrogens and progesterone

Thymus gland, important during childhood and puberty, produces a substance that enables the lymphocytes to become plasma cells that manufacture antibodies; it atrophies after puberty.

CLINICAL AND PATHOLOGICAL CONDITIONS

Diseases of the adenohypophysis

Hyposecretion of growth hormone (GH). (a) *Dwarfism.* Body height is abnormally short. This situation occurs before growth is complete. (b) *Simmonds' disease.* The atrophy of the pituitary gland and the resulting lack of growth hormone produce a general state of poor health called *pituitary cachexia*, senility, the atrophy of the sex organs, and the loss of secondary sex characteristics. Decreased pituitary secretion is most frequently associated with glandular destruction or atrophy.

Hypersecretion of growth hormone (GH). (a) *Gigantism.* Body height is abnormally tall, sometimes exceeding 8 feet. This situation occurs before skeletal growth is complete. (b) *Acromegaly.* In adults the bones of the hands, feet, and face, especially the jaw, become enlarged and elongated. Both gigantism and acromegaly are frequently caused by tumors called *acidophil adenomas.* Although benign, these tumors may put pressure on the optic tract and cause tunnel vision and even blindness.

Disease of the neurohypophysis

Diabetes insipidus (in-sip'i-dus). This disease is the result of a lack of (hyposecretion) antidiuretic hormone. Water is not reabsorbed by the kidneys. Frequent urination (polyuria) and abnormal thirst (polydipsia) occur as a result of water not being reabsorbed by the kidneys.

Diseases of the thyroid gland

Hypothyroidism. The lack of thyroid hormones causes a low basal metabolism rate, a bloated face, general weakness, and mental dullness. *Myxedema* (miks-e-dee'ma, MYX/O mucous) is extreme hypothyroidism. The injection of thyroid hormones is used to treat thyroid deficiencies.

Cretinism (kree'tin-izm). Extreme hypothyroidism in infants inhibits physical and mental development. Poorly developed muscles, bloated abdomen, goiter, and mental retardation are characteristic of a child affected with cretinism.

Hyperthyroidism (Grave's disease). Most commonly occurring in women, hyperthyroidism causes nervousness, irritability, insomnia, and a marked protrusion of the eyeballs (exophthalmos). Antithyroid drugs can be used to inhibit thyroid secretions.

Goiter (goi'ter). This is an enlargement of the thyroid gland caused by a lack of iodine that it needs to produce its secretions. Iodine supplements can be used to treat goiter in early stages. A portion of the thyroid is removed in cases of extremely large goiters.

Thyroid neoplasms. (a) One type of thyroid neoplasm is an *encapsulated adenoma.* This benign tumor does not normally interfere with hormonal secretion. (b) *Thyroid cancers*, especially papillary carcinomas, occur more commonly in women than in men. They usually don't metastasize too far from their origin and can be easily removed. The use of radiation to treat skin disease or tonsillitis has been linked to thyroid cancer.

Diseases of the parathyroid glands

Hyperparathyroidism. Oversecretion of parathyroid hormone is generally caused by a parathyroid adenoma. As a result of hyperparathyroidism, the levels of calcium and phosphate in the blood rise, calcium is drawn from the bones, leaving them weak and prone to fracture, and kidney stones may develop. *Secondary hyperparathyroidism* is caused by chronic renal disease in which excessive amounts of calcium are excreted and parathyroid hyperplasia develops in an effort to offset this loss.

Hypoparathyroidism. This is a parathyroid insufficiency caused by the destruction of the parathyroid glands. The low level of calcium in the blood causes *tetany* (spasms, uncontrollable muscle contractions).

Diseases of the adrenal cortex

Hypersecretion of aldosterone (Conn's syndrome). Aldosterone controls the excretion of sodium by the kidneys. In *aldosteronism* there is a high concentration of sodium in the blood and a low level of potassium, which causes a general muscle weakness. High blood pressure occurs and arteriosclerosis of the kidneys may develop. A benign tumor is the most common cause of this disease.

Cushing's syndrome (hypersecretion of ACTH or hyperadrenocorticalism). Hyperplasia of the adrenal cortex causes a hypersecretion of cortisol. Muscle and skeletal weakness, obesity characterized by stretch marks (*striae* stry'ay, striations), and high blood pressure occur in adults suffering from hyperadrenocorticalism.

Androgenital syndrome. This disease is also caused by an excessive secretion of the adrenal cortex—in this case, a hypersecretion of androgens. Young females may develop masculine traits (called *virilization*), such as a deep voice and the growth of facial hair. Infant females have an enlarged penislike clitoris and labia resembling a scrotum. In young males oversecretion of androgens by the adrenal cortex causes *precocious puberty*, characterized by enlargement of the penis and the appearance of pubic hair.

Adrenal cortex insufficiency (hypoadrenocorticalism). Adrenocorticoid deficiency develops as a result of the destruction or atrophy of the adrenal cortex. General weakness, low blood pressure (hypotension), hemorrhaging into the skin, and patches of brown pigment on the lips and gums are the symptoms of hypoadrenocorticalism. Chronic adrenal insufficiency is called *Addison's disease.*

Diseases of the adrenal medulla

A benign tumor called *pheochromocytoma* (fee-o-kromo-sy-toe'ma, PHE/O dark) can occur in the chromaffin cells of the medulla. As a result of an increase of the secretion of norepinephrine (due to the tumor), headaches, sweating, palpitation, and high blood pressure develop. Usually the tumor is surgically removed.

Diseases of the pancreas

Diabetes mellitus (dy-a-bee'tez mel-le'tus).   Insulin enables the body tissues to utilize glucose. If insulin is absent or in an insufficient amount, the level of glucose in the blood increases (hyperglycemia) and is concentrated in the kidneys, where it is excreted in the urine (glycosuria). The symptoms of diabetes mellitus are *polyuria, polyphagia,* and *polydypsia.* There are two forms of diabetes mellitus: *juvenile diabetes* and *maturity-onset diabetes.* Juvenile diabetes occurs in young people from infancy to 20 years of age; maturity-onset diabetes usually appears after age 40.

Two tests are commonly used to determine the level of blood sugar. In the *glucose tolerance test* the individual is given specific amounts of glucose orally or intravenously and blood samples are taken periodically to determine how much glucose has remained in the blood. The *fasting blood sugar test* is used to determine the blood sugar level in an individual who has not eaten for a predetermined period.

Diabetes mellitus is caused by a lack of *insulin.* For some reason, the *islets* (cells of the pancreas) don't function, are injured, or atrophy. Many diabetics have other members of the family who are diabetic, which points to an hereditary factor. Diabetes can be controlled by hypoglycemics administered orally or by injection.

Several complications result from diabetes. Arteriosclerosis develops more quickly and early in diabetics. The blood vessels of the eye, kidneys, and heart are especially susceptible to diabetic-induced arteriosclerosis. Impaired renal function and overproduction of ketone bodies by the liver (ketosis) also occur. In the elderly poor circulation frequently causes gangrene in the lower extremities, especially the toes.

Hyperinsulinism.   Hypoglycemia is caused by an excessive secretion of insulin by the pancreas. Hyperinsulinism may be caused by a tumor, extreme sensitivity to the level of blood sugar, or an overdosage of insulin. Excessive insulin can cause *insulin shock*, which is characterized by convulsions and unconsciousness.

EXERCISES

I.   Give the meaning for each of the following medical words. Divide each word into base(s), prefix, and suffix; underline the letter(s) that has the primary stress. *Example:*

ADRENALITIS   inflammation of the adrenal glands   adren/al/<u>it</u>is

....

1. ISOCOLLOID (IS/O equal) ....

2. HYPERCALCEMIA ....

3. CHROMODERMATOSIS ....

4. STEROID ....

5. APOPHYSIS ....

6. SOMATASTHENIA ....

7. THYROLYTIC ....

8. PARATHYROPRIVIA (-PRIVIA deprived of) ....

9. ACROEDEMA ....

10. ANADIPSIA ....

11. THYROTOXICOSIS (TOXIC/O poison) ....

12. HYPERKALEMIA ....

13. CORTICOTROPIN ....

14. ADRENOPATHY ....

15. NATIURESIS ....

16. PINEALOMA ....

    II. Make medical words for the following phrases. Indicate the primary stress by underlining the stressed letter(s).

inflammation of the thyroid gland

thyroid<u>i</u>tis
....

1. having a gluelike substance

....

2. excision of the thyroid

....

3. removal of the pituitary gland

....

4. excision of an adrenal gland

....

5. decrease of calcium in the blood

....

6. staining easily with both acid and base dyes

. . . .

7. inflammation of the joints of the extremities

. . . .

8. pertaining to a state of poor health

. . . .

9. a growing together or fusion of two bones

. . . .

10. a hormone that stimulates the thyroid gland

. . . .

11. decrease of potassium in the blood

. . . .

12. abnormal thirst

. . . .

13. removal of the parathyroid glands

. . . .

14. stimulating the adrenal glands

. . . .

15. pertaining to the body

. . . .

16. surgical removal of the thyroid and parathyroid glands

. . . .

III.   Match the following descriptions with their medical names.

1. ductless glands . . . .   a. catecholamines

2. substances that activate target organs . . . .   b. interstitial cells of
                                                                           the testes
3. the pituitary gland . . . .

4. the glandular lobe of the pituitary ....

5. lobe of the pituitary composed of nervous

    tissue ....

6. gland located in front of the trachea ....

7. set of glands located within the lobes of another

    gland ....

8. hormone produced by the adrenal medulla ....

9. hormones composed of amino acids that imitate the

    sympathetic division of the ANS ....

10. hormones of the adrenal cortex ....

11. hormone produced by the kidney ....

12. insulin is produced here ....

13. has the opposite effect of insulin ....

14. testosterone is produced here ....

15. a group of female sex hormones ....

16. a hormone produced by the pineal body that regulates the

    menstrual cycle ....

17. a gland that atrophies shortly after birth ....

18. hormone produced by the intestines, promotes the

    production of bile and pancreatic enzymes ....

19. produces the hormone gastrin ....

20. produces chorionic gonadotropin during

    pregnancy ....

c. thyroid

d. secretin

e. placenta

f. mineralocorticoids

g. hormones

h. parathyroid glands

i. endocrine glands

j. renin

k. thymus

l. neurohypophysis

m. epinephrine

n. stomach

o. hypophysis

p. isles of Langerhans

q. adenohypophysis

r. estrogens

s. glucagon

t. melatonin

IV. For each abbreviation write out the hormone, its source, and its function.

	Hormone	*Source*	*Function*

1. FHS ....

2. LTH ....

3. ACTH ....

4. ADH ....

5. LH ....

6. GH ....

7. TSH ....

8. ISCH ....

9. MSH ....

V. Multiple choice: Circle the correct letter.

1. A lack of growth hormone produces
   (a) gigantism
   (b) acromegaly
   (c) dwarfism
   (d) diabetes insipidus

2. Simmonds' disease is caused by
   (a) hyposecretion of the adenohypophysis
   (b) hypersecretion of the adenohypophysis
   (c) hyposecretion of the neurohypophysis
   (d) hypersecretion of the neurohypophysis

3. Caused by a hyposecretion of ADH
   (a) acromegaly
   (b) gigantism
   (c) pituitary cachexia
   (d) diabetes insipidus

4. Myxedema is
   (a) cretinism
   (b) extreme hypothyroidism
   (c) extreme hyperthyroidism
   (d) mild hyperthyroidism

5. Exophthalmia is a symptom of
   (a) myxedema
   (b) cretinism
   (c) hypothyroidism
   (d) hyperthyroidism

6. A high concentration of sodium in the blood is caused by
   (a) hypersecretion of ACTH
   (b) adrenal cortical insufficiency
   (c) hypersecretion of aldosterone
   (d) hyposecretion of aldosterone

7. A disease characterized by general weakness, obesity with prominent stretch marks, and hypertension; it is caused by a hypersecretion of cortisol.
   (a) Conn's syndrome
   (b) Cushing's syndrome
   (c) Addison's disease
   (d) adrenal cortical insufficiency

8. In young boys excessive secretions of androgens by the adrenal cortex causes
   (a) virilization
   (b) Addison's disease
   (c) Cushing's syndrome
   (d) precocious puberty

9. A disease characterized by the lack of insulin
   (a) diabetes insipidus
   (b) diabetes mellitus
   (c) hypoglycemia
   (d) insulin shock

10. Symptoms of diabetes mellitus
    (a) polyuria
    (b) polydipsia
    (c) polyphagia
    (d) all of the above

VI. Match the disease with its cause.

1. cretinism ....   a.   hypersecretion of cortisol

2. goiter ....   b.   hypersecretion of GH

3. acromegaly ....   c.   hyposecretion of insulin

4. parathyroid insufficiency ....   d.   extreme hypothyroidism

5. tetany ....   e.   hyposecretion of ADH

6. Cushing's syndrome ....,   f. chronic hyposecretion of the
                                          adrenal cortex

7. virilization ....   g. low level of blood calcium

8. Addison's disease ....   h. hypoparathyroidism

9. diabetes mellitus ....   i. hyperthyroidism

10. diabetes insipidus ....   j. hyperadrenocorticalism

ANSWERS TO EXERCISES

I.

1. equal glue, a colloid that retains its composition, is/o/<u>coll</u>/oid
2. excessive amount of calcium in the blood, hyper/calc/<u>emia</u>
3. any skin disease characterized by pigmentation, chrom/o/dermat<u>/osis</u>
4. a substance having a complex carbon ring molecule, especially adrenal cortex and sex
   hormones, <u>ster</u>/oid
5. a growing away, offshoot or tubercle, apo/<u>phys</u>/is
6. bodily weakness, somat/as<u>then</u>/ia
7. destroying thyroid tissue, thyr/o/<u>ly</u>/tic
8. absence of the parathyr/o/<u>privia</u>
9. swelling of the extremities, acr/o/ed<u>ema</u>
10. severe thirst, ana/<u>dips</u>/ia
11. toxic condition caused by hyperfunction of the thyroid gland, thyr/o/toxic<u>/osis</u>
12. excessive potassium in the blood, hyper/kal<u>/emia</u>
13. a substance that stimulates the adrenal cortex, cortic/o/<u>trop</u>/in
14. any disease of the adrenal glands, adren/<u>o/</u>pathy
15. excretion of sodium in the urine, nati/ur<u>/esis</u>
16. tumor of the pineal body, pineal<u>/</u>oma

II.

1. coll<u>oi</u>dal;   2. thyroid<u>ect</u>omy;   3. hypophy<u>sect</u>omy;   4. adrenal<u>ect</u>omy;
5. hypocal<u>cem</u>ia;   6. di<u>chr</u>omophil;   7. acroar<u>thr</u>itis;   8. ca<u>chec</u>tic;
9. sym<u>phys</u>is;   10. thyro<u>trop</u>in;   11. hypoka<u>lem</u>ia;   12. dip<u>sos</u>is;
13. parathyroid<u>ect</u>omy;   14. adreno<u>trop</u>ic;   15. so<u>mat</u>ic;
16. thyroparathyroid<u>ect</u>omy.

III.

1. i;   2. g;   3. o;   4. q;   5. l;   6. c;   7. h;   8. m;
9. a;   10. f;   11. j;   12. p;   13. s;   14. b;   15. r;   16. t;
17. k;   18. d;   19. n;   20. e.

IV.

Hormone	*Source*	*Function*
1. follicle-stimulating hormone	adenohypophysis	in male—growth of seminiferous tubules; in female—growth of ovarian follicles
2. lactogenic hormone	adenohypophysis	stimulates the production of milk by mammary glands
3. adrenocorticotropic hormone	adenohypophysis	stimulates adrenal cortex
4. antidiuretic hormone	neurohypophysis	stimulates reabsorption of water by the kidney
5. luteinizing hormone	adenohypophysis	stimulates development of the ovarian follicle
6. somatotropin or growth hormone	adenohypophysis	stimulates body growth
7. thyroid-stimulating hormone	adenohypophysis	stimulates the thyroid
8. interstitial cell stimulating hormone	adenohypophysis	secretion of androgens by testes
9. melanocyte-stimulating hormone	adenohypophysis	stimulates melanin deposits on the skin

V.

1. (c);   2. (a);   3. (d);   4. (b);   5. (d);   6. (c);   7. (b);
8. (d);   9. (b);   10. (d).

VI.

1. d;   2. i;   3. b;   4. h;   5. g;   6. a;   7. j;   8. f;
9. c;   10. e.

17 Pharmacology

COMBINING FORMS

	Meaning	Example
PHARMAC/O (far'ma-ko)	drug	PHARMACOGNOSY (far-ma-kog'no-se), study of natural sources of drugs and their particular properties
TOXIC/O (toks'i-ko)	poison	TOXICOLOGY (toks-i-kol'o-je), study of poisonous substances and their actions in the body
TOX/O (toks'o)	poison	TOXIN (toks'in), poisonous substance produced by a plant or animal
CHEM/O (kee'mo)	chemical, drug	CHEMOTHERAPY (kee-mo-ther'a-pe), use of chemicals to treat a disease
-PHYLAXIS (fi-laks'is)	guard, protection	ANAPHYLACTIC (an-a-fi-lak'tik), pertaining to the body's overprotective reaction
ESTHESI/O (es-thee'ze-o)	perception, feeling	ANESTHESIA (an-es-thee'se-a), lack of perception or feeling
IDI/O (id'e-o)	own, individual	IDIOSYNCRACY (id-e-o-sin'kra-se), individual reaction to a drug
ERG/O (er'go)	work	ADRENERGIC (ad-ren-er'jik), substance that acts like adrenalin (epinephrine)
ALGES/I (al-jee'ze)	sensitivity to pain	HYPERALGESIA (hy-per-al-jee'ze-a), excessive sensitivity to pain
NARC/O (nar'ko)	numbness, narcotic	NARCOSIS (nar-ko'sis), numb or unconsciousness state caused by narcotics
PYR/O (py'ro)	heat, fever	PYROGENIC (py-ro-jen'ik), fever producing
HYPN/O (hip'no)	sleep	HYPNOTIC (hip-not'ik), sleep producing
SOMN/I (som'ne)	sleep	INSOMNIA (in-som'ne-a), sleeplessness

	Meaning	*Example*
SOPOR/I (so'por-i)	deep sleep	SOPORIFIC (so-po-rif'ik), producing a deep sleep
TON/O (toe'no)	tension, stretching	ATONY (at'o-ne), lack of muscle tone
TUSS/I (tus'si)	cough	ANTITUSSIVE (an-ti-tus'iv), a drug that supresses coughing
SPASM/O (spaz'mo)	spasm, convulsion	SPASMODIC (spaz-mod'ik), characterized by a spazm
HIST/O (his'to)	tissue	HISTOLOGY (his-tol'o-je), study of tissue
-THERAPY (ther'a-pe)	treatment	THERMOTHERAPY (ther-mo-ther'a-pe), use of heat to treat a disease

Pharmacology is the study of drugs and their effects. Drugs may be used for their preventative, diagnostic, therapeutic, or palliative value. There are several sources of drugs. They may be derived from plant, animal, or mineral sources; they may also be manmade or synthetic by combining various chemicals. The science of drugs has branched out into several specialized fields. Toxicology, pharmacodynamics, and chemotherapy all are branches of pharmacology. *Toxicology* deals with the identification and study of poisonous substances, their effects on the body, and the preparation of antidotes. *Pharmacodynamics* is the study of the actions of drugs on living organisms,—for example, their rates of absorption and excretion. *Chemotherapy* is the branch of pharmacology dealing with the use of chemicals to destroy microorganisms and cancerous cells.

DRUG NOMENCLATURE (no-men-klay'chur, system for naming) AND STANDARDS

Drugs have three names. The *chemical name* gives the chemical structure of the drug. The *generic name* is the nonproprietary (nonbrand name) name for the drug. The *brand name* is the trade name of a drug established by each manufacturer. The first letter of a brand name is always capitalized.

Here are some examples of how drugs are classified.

Chemical name	*Generic name*	*Brand name*
Acetylsalicylic acid	Aspirin	Bayer
A sulfonamide compound ($C_{12}H_{18}N_2O_3S$)	Tolbutamide	Orinase (used to treat diabetics)
Synthetic T_4 (a synthetic preparation of an active principle of the thyroid gland)	Levothyroxine sodium	Levoid (used to treat hypothyroidism)

The question of whether a brand name drug and a generic drug are equivalent often arises. Although both drugs are chemically equivalent, they may differ in other respects, such as the agent (method of dispensing the drug—e.g., quality of the substance that binds the pill), particle size, purity, and overall quality.

The identification and quality standards for a drug are established by the *United States Pharmacopeia* (USP), a committee of pharmacologists, pharmacists, physicians, and chemists. A *pharmacopeia* is an official list of drugs and their formulations that is published every five years. Drugs on the market that have USP after their brand name have met the standards established by the pharmacopeia for that particular drug. The *National Formulary* (NF) is a supplementary list of drugs put out by the U.S. Pharmacopeia. The federal government regulates drugs through the *Food and Drug Administration* (FDA).

THE EFFECTS OF DRUGS

A drug is prescribed by a physician on the basis of its ability to treat the condition under consideration. There are, however, other effects that a drug or combination of drugs may have on the body. Some are beneficial; others are unwanted and may cause a mild allergic reaction or a severe reaction known as *anaphylatic shock*. The following terms are used to describe the effects that drugs have.

Side effect.   Any effect other than that for which the drug was prescribed is called a side effect.

Hypersensitivity (also called *anaphylaxis*).   This is an allergic reaction to a drug.

Idiosyncracy.   This is an individual's personal reaction to a drug. Sometimes a large dose of a drug will produce an allergic reaction in an individual who had been previously been given a smaller quantity of the same drug.

Additive action.   Two or more drugs are used to increase the desired effect.

Synergism (also called *potentiation*).   Two or more drugs interact to provide an effect greater or different from the effect produced when each drug is given without the other.

Cumulation.   This is the buildup of a drug in the body tissues as a result of the frequent administration of the same drug.

Tolerance.   The body builds up a resistance to a drug so that larger doses are needed to produce the same reaction that was previously obtained by a smaller dose.

Addiction.   The individual becomes physically or mentally, or both, dependent on a specific drug.

Toxicity.   Sometimes the nontherapeutic effects of a drug may be harmful and even poisonous.

The *Physician's Desk Reference* provides information on a drug's uses and side effects.

DRUG PREPARATIONS

Drug preparations are the substances that drugs are mixed with so that they may be easily and effectively administered. Here are some common preparations.

Solution.   The drug is dissolved in a liquid. Examples are aqueous solutions, tinctures and spirits, and extracts. In an *aqueous solution* the drug is dissolved in water. *Tinctures* are drugs dissolved in alcohol. Alcohol itself is a compound that is a hydroxyl (having one atom of hydrogen and one of oxygen) derivative of a hydrocarbon. It is used extensively in medicinal preparations (e.g., tinctures and extracts). A 70% solution of alcohol is used externally as an antiseptic; isopropyl alcohol is used externally as a rubbing compound. *Spirits* are concentrated alcoholic solutions. An *extract* is a concentrated drug obtained by extracting the drug, using solvents and then eliminating the solvents.

Suspension.   The drug is mixed with a substance but not dissolved in it. Examples are gels and emulsions.

Tablet.   The drug is compressed into a small mass.

Capsule.   The drug is enclosed in a gelatin capsule.

Ointment.   The drug is dispersed in a fatty base. A salve is an example of an ointment.

ADMINISTRATION OF MEDICATION

There are several methods of administering drugs, depending on the type of drugs and the effect desired. Several factors determine how a drug is to be administered. Dose, absorption, elimination, area of distribution (systemic or local) are important considerations in drug administration. The methods are as follows.

Oral

The medication is swallowed with water, which serves to dilute the medicine. In addition to swallowing the medicine, there are two other types of oral administration: sublingual and buccal administration. In *sublingual administration* the medication is placed under the tongue where it dissolves. In *buccal administration* the medication is placed between the cheek and the teeth until it dissolves.

Parenteral

Parenteral administration of a drug is any form of injection. Below are the forms of parenteral injections.

Subcutaneous (hypodermic).   The medication is injected into the subcutaneous layer of skin. The upper arm or the thigh is commonly used for subcutaneous injections.

Intramuscular.   Some substances, such as penicillin, are not absorbed well by the subcutaneous tissue and so they are injected into muscular tissue. An intramuscular injection is commonly given at the following sites:

1. The upper quadrant of the buttocks (*gluteus maximus*).
2. The midarea of the thigh (*vastus lateralis*).
3. The ventrogluteal site (*gluteus medius* and *miniumus*).

Intradermal.   The medication is injected into the dermis. This type of injection is used when the medication is to be absorbed slowly. The inner surface of the forearm is commonly used in this case.
Intravenous.   The medication is injected into the vein.

Topical
Topical medications are applied to the body surface and their effect is frequently limited (local) to the area treated. Ointments, creams, and lotions are examples of topical medications.

Instillations
The administration of medication by instillation is through drops or pouring. Eye, ear, and nose drops are examples of instillations.

Suppository
A cylindrical solid is inserted into the rectum or vagina. As the suppository melts, the medication is released.

Inhalation
Drugs are dispersed into the air in a gas or vapor form. Aerosols and ampules (small breakable tubes) are common methods of administering drugs by inhalation.

DRUG GROUPS

The following groups of drugs are listed according to the structures of the body affected. This list is selective and does not include all classes of drugs.

Central Nervous System Drugs

Stimulants
They increase the activity of the central nervous system. Each stimulant affects one or more areas of the CNS. The effects of stimulants are increased alertness, restlessness and insomnia, rapid heartbeat, and, in extreme cases, convulsion. Caffeine and amphetamines (used in weight reduction) are examples of stimulants.

Depressants
They cause a decrease in the activity of the CNS. As a result, the individual experiences decreased alertness, dulled senses, and sometimes sleep. Groups of depressants are listed below.

Analgesics are drugs that relieve pain by decreasing one's sensitivity to pain or by interrupting one's perception of pain. Both *narcotic* (e.g., morphine and codeine) and nonnarcotic (e.g., aspirin) analgesics exist. In addition to reducing sensitivity to pain, some analgesics (e.g., aspirin) also reduce fever. These substances are called *antipyretics*.

Hypnotics, Sedatives, and *Barbiturates: Hypnotics* are drugs that produce sleep. They are commonly referred to as *somnifacient* or *soporific agents* (*agents* are drugs). A *sedative* (SED/O calm) is a drug that has a calming, tranquilizing effect. Barbiturates (bar-bit′ou-rayts) are barbituric acid derivatives (e.g., pheno*barbital* and amo*barbital*). They are used as both sedatives and hypnotics.

Anesthetics produce a loss of awareness and sensation. A *local anesthetic* causes a loss of sensation in a limited area of the body. Anesthetics are administered in several ways—intravenously, topically, by inhalation, or by injection.

Tranquilizers reduce mental tension and anxiety. They are used extensively in psychotherapy.

Autonomic Drugs

These drugs affect the autonomic nervous system, which controls involuntary body functions.

Adrenergic drugs

These are substances that work like epinephrine. They cause the constriction of the peripheral blood vessels, increased heart rate and output, stimulation of the CNS, and the relaxation of the visceral muscles. Since the drugs (epinephrine preparations) imitate the actions of the sympathetic division of the ANS, they are called *sympathomimetic*.

Adrenergic blocking drugs

These are substances that have an effect that is opposite to that of epinephrine. Vasodilatation, hypotension, increased gastrointestinal activity, and decreased heart rate and output are characteristic of their actions. Adrenergic blocking drugs are also called *sympatholytic* drugs because they block the actions of the sympathetic division of the ANS.

Cholinergic drugs

They work like acetylcholine, the substance permitting the transmission of nerve impulses. The effects of cholinergic drugs are increased gastrointestinal activity, increased contraction of the urinary bladder, vasodilatation of the peripheral blood vessels, increased skeletal muscle tone, and slower heart rate. Cholinergic agents are called *parasympathomimetic drugs* because they imitate the effects of the parasympathetic division of the ANS.

Cholinergic blocking agents

They have an effect opposite to that of the cholinergic agents. For this reason, they are called *parasympatholytic drugs*.

Cardiovascular Drugs

Cardiac drugs

Cardiotonic agents stimulate heart muscle and strengthen the contractions of the heart.

Cardiac depressants slow the heart rate and reduce quick, irregular heartbeats to slow, normal beats. For this reason, cardiac depressants are called *antiarrhythmic agents*.

Vascular drugs

Vasoconstrictors raise blood pressure and increase heart rate by constricting the blood vessels. They are used to control superficial bleeding.

Vasodilators expand blood vessels by relaxing vessel walls. Hypertension and both coronary and vascular diseases are treated with vasodilators.

Anticoagulants are drugs that prevent clotting. They are especially useful in preventing the formation of thrombi and emboli.

Respiratory Drugs

Antitussives are drugs that suppress coughing.
Antispasmodic drugs are used to relieve bronchial spasms.

Histamines and Antihistamines

Histamines are substances produced by body tissues, especially the skin and lungs. These substances are released when foreign substances (*antigens*) enter the body. Redness, rash, watery eyes—all are allergic symptoms produced by histamines.

Antihistamines are drugs that relieve allergic symptoms by inhibiting histamine activity.

Gastrointestinal Drugs

Antacids are substances that reduce acidity, usually by absorbing or neutralizing the excess acid.

Digestants aid digestion.

Cathartics (ka-thar'tics) are *purgatives*, substances that stimulate bowel movement. There are several types of cathartics.

1. Emollients (softeners)
2. Saline agents
3. Bulk-forming agents
4. Chemical agents

Laxatives are mild cathartics.
Antidiarrheal agents control diarrhea.

Drugs Used on the Skin and Membranes

Anti-inflammatory agents are topical agents that reduce inflammation.
Anti-infectives halt and reduce infection. Antibiotics and fungicides are examples of anti-infectives.
Emollients (MOLLI/O soften) and *demulcents* (dee-mul'sents, MULC/O soothe) are softening agents.

Urogenital Drugs

Diuretics increase the production of urine.
Antidiuretics decrease the production of urine.
Oxytocins cause uterine contractions.
Sex hormones are used to treat a variety of conditions affecting the genitals and secondary sex characteristics.

ANTIBIOTICS

Antibiotics are drugs that are produced from bacteria or molds or are synthetically produced. They destroy harmful microorganisms by killing them (*bacteriocidal* function), by inhibiting their growth (*bacteriostatic* function), or by both methods. A *broad spectrum antibiotic* destroys several types of bacteria. The most commonly used antibiotics are classified according to the following types: penicillins, streptomycins, tetracyclines, and erythromycin.

VITAMINS AND MINERALS

Vitamins are organic substances that are necessary for maintaining normal body functions by working with enzymes in regulating metabolic processes. Minerals are inorganic substances that are also essential for life.

Table 16-1 lists several vitamins and minerals, their sources, and examples of disorders caused by the deficiency or excess of a certain vitamin or mineral.

Table 16-1

Vitamin	Examples of food sources	Examples of conditions produced by a deficiency (hypovitaminosis)	Examples of conditions produced by an excess (hypervitaminosis)
A	Organ meats, eggs, yellow and leafy green vegetables	Dry skin, night blindness	Skin rash, weight loss, hair loss, hypercalcemia, heptatomegaly, splenomegaly, anemia
B_1 (thiamine)	Organ meats, whole grains, legumes, wheat germ	Muscle tenderness, ataxia, anorexia; severe symptoms (beriberi) include paralysis, edema, dyspnea, tachycardia	
B_2 (riboflavin)	Organ meats, green vegetables, dairy products, eggs	Oily skin, paleness, conjunctivitis, sensitivity to light; severe symptoms include vascularization of the cornea, anemia, edema	
B_6 (pyridoxine)	Egg yolk, milk, legumes, pork	Anemia	
B_{12} (cyanocobalamin)	Organ meats, dairy products, eggs	Anemia, jaundice, achlorhydria	
C (ascorbic acid)	Citrus fruits	Bleeding gums, edema; severe symptoms include anemia, bone degeneration and swollen joints, bleeding	
D	Vitamin D milk	Rickets in children, osteomalacia in adults	Hypercalcemia, kidney damage
E	Green vegetables	Increase in red blood cell destruction (Deficiencies are not common.)	
Folic acid (folacin)	Organ meats, green leafy vegetables, wheat, eggs	Anemia, abortion of fetus	
Niacin (nicotinic acid)	Grains, meat, liver, fish	Eruptions on the surface of the skin (pellagra), mental depression, gastrointestinal disorders	
Mineral		*Hypomineralosis*	*Hypermineralosis*
Iron	Meats, organ meats, grains	Iron-deficiency anemia	
Iodine	Seafood, iodized salt	Goiter, cretinism	Goiter
Magnesium	Fruits, vegetables, grains	Tetany, mental depression	
Copper	Vegetables, meats	Anemia, poor growth, inability to utilize iron	
Manganese	Leafy vegetables, grains, bananas	Lack of certain enzyme functions (Deficiencies are not common.)	

ABBREVIATIONS USED IN PRESCRIPTION WRITING

Prescription writing uses several abbreviations. Here is a table of some of the Latin abbreviations that you should know.

Abbreviation	Word/Phrase	Meaning
āa	ana (Greek)	of each
ac	ante cibum	before meals
ad	ad	to, up to
ad lib.	ad libitum	freely, as desired
agit.	agita	shake, stir
ante	ante	before
aq.	aqua	water
aq. dest.	aqua destillata	distilled water
bis	bis	twice
b.i.d.	bis in die	twice daily
c̄	cum	with
cap(s).	capsula(e)	capsule(s)
collyr.	collyrium	eyewash
comp.	compositus	compound
dil.	dilutus	dilute, dissolve
elix.	elixir	elixir
ft.	fac, fiat, fiant	make
g	gramme	gram
gr.	granum	grain
gt.	gutta(e)	drop(s)
h.	hora	hour
h.s., hor. som.	hora somni	at bedtime
in d.	in die	in a day
inf.	infusum	an infusion
inj.	injectio	an injection
liq.	liquor	a solution
m.	misce	mix
min.	minimum	a minim/drop
noct.	nocte	at night
non rep.	non repetatur	do not repeat
no.	numerus	number
o.d.	oculus dexter	the right eye
o.h.	omni hora	every hour, hourly
o.s.	oculus sinister	the left eye
o.u.	oculus uterque	each eye
p.c.	post cibum	after meals
p.o.	per os	orally
p.r.n.	pro re nata	when needed, as the occasion arises
q.d.	quaque die	daily, everyday

Abbreviation	Word / Phrase	Meaning
q.h.	quaque hora	hourly, every hour
q.i.d.	quater in die	four times a day
q.s.	quantum sufficiat	a sufficient quantity
Rx	recipe	take
rept.	repetatur	let it be repeated
s̄	sine	without
s.o.s.	si opus est	if it is needed
s̄s̄.	semis	a half
sig., s.	signa	(you) label
stat.	statim	at once, immediately
ti., tinct.	tinctura	a tincture
ut dict.	ut dictum	as directed

EXERCISES

I. Give the meaning for each of the following medical words. Divide each word into base(s), prefix, and suffix; underline the letter(s) that has the primary stress. *Example:*

AHYPNIA   sleeplessness   a/hypn/ia
....

1. NARCOANESTHESIA ....

2. ACTINOTHERAPY (ACTIN/O ray) ....

3. PHARMACODYNAMICS ....

4. DYSTONIA ....

5. HYPERPYREXIA ....

6. PERTUSSIS ....

7. HISTOLYSIS ....

8. PHARMACOKINETICS ....

9. TOXICOSIS ....

10. SYNEXTHESIA ....

11. HYPALGESIA ....

12. SOMNAMBULISM (AMBUL/O walk) ....

13. SPASMOPHILIA ....

14. ANTITOXIN ....

15. IDIOPATHY ....

16. CHOLINERGIC ....

17. SOPOROUS ....

18. ALLERGY (ALL/O other) ....

19. TOXICOPATHY ....

20. PARESTHESIA ....

II. Make medical words from the following phrases. Indicate the primary stress by underlining the stressed letter(s). *Example:*

instrument for measuring tension or pressure

tonometer
....

1. pertaining to a chemical substance used to treat a disease

....

2. producing toxins

....

3. study of diseased tissues

....

4. absence of the sense of cold

....

5. working together

....

6. treatment of a disease with light

....

7. pertaining to a substance that relieves pain

....

8. drug causing numbness

. . . .

9. use of drugs to treat disease

. . . .

10. overprotective reaction of the body

. . . .

11. lacking tension

. . . .

12. producing sleep

. . . .

13. acting to arrest a spasm

. . . .

14. fever reducing

. . . .

15. presence of toxins in the blood

. . . .

III. Fill in the blanks in the following statements.

1. . . . . is the physical or mental dependence on a drug.

2. . . . . is a serious overreaction of the body to a certain drug or combination of drugs.

3. The interaction of two or more drugs to produce an effect greater or different from the administration of a single drug is called . . . .

4. Drugs have three names. The . . . . name is the nonproprietary name for the drug. The . . . . name is the drug's scientific name. The chemical structure of a drug is its . . . . name.

5. Resistance to a drug is called . . . .

6. The study of drugs and their effects is called .... It is subdivided into several specialties such as ...., the study of poisons; ...., the use of chemicals to treat diseases; and ...., the study of how drugs act inside the body.

7. The committee that establishes standards for each drug is called the .... A supplementary drug list put out by this committee is the ....

8. The poisonous effects of a drug is its ....

9. An individual's sensitivity to a drug and subsequent reaction is called an ....

10. .... is the combining of two or more drugs to increase the desired effect.

11. A .... is any effect of a drug other than the one for which it was prescribed.

12. The buildup of a drug in the body tissues is known as ....

    IV. Match the following descriptions with their medical words.

1. dissolution of a drug in a liquid	a.	suspension
2. dissolution of a drug in alcohol	b.	ointment
3. concentrated alcoholic solutions	c.	tablet
4. concentrated form of a drug from which the solvent has been removed	d.	solution
	e.	extract
5. drug is mixed with a substance but not dissolved in it	f.	spirits
	g.	capsule
6. compression of a drug into a small mass	h.	tincture
7. drug in a gelatin container		
8. drug is mixed with a fatty base		

V.   Circle the correct answer for each of the following statements.

1. swallowing medication with water
    buccal administration   oral administration   parenteral administration

2. administration of a medication by injection
    buccal   instillation   parenteral

3. injection of medication into the skin
    intradermal   subcutaneous   topical

4. an example of an inhalation
    ear drops   ointment   aerosol

5. an example of a topical medication
    nose drops   cream   suppository

6. Medication is injected directly into the bloodstream.
    intramuscular   intradermal   intravenous

VI.   Match the following descriptions with their medical terms.

1. drugs that work like epinephrine ....   a. tranquilizers

2. vascular drug that raises blood pressure ....   b. antiarrhythmic
                                                                     agents

3. counters the effects of histamines ....
                                                                 c. antitussives

4. increase CNS activity ....
                                                                 d. oxytocins

5. another name for a drug ....
                                                                 e. hypnotics

6. reduce mental tension ....
                                                                 f. stimulants

7. drugs that stimulate heart action ....
                                                                 g. adrenergic blocking
8. increase the production of urine ....   agents

9. drugs produced from bacteria and molds, used to destroy
                                                                 h. antibiotics
    harmful microorganisms ....
                                                                 i. cathartic

10. strong purgative ....
                                                                 j. anesthetic

11. decrease CNS activity ....
                                                                 k. depressants

12. has a calming, tranquilizing effect ....
                                                                 l. cardiotonic agents

13. parasympatholytic drugs ....

14. drugs that prevent the formation of thrombi and

emboli ....

15. drugs that reduce excess acidity ....

16. soften the skin ....

17. pain-relieving drugs ....

18. causes a loss of awareness and sensation ....

19. cardiac depressants ....

20. suppress coughing ....

21. drugs that produce sleep ....

22. cause uterine contractions ....

23. sympatholytic drugs ....

24. vascular drug that reduces blood pressure ....

25. parasympathomimetic drugs ....

26. used as a drug preparation and also as a

bacteriocide ....

m. anticoagulants

n. antacids

o. analgesics

p. emollients

q. agent

r. cholinergic-blocking
    agents

s. vasodilator

t. diuretics

u. sedative

v. alcohol

w. adrenergic

x. vasoconstrictor

y. cholinergic drugs

z. antihistamines

VII. Below is a select list of pharmaceutical abbreviations. Write out each abbreviation and its meaning.

Word/Phrase   *Meaning*

1. ad lib. ....

2. o.s. ....

3. c̄ ....

4. p.r.n. ....

5. s̄ ....

6. aq. dest. ....

7. non rep. ....

8. q.h. ....

9. ut dict. ....

10. ac ....

11. gt. ....

12. o.u. ....

13. s.o.s. ....

14. q.i.d. ....

15. agit. ....

ANSWERS TO EXERCISES

I.

1. loss of sensation-produced by a narcotic, narc/o/an/esthesi/a
2. treatment of a disease by using rays (light, x rays, etc.), actin/o/therapy
3. study of drugs and their actions in living organisms, pharmac/o/dynam/ics
4. poor or impaired muscle tension, dys/ton/ia
5. abnormally high body temperature, hyper/pyr/ex/ia
6. intensive cough, whooping cough, per/tuss/is
7. destruction of tissue, hist/o/ly/sis
8. study of the action of drugs inside the body, pharmac/o/kine/tics
9. condition caused by poisoning, toxic/o/sis
10. stimulation of one area of the body causes stimulation of another area, syn/esthesi/a
11. decrease in sensitivity to pain, hyp/alges/ia
12. sleepwalking, somn/ambul/ism
13. tendency toward spasms or convulsions, spasm/o/phil/ia
14. substance that acts against a toxin, anti/tox/in
15. disease peculiar to an individual, idi/o/pathy
16. substance that acts like acetylcholine, cholin/erg/ic
17. characterized by a deep sleep, sopor/ous
18. altered action of a body tissue to a substance, all/erg/y
19. any disease caused by a poison, toxic/o/pathy
20. abnormal sensation, par/esthesi/a

II.

1. chemothera<u>peu</u>tic;   **2.** toxi<u>gen</u>ic;   **3.** histopath<u>olo</u>gy;   **4.** cryanes<u>the</u>sia;
5. syn<u>er</u>gism;   **6.** photo<u>ther</u>apy;   **7.** anal<u>ges</u>ic;   **8.** nar<u>cot</u>ic;
9. pharmaco<u>ther</u>apy;   **10.** anaphy<u>lax</u>is;   **11.** at<u>on</u>ic;   **12.** som<u>nif</u>erous;
13. antispas<u>mod</u>ic;   **14.** antipy<u>ret</u>ic;   **15.** tox<u>e</u>mia.

III.

1. addiction;   **2.** anaphylactic shock;   **3.** synergism or potentiation;
4. brand, generic, chemical;   **5.** tolerance;
6. pharmacology, toxicology, chemotherapy, pharmacodynamics;
7. U.S. Pharmacopeia, National Formulary;   **8.** toxicity;   **9.** idiosyncracy;
10. additive action;   **11.** side effect;   **12.** cumulation.

IV.

1. d;   **2.** h;   **3.** f;   **4.** e;   **5.** a;   **6.** c;   **7.** g;   **8.** b.

V.

1. oral administration;   **2.** parenteral;   **3.** intradermal;   **4.** aerosol;
5. cream;   **6.** intravenous.

VI.

1. w;   **2.** x;   **3.** z;   **4.** f;   **5.** q;   **6.** a;   **7.** l;   **8.** t;   **9.** h;
10. i;   **11.** k;   **12.** u;   **13.** r;   **14.** m;   **15.** n;   **16.** p;   **17.** o;
18. j;   **19.** b;   **20.** c;   **21.** e;   **22.** d;   **23.** g;   **24.** s;
25. y;   **26.** v.

VII.

	Word/Phrase	*Meaning*
1.	ad libitum	freely, as desired
2.	osulus sinister	left eye
3.	cum	with
4.	pro re nata	when needed
5.	sine	without
6.	aqua destillata	distilled water
7.	non repetatur	do not repeat
8.	quaque hora	hourly
9.	ut dictum	as directed
10.	ante cibum	before meals
11.	gutta(e)	drop(s)
12.	oculus uterque	each eye
13.	si opus est	if it is needed
14.	quater in die	four times a day
15.	agita	stir, shake

18 Oncology

COMBINING FORMS

	Meaning	*Example*
TUM/O (tou'mo)	swelling	TUMOR (tou'mor), a swelling
ONC/O (ong'ko)	mass, tumor	ONCOGENIC (ong-ko-jen'ik), tumor producing
-PLASM (plaz'im)	something formed	NEOPLASM (nee-o-plaz'im), abnormal formation of new tissue, a tumor
NE/O (nee'o)	new	NEONATE (nee'o-nayt), newborn
CARCIN/O (kar'si-no)	cancer	CARCINOGENIC (kar-si-no-jen'ik), cancer producing
-CARCINOMA (kar-si-no'ma)	malignant tumor developing from epithelial tissue	ADENOCARCINOMA (ad-e-no-kar-si-no'ma), malignant tumor developing from glandular tissue
SARC/O (sar'ko)	flesh	SARCOPOIETIC (sar-ko-poy-et'ik), producing flesh or connective tissue
-SARCOMA (sar-ko'ma)	malignant tumor developing from connective tissue	LIPOSARCOMA (lip-o-sar-ko'ma), malignant tumor containing fat
MUT/O (mu'to)	change	MUTAGEN (mu'ta-jen), an agent that produces change
VIR/O (vy'ro)	virus	VIRAL (vy'ral), pertaining to a virus
META- (me'ta)	beyond, after	METASTASIS (me-tas'ta-sis), movement of cancer cells beyond their original place of development
-GNOSIS (no'sis)	knowledge	PROGNOSIS (prog'no'sis), determining the outcome of a disease

Oncology is the study of tumors and their treatment. A *tumor*, also called a *neoplasm*, is a mass of abnormal cells or tissues that grow uncontrollably. Each neoplasm develops from a single cell that has undergone a genetic alteration. Tumors

333

are generally classed into two groups. *Benign tumors* are noncancerous neoplasms; *malignant tumors* are cancerous and hence life threatening.

Benign and malignant growths differ in several ways. Malignant neoplasms grow rapidly; benign neoplasms, on the other hand, grow slowly and the number of cell divisions (mitoses) is far less in comparison with malignant neoplasms. Benign neoplasms are *encapsulated* and do not do much damage to surrounding tissue. Malignant growths, however, are *invasive* (spread to surrounding tissue). Not only do malignant neoplasms destroy surrounding tissue, but they also infiltrate blood and lymph vessels from which they spread to other areas of the body. This migration to other areas of the body is called *metastasis.*

Cancer cells show a high degree of *anaplasia* (reversion to a more primitive form). These anaplastic cells resemble primitive, fetal-like cells. They grow rapidly (hyperplasia) and do not *differentiate*—that is, function like normal cells and join with other cells to form normal tissue.

TYPES OF TUMORS

All tumors are named according to the type of tissue from which they develop. Noncancerous tumors have the suffix *-oma* added to the tissue type. For example, an aden*oma* is a benign tumor originating in the glandular epithelium. The suffixes *-carcinoma* and *-sarcoma* indicate malignant tumors. *Carcinomas* are the most common form of cancer. They can arise from both external and internal epithelial tissue. They readily infiltrate surrounding tissue and quickly metastasize. The word adeno*carcinoma* indicates cancer of the glandular epithelium. *Sarcomas* are malignant tumors developing from connective tissue (bone, fat, muscle, blood, etc.). Lympho-*sarcoma*, for instance, is cancer of lymphatic tissue. A third type of cancerous tumor is a combination of epithelial and connective tissue. These tumors are called *mixed tissue tumors. Wilms' tumor*, which occurs in children, is an example of a mixed tissue tumor. Here are some examples of various types of tumors.

Origin	*Benign Form*	*Malignant Form*
Squamous epithelium	Papilloma	Squamous carcinoma
Blood vessels	Hemangioma	Hemangiosarcoma
Smooth muscle	Leiomyoma	Leiomyosarcoma
Striated muscle	Rhabdomyoma	Rhabdomyosarcoma
Bone	Osteoma	Osteosarcoma
Cartilage	Chondroma	Chondrosarcoma

In addition to their histologic classification, tumors are also classified according to stage of development. In the *TNM* classification tumors are classed according to their size (*T*umor), the degree of lymph node invasion (lymph *N* odes), and their spread to other areas of the body (*M*etastasis). Here is a list of the stages of tumor development.

Stage 0. The tumor is limited to a small area. This is frequently referred to as *carcinoma in situ.*

Stage I. The tumor spreads but does not seriously infiltrate surrounding tissue.

Stage II. Surrounding tissue is infiltrated extensively.

Stage III. The tumor invades surrounding lymph and blood vessels.

Stage IV. Metastasis has occurred.

The microscopic evaluation of tumor cells is called *grading.* Unlike *staging,* grading is concerned with the degree of anaplasia of the malignant cells. Grade I cells are much like normal cells in their degree of differentiation. With each succeeding grade, differentiation is reduced and anaplasia becomes more prominent. The size and type of the tumor and the stage of development are the most important factors for a favorable prognosis.

ETIOLOGY OF CANCER

Whatever factors are given as the causes of cancer, the underlying cause of all cancer is DNA or RNA *mutation.* DNA is the substance of genes that contains the hereditary traits of an organism. DNA's two basic functions are *cellular replication* and *protein synthesis.* When cell division occurs, each DNA molecule, which resembles a double spiral (called a *helix,* HELIC/O spiral), unwinds, and each DNA strand serves as a pattern or mold called a *template* for the formation of a new DNA strand. The result is two pairs of spirals. This replication occurs in all genes and results in the formation of a double set of chromosomes, one set for each new cell. The other function of DNA is protein synthesis. DNA itself is made from a sequence or pattern of four bases. These bases are *adenine, quanine, cytosine,* and *thymine.* The arrangement of these bases on the DNA molecule determines the proteins that each cell can produce. We call this arrangement of bases on DNA the *genetic code.* To carry out protein synthesis, DNA manufactures a messenger, RNA (ribonucleic acid), which enters the cytoplasm and attaches itself to the ribosomes (where protein is synthesized) located on the endoplasmic reticulum. The sequence of the bases on the messenger RNA establishes the pattern for the arrangement of *amino acids* (substances that make up proteins), thus determining the type of protein and enzymes (complex proteins that each cell can manufacture. Therefore any mutation of the DNA molecule or RNA messenger alters the arrangement of the amino acids, which results in the production of different proteins by the cell. Consequently, the affected cells grow differently and lack the differentiation characteristic of normal cells.

Several factors are known to cause cellular mutation.

Heredity

A definite pattern of inherited cancers has not been established for most cancers; because some families have a higher incidence of cancer than others, however, the likelihood of inheriting a predisposition to cancer is increased. Retinoblastoma, cancer of the eye occurring in childhood, adenomas of the thyroid and parathyroids, and colonic polyposis are considered inheritable neoplasms.

Precancerous disorders

Several nonneoplastic disorders have been linked to cancer. The increased and extensive cellular growth caused by these disorders may predispose them to form neoplasms. Some examples of precancerous disorders are listed below.

Precancerous Disorder	*Cancer*
Leukoplakia	Squamous cancer of the mouth
Cirrhosis of the liver	Hepatic cell adenocarcinoma
Chronic ulcerative colitis	Colonic adenocarcinoma
Chronic cervicitis	Squamous cancer of the cervix
Chronic balanitis	Squamous cancer of the penis
Paget's disease of the bone	Osteosarcoma
Aplastic anemia	Acute leukemia

Viruses

Viruses are minute organisms consisting of a strand of RNA or DNA covered by a protein shell. Since viruses are *parasites*, they cannot carry on life processes and reproduce unless they are in a *host* organism. Viruses cause cell mutation by injecting themselves into the DNA or RNA of a cell. Although viruses can cause cancer in laboratory animals, their link to cancer in humans has not been fully established. We do know, however, that certain viruses can cause cancer in humans. The virus that causes infectious mononucleosis, for example, is also the cause of Burkitt's lymphoma, a malignant tumor of the jaw.

Environmental factors

Several cancer-producing or *carcinogenic* agents exist in our environment, naturally or artificially, as a result of industrialization and technology. Several chemical substances are known carcinogens, and the people most frequently affected are the workers who are exposed daily to these substances. Below are examples of carcinogens produced by man.

1. Aromatic amines, such as *b*-naphthylamine, produce papillomas and bladder cancer. Workers in dye and pesticide plants can inhale or absorb these substances.
2. Petroleum products, waxes, tars, and similar items cause skin cancer in those working in such industries as refineries and asphalt companies.
3. Chromium and nickel produce cancer of the nasal cavity, sinus, and bronchus in workers mining and refining these substances.

4. Coal derivatives, such as coal tar, pitch, and creosote, produce skin cancer and cancer of the larynx and bronchus in coke oven workers, coal tar distillers, and those working in certain areas of the lumber and chemical industries.
5. Radiation is a potent carcinogen. Radiologists and others working near radiation have a high incidence of leukemia and skin and bone cancer.

Besides job-related carcinogens, most people are exposed to several potent cancerous agents. The hydrocarbons produced by automobiles and cigarette smoke cause cancer of the skin, bladder, and respiratory tract and organs. Food additives, such as nitrates in bacon and other meats, have been linked to gastrointestinal cancer. Chemicals like vinyl chloride are widely used in homes and are now considered carcinogenic. Several potent carcinogens also exist in nature. Overexposure to sunlight is the most common cause of skin cancer. *Mycotoxins* produced by molds are also potent carcinogens. Food contaminated with molds has been linked to liver cancer.

DIAGNOSIS OF CANCER

Several methods exist for diagnosing malignancies. The earlier the diagnosis, the more positive the prognosis.

Self-examination
Every individual should be aware of the warning signs of cancer:

1. Unusual bleeding or discharge.
2. A lump.
3. A sore that does not heal.
4. A change in bowel or bladder habits.
5. A cough or hoarseness that persists.
6. Difficulty in swallowing or indigestion.
7. Any change in a wart or mole.
8. Weight loss for no apparent reason.

X ray
X rays are used to detect tumors in several areas of the body. Sometimes dyes are injected into blood vessels or substances are swallowed so that any obstruction (i.e., a tumor) to the paths left by these substances will appear on the x ray.

Exfoliative cytology
Cells are scrapped off the body surface or internal lining and examined microscopically for tumor cells. The Pap smear is an example of exfoliation.

Biopsy
Living tissue is removed for microscopic examination by a pathologist. In a *needle biopsy* a needle is injected into the suspected area and a tissue sample is removed for

microscopic evaluation. A *frozen section* is taken when a lump is surgically removed. A thin portion of the tumor is sliced, dyed, and quickly frozen. Next, it is examined microscopically to determine whether it is benign or malignant.

Biochemical diagnosis

Because cancer cells are highly anaplastic (undifferentiated and primitive), tumors produce *oncofetal antigens* that can be identified by a blood test or urinanalysis. For example, a *carcinoembryonic antigen* (CEA) is produced by colon cancers; *alpha-fetoprotein* (AFP) is produced by liver cancers.

TREATMENT

The method or combination of methods used to treat cancer depends on several factors, such as stage of tumor development, site of malignancy, and the general health of the individual.

Surgery

Surgery is used to remove a cancerous lesion or tumor. In their early stages, malignant tumors or skin cancers can be cured by surgery. Surgery is frequently used to relieve the effects of cancers. For example, obstructions caused by tumors or lesions can be surgically bypassed. Surgery to relieve the effects of cancer is called *palliative* (pal'le-a-tiv) *surgery*. Surgery is also used to remove tissue samples for biopsy.

Radiotherapy

Radiotherapy is the use of radiation to treat malignant tumors. Tumor tissue is destroyed by the *ionization* of the tissue cells. Since cancer cells grow at a faster rate than normal cells, they are more susceptible to the effects of radiation. *Irridation*, treatment by radiation, is given in small, frequent doses until a lethal dosage (about 300 radians) for most tumors is obtained. Radiation is especially effective in treating uterine and gonadal carcinomas, squamous carcinoma of the mouth and oropharynx, and Hodgkin's lymphoma. Some of the more common cancers, such as tumors of the breast and colon, are not effectively treated with radiation. Sometimes radiotherapy is used before surgery to shrink tumors so that they are more easily removed. After surgery, radiotherapy is used to destroy any remaining cancer cells. Unfortunately, several side effects accompany radiation treatment. Bone marrow is sometimes damaged, causing immunosuppression, which leaves an individual susceptible to various diseases. Also, surrounding tissue can be severely damaged by exposure to radiation, and there is the constant danger of producing cancer from exposure to radiation.

Chemotherapy

Antitumor drugs are effective in curing some tumors (e.g., placental and testicular tumors, Wilms' tumor, and Hodgkin's disease) and are also used to prolong the lives of patients with other types of malignancy. There are two types of antitumor drugs: *polyfunctional alkylating* (al'ki-lay-ting) *agents* and *metabolic antagonists. Nitrogen mustards* and *sulfonic acid esters* (An ester is a compound derived from an organic acid and alcohol.) are examples of alkylating agents; purine, pyrimidine analogs, and folic acid antagonists are examples of *antimetabolites. Combined chemotherapy*, the use of many drugs, has been successful in treating the more common tumors, such as breast cancer.

Antitumor drugs work in several ways to destroy cancer cells.

1. They prevent the formation of DNA.
2. They inactivate DNA.
3. They prevent RNA synthesis and protein synthesis.
4. They prevent cell division (mitosis).

As with radiotherapy, chemotherapy has several undesirable side effects. Injury to bone marrow, resulting in the reduction of white blood cells, the destruction of lymphocytes, and the reduction in the number of blood platelets (responsible for clotting) are the serious side effects. Vomiting, nausea, and diarrhea are some of the minor side effects.

Hormones have also been found useful in treating certain forms of cancer. For example, estrogen is used to treat cancer of the prostate. *Immunotherapy*, an offshoot of chemotherapy, aims at stimulating the patient's immune response against the tumor.

EXERCISES

I. Give the meaning for each of the following medical words. Divide each word into base(s), prefix, and suffix; underline the letter(s) that has the primary stress. *Example:*

CHONDROCARCINOMA   cartilaginous cancer   chondr/o/carcin/oma
....

1. ARTHRONCUS   ....

2. CARCINOEMBRYONIC   ....

3. RHABDOMYOSARCOMA   ....

4. VIREMIA   ....

5. METABOLISM   ....

6. RADIOPHARMACEUTICALS   ....

7. ACROGNOSIS   ....

8. TUMEFACIENT ....

9. ONCOSIS ....

10. NEOPLASIA ....

11. CARCINOGEN ....

12. PHLEBOCARCINOMA ....

13. MUTAGENESIS ....

14. SARCOMPHALOCELE ....

15. RADIODERMATITIS ....

16. METAMORPHOSIS (MORPH/O form) ....

17. INTUMESCENCE ....

18. NEONATAL (NAT/O birth, born) ....

19. PROTOPLASM ....

20. VIRICIDAL ....

II. Make medical words from the following phrases. Indicate the primary stress by underlining the stressed letter(s). *Example:*

producing a tumor

tumorigenic
....

1. the study of tumors and their treatment

....

2. malignant tumor developing from epithelial tissue

....

3. pertaining to the formation of new, abnormal tissue

....

4. surgical formation of a *new* opening

....

5. fleshlike

. . . .

6. study of viruses and viral diseases

. . . .

7. malignant tumor developing from smooth muscle

. . . .

8. destruction of tissue by radiation

. . . .

9. containing a tumor(s)

. . . .

10. cellular protoplasm

. . . .

11. malignant bone tumor

. . . .

12. a fleshy tumor (of the testicle)

. . . .

13. tumor of the breast

. . . .

14. pertaining to a substance that destroys cancer cells

. . . .

15. one who treats and diagnoses cancer

. . . .

III. Identify each term below as the quality of a benign (B) or a malignant (M) tumor.

1. metastasize . . . .

2. frequent mitoses . . . .

3. slow growth . . . .

4. rapid growth ....

5. encapsulated ....

6. invasive ....

IV. Match the descriptions with their medical terms.

1. formation of new and abnormal cells ....   a. mixed tissue tumor

2. primitive, dedifferentiated type of cells ....   b. grading

3. rapid, abnormal growth ....   c. sarcoma

4. normal cellular function and specialization ....   d. metastasis

5. malignancy of epithelial origin ....   e. anaplasia

6. malignancy arising from connective tissue ....   f. hyperplasia

7. malignancy arising from both epithelial and connective

    tissue ....   g. neoplasm

                                              h. carcinoma

8. cancer in its earliest stage ,.........   i. differentiation

9. spread of cancer to other areas of the body ....   j. carcinoma in situ

10. microscopic evaluation of a tumor ....

V. Give the names for both the benign and malignant tumors arising from the tissues listed below.

Tissue	Benign Tumor	Malignant Tumor
1. skeletal muscle	....	....
2. bone	....	....
3. glandular epithelium	....	....
4. blood vessels	....	....
5. fat	....	....

6. fibrous tissue ....

7. visceral muscle ....

8. cartilage ....

      VI. Fill in the blank spaces for the following statements.

1. The two basic functions of DNA are .... and

    ....

2. .... of DNA is the cause of cancerous growth.

3. Each DNA strand serves as a pattern called a .... for the formation of a new DNA strand.

4. ...., ..., ..., and ....

    are the bases of DNA.

5. The arrangement of the bases on DNA is called the ....

6. .... functions as a messenger from DNA to the ribosomes on the endoplasmic reticulum.

7. .... occurs in the ribosomes.

8. .... are the substances that make up protein.

9. Specialization characteristic of normal cells is called ....

10. .... is an inheritable cancer of the eye that occurs in childhood.

11. Name the precancerous disorders that cause each of the following cancers:

    squamous cancer of the mouth ....

    hepatic cell adenocarcinoma ....

    acute leukemia ....

    squamous cancer of the cervix ....

12. Viruses are .... that carry on their vital functions inside a ....

    organism.

13. Environmental agents capable of producing cancer in man or laboratory animals are

     referred to as ....

14. .... are cancer-causing substances produced by molds.

VII.   Briefly respond to the following questions or statements.

1. List the eight warning signs of cancer.

(a) ....

(b) ....

(c) ....

(d) ....

(e) ....

(f) ....

(g) ....

(h) ....

2. How are dyes used to detect cancer?

3. Scraping cell samples from the body surface or internal lining is called ....

     ....

4. Name and briefly describe the two types of biopsy.

(a) ....

(b) ....

5. How is cancer diagnosed, using a biochemical analysis?

6. List three reasons for performing surgery on a cancer patient.

(a) ....

(b) ....

(c) ....

7. What aspect of cancerous cells makes them more susceptible to the effects of radiation than normal cells?

8. How is radiation effectively used before and after cancer surgery?

9. What are the two types of antitumor drugs?

    (a) ....

    (b) ....

10. List the four ways by which antitumor drugs destroy cancer cells.

    (a) ....

    (b) ....

    (c) ....

    (d) ....

ANSWERS TO EXERCISES

I.

1. tumor of a joint, arthr/onc/us
2. pertaining to embryonic substances (antigens) secreted by cancerous tissue, carcin/o/embryon/ic
3. cancerous tissue developing from striated (skeletal) muscle, rhabd/o/my/o/sarc/oma
4. presence of viruses in the blood, vir/emia
5. transformation of substances into energy and wastes, meta/bol/ism
6. radioactive substances administered to a patient so their course through a hollow structure of the body can be traced, radi/o/pharmc/eutic/als
7. awareness of one's limbs, acr/o/gnosis
8. producing a swelling, tum/e/fac/i/ent
9. condition giving rise to tumors, onc/osis
10. abnormal formation of new tissues, ne/o/plas/ia
11. cancer-producing agent, carcin/o/gen
12. cancer of a vein, phleb/o/carcin/oma
13. the process of producing a change, mut/a/gen/esis
14. fleshy tumor of the umbilicus, sarc/omphal/o/cele
15. inflammation of the skin caused by x rays or other forms of radiation, radi/o/dermat/itis
16. change in for, transformation, meta/morph/osis
17. a swelling or the process of swelling, in/tum/esc/ence
18. pertaining to a newborn infant or the first four weeks after birth, ne/o/nat/al
19. thick, colloidal substance that is the basis for all life, prot/o/plasm
20. destructive to viruses, vir/i/cid/al

II.

1. on<u>col</u>ogy;   **2.** carci<u>nom</u>a;   **3.** neo<u>plas</u>tic;   **4.** ne<u>os</u>tomy;   **5.** <u>sar</u>coid;
6. vi<u>rol</u>ogy;   **7.** leiomyosar<u>com</u>a;   **8.** radione<u>cros</u>is;   **9.** <u>tum</u>orous;
10. <u>cy</u>toplasm;   **11.** osteosar<u>com</u>a;   **12.** <u>sar</u>cocele;   **13.** mast<u>on</u>cus;
14. carcino<u>lyt</u>ic;   **15.** on<u>col</u>ogist.

III. 1. M;   **2.** M;   **3.** B;   **4.** M;   **5.** B;   **6.** M.

IV.

1. g;   **2.** e;   **3.** f;   **4.** i;   **5.** h;   **6.** c;   **7.** a;   **8.** j;
9. d;   **10.** b.

V.

Benign Tumor   *Malignant Tumor*
1. rhabdomyoma   rhabdomyosarcoma
2. osteoma   osteosarcoma
3. adenoma   adenocarcinoma
4. hemangioma   hemangiosarcoma
5. lipoma   liposarcoma
6. fibroma   fibrosarcoma
7. leiomyoma   leiomyosarcoma
8. chondroma   chondrosarcoma

VI.

1. cellular replication, protein synthesis
2. mutation
3. template
4. adenine, quanine, cytosine, thymine
5. genetic code
6. RNA (ribonucleic acid)
7. protein synthesis
8. amino acids
9. differentiation
10. retinoblastoma
11. leukoplakia
cirrhosis of the liver
aplastic anemia
chronic cervitis
12. parasites, host
13. carcinogenic
14. mycotoxins

VII.

1. (a) unusual bleeding or discharge
(b) a lump

    (c) a sore that doesn't heal
    (d) a change in bowel or bladder habits
    (e) a cough or hoarseness that is persistent
    (f) difficulty in swallowing or indigestion
    (g) any change in a wart or mole
    (h) weight loss for no apparent reason

2. They enable an obstruction of a vessel or hollow structure to show up on an x ray.

3. exfoliative cytology

4. (a) Needle biopsy. A needle is injected into the tumor and a tissue sample is removed for microscopic examination.
    (b) Frozen section. After a tumor is surgically removed, a portion of it is sliced, dyed, and frozen so that it can be examined microscopically.

5. Malignant tumors produce oncofetal antigens that appear in both the blood and the urine.

6. (a) to remove the tumor to obtain a full or partial cure
    (b) to relieve the effects of cancer (palliative surgery)
    (c) to remove a tissue sample for biopsy

7. their growth rate

8. before—to shrink a tumor so that it can be removed more easily
after—to destroy remaining cancerous cells

9. (a) polyfunctional alkylating agents
    (b) metabolic antagonists or antimetabolites

10. (a) prevent the formation of DNA
    (b) inactivate DNA
    (c) prevent RNA formation
    (d) prevent cell division (mitosis)

19 Radiology and Surgery

COMBINING FORMS

	Meaning	*Example*
RADI/O (ray'de-o)	ray, radioactive substance	RADIOLOGY (ray-de-ol'o-je), branch of medicine that uses x rays or radiation to diagnose and treat disease
ROENTGEN/O (rent-gen'o)	x rays	ROENTGENOGRAM (rent-gen'o-gram), an x ray
LUC/O (lu'ko)	light	RADIOLUCENT (ray-de-o-lu'sent), pertaining to a substance through which x rays are able to pass
PHOT/O (fo'to)	light	PHOTOFLUOROGRAM (fo-to-flur'o-gram), picture of a fluoroscopic image
CINE/O (sin'e-o)	motion, movement	CINERADIOGRAPHY (sin-er-a-de-og'ra-fe), a series of x rays
TERAT/O (ter'a-to)	extremely deformed fetus	TERATOMA (ter-a-toe'ma), congenital tumor
IS/O (eye'so)	equal	ISOTOPE (eye'so-toep), a group of chemical substances having the same atomic number but different atomic weights
TOP/O (top'o)	place	TOPICAL (top'ik-al), pertaining to a specific place, local
ION/O (eye'o-no)	ion, an atom that has given up or gained an electron	ANIONS (an'eye-ons), negatively charged ions
IONT/O (eye-on'to)	ion, an atom that has given up or gained an electron	IONTORAIOMETER (eye-on-to-ray-de-om'i-ter), an instrument for measuring the amount and intensity of x rays

	Meaning	*Example*
TEL- (tel′) TELE- (tel′e)	far, distant	TELETHERAPY (tel-e-ther′a-pe), treatment in which the radio-active substance is kept at a distance from the patient
SURGIC/O (sur′ji-ko)	surgery	SURGICAL (sur′ji-kal), pertaining to surgery
-SURGERY (sur′jur-e)	surgery	NEUROSURGERY (nu-ro-sur′jur-e), surgery of the nervous system, especially the brain
SEC/O (sek′o)	cut	RESECTION (ree-sek′shun), excision of a part of a structure
PALLI/O (pal′e-o)	relief, alleviation	PALLIATIVE (pal′e-a-tiv), relieving, alleviating
RADIC/O (rad′i-ko)	root	RADICAL (rad′i-kal), pertaining to the root, extensive surgery
OBSTETRIC/O (ob-ste′trik-o)	midwife, obstetrician obstetrics	OBSTETRICIAN (ob-ste-trish′an), a physician who specializes in treating women during pregnancy and childbirth
SEPT/O (sep′to)	rotting, putrefaction	ANTISEPTIC (an-ti-sep′tik), preventing putrefaction by destroying or inhibiting microorganisms
HAL/O (hal′o)	salt	HALOGEN (hal′o-jen), substance that produces salt
VIT/O (vy′to)	life	VITAL (vy′tal), pertaining to life
STERE/O (ster′e-o)	solid, having three dimensions	STEREOTACTIC (ster-e-o-tak′tik), pertaining to three-dimensional x rays
-TAXIS (tak′sis)	arrangement, regulation	THERMOTAXIS (ther-mo-taks′is), regulation of body temperature
CRY/O (kry′o)	cold	CRYOSURGERY (kry-o-sur′jur-e), the surgical use of substances that produce extremely low temperatures
SON/O (soo′no)	sound	ULTRASONIC (ul-tra-son′ik), beyond the ability of the human ear to hear
ULTRA- (ul′tra)	beyond	ULTRAMICROBE (ul-tra-my′krob), a microorganism that is beyond the range of the microscope
CAUTER/O (kaw′ter-o)	burn	CAUTERY (kaw′ter-e), the destruction of tissue by burning with an instrument, the instrument itself

RADIOLOGY

Radiology is the area of medicine that uses radiation to diagnose and treat diseases.

X Rays

X rays, also called *roentgens* after their founder Wilhelm Roentgen, are electromagnetic waves that penetrate solid objects, such as an area of the body, and produce an image on photographic film. X rays are based on the principle that atoms give off energy in the form of rays or particles. These rays or particles have been named *alpha* (α), *beta* (β), and *gamma* (γ) rays or particles. This shedding of energy is called *radiation*. X-ray machines produce radiation in a vacuum tube. Here electrically produced electrons are sent out from the negative pole called a *cathode*. These electrons bombard the positive pole called the *anode*, resulting in the production of x rays (Figure 19-1).

A high-voltage emission of electrons results in shorter, more penetrating waves called *hard radiation*. X rays produced by low-voltage electrons (*soft radiation*) are longer, softer waves that are more easily absorbed by tissue. The extent to which body tissues absorb x rays provides the varying degrees of contrast that appear on x-ray negatives. Three factors determine the absorption capability of an object: (a) its atomic

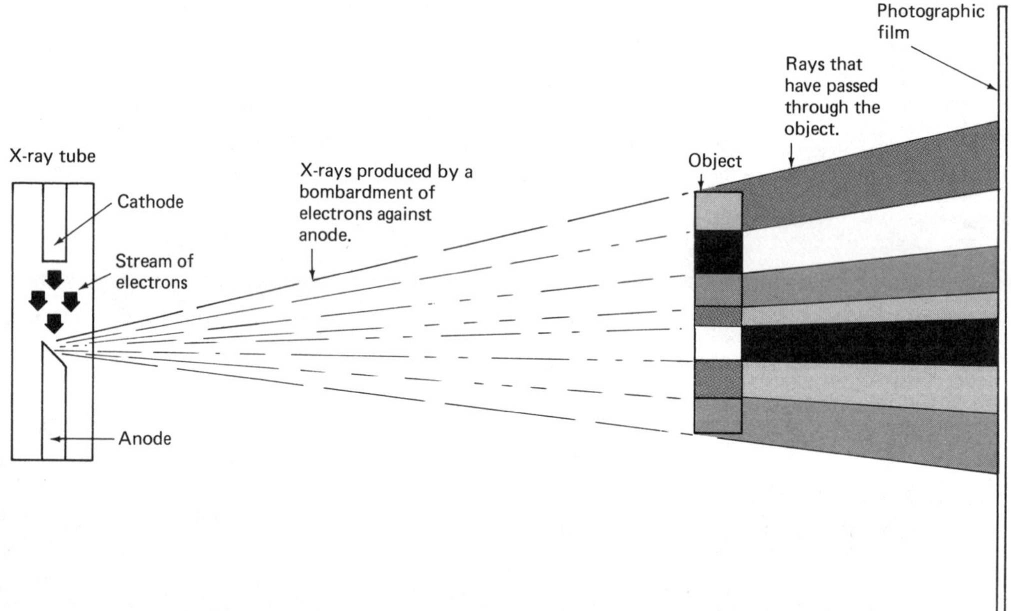

Figure 19-1 Diagram illustrating the differential absorption of x rays by various tissues. (Harvey, Johns, McKusick *et al.*, *The Principles and Practice of Medicine*, © 1980, Figure 2-2, p. 28. Adapted by permission of Appleton-Century-Crofts.)

number (number of protons in the nucleus of an atom), (b) its thickness, and (c) its overall density. Areas of low density readily transmit x rays and are referred to as *radiolucent* areas. A lung filled with air, for example, is radiolucent. Because areas of great density absorb the x rays, they are called *radiopaque*. Bones are radiopaque; therefore they will appear as light areas on an x-ray film called an *x ray*, an *x-ray plate*, or a *roentgenogram*. Soft tissue, because of its low density, will appear dark on an x ray.

X rays are a useful diagnostic tool only if they produce pictures that show body tissues clearly distinct from one another. When the tissues of an area of the body (e.g., the abdomen) provide little contrast for effective examination, certain substances are introduced to the area to provide greater contrast between the various tissues. These substances are called *contrast mediums*. *Barium* and *iodine* compounds are high-density contrast mediums; so they will appear light on x-ray films. Air, on the other hand, will absorb few x rays and will appear dark on the film. For example, in an *angiography*, a series of x rays to determine the condition of blood vessels, an opaque dye is injected into blood vessels to provide clear contrast. Contrast mediums are commonly used in x rays of the cardiovascular, lymphatic, digestive, and genitourinary systems and the spinal canal and bronchial tree (see Table 19-1 for additional uses of contrast media).

The following are special applications of x-ray technology.

Fluoroscopy (flur-os′ko-pe)

The individual is placed between the x-ray unit and a screen. The area x-rayed is reflected onto the screen, not x-ray film. The movements of the internal structures can be observed; the image produced by a *fluoroscope*, however, is dull and lacks the sharp contrast of an x-ray film. Devices called image intensifiers are used to improve the quality of the image. *Photofluorograms* are pictures taken during fluoroscopy.

Tomography

The x-ray tube and the film plate are moved according to a predetermined pattern during exposure so that, with the exception of the tissue under examination, all other tissue is blurred out. This procedure gives several views of the tissue being examined at different depths. Tomography is especially useful in focusing on tissues or areas that may be difficult to observe when placed within the surrounding tissue. For example, lesions of the ventricles of the brain are easier to detect by tomography (taken during *pneumoencephalography*). *Tomograms*, also called *laminograms* or *body section roentgenograms*, are the x-ray films produced in tomography.

Cineradiography

Cineradiography, also called *serial radiography*, is the production of a series of x rays like a motion picture to observe the functioning of an organ. For example, cineradiography is used to observe the actions of the heart valves and to note any defects. Also, by using cineradiography to record joint movements, orthopedic disorders can more easily be identified.

Table 19-1 Examples of X-ray Procedures Using Contrast Mediums or Tracer Substances

X Ray	Procedure	Diagnostic Purpose
Intravenous pyelogram (IVP)	A radiopaque dye is injected intravenously and x-ray films are taken at various intervals.	Decrease in kidney function, damage caused by hypertension, urinary tract obstruction
Myelogram	A contrast substance is injected into the sub-arachnoid space of the spinal cord (provides contrast for the cord, spinal canal, spinal roots).	Obstruction of the spaces of the spinal cord
Upper GI (gastrointestinal) series	Barium sulfate is swallowed and a series of x-ray films are taken as the barium passes through the GI tract.	Obstructions, such as tumors or abnormalities of the esophagus, stomach, and upper portion of the small intestines
Lower GI series (barium enema)	A barium enema is given so that the colon can be x-rayed.	Ulcerative colitis, tumors, diverticula
Arteriogram	A contrast substance is injected into the arteries.	Arterial obstruction
Lymphangiography	An oily contrast substance is injected into the lymph vessels to produce x-ray films of the lymph system, especially the pelvic and retroperitoneal lymph nodes.	Useful in determining Hodgkin's disease
Liver scan	By using a radioactive substance, a *photoscan* (also called a *scintiscan*) of the liver is produced. This gives an x-ray film of the shape and size of the liver.	Provides a map for liver biopsy, which is used to study more serious liver diseases, such as chronic hepatitis, cirrhosis, and cancer
Brain scan	The radioisotope technetium-99 is injected to reveal any abnormal brain lesions.	Used to detect vascular tumors, such as meningiomas and gliomas

Radiotherapy

Radiotherapy is the use of radiation to treat certain diseases. Malignant tumors are often treated by *irradiation*, the application of radiation to the tumor. When radiation is applied to a cell, the atoms of that cell become *ionized*—that is, they either gain or lose electrons. As a result, cellular functions become disrupted. Because they divide frequently, malignant cells are highly susceptible to irradiation. Radiation is applied in frequent, small doses until a level lethal to the tumor has been reached. Leukemias, lymphomas, embryonic-type tumors called *teratomas*, skin cancers, and cancers of the lips, tongue, and nasopharynx respond favorably to radiation treatment. Tumors originating from muscle, bone, and nerve tissues don't respond as well to radiotherapy. Radiation is also used to shrink a tumor prior to surgery or to destroy any cancerous cells that may remain after surgery. Unfortunately, some side effects accompany radiation treatment. The skin of the area being irradiated becomes irritated, and nausea, vomiting, malaise, and even fever frequently accompany treatment.

Radioisotopes

In addition to x-ray therapy, radioactive substances called *radioisotopes* are used in several ways to treat cancer. The use of radioactive substances to treat cancer or as tracer substances in an organ (called *tagged* substances) has become a specialized field within radiology known as *nuclear medicine*. Radioisotopes have two significant advantages over conventional x-ray therapy. First, the powerful emission produced by a radioisotope is without any electrical equipment. Secondly, skin and bone damage— common in x-ray therapy—is significantly reduced by using radioisotopes. Here are some forms of treatment employing radioisotopes.

Teletherapy. The radioactive substance is kept in a protective container at a distance (6 to 7 feet) from the patient. Gamma rays are emitted from the radioisotope, such as cobalt-60 or cesium-137, and absorbed by the patient.

Radioisotope molds. The radioactive substance is either sealed in a small container and placed directly onto the affected area or it is dispersed onto some material, such as plastic or paper, that is attached directly to the skin.

Intracavitary isotope therapy. The radioisotope is placed directly into a body cavity or hollow organ. For example, radioactive colloidal gold or sodium is placed in a balloon inside the bladder. Encapsulated radioactive substances are placed directly into certain hollow areas of the body—for example, the uterus.

Interstitial isotope therapy. Radioisotopes in the form of needles called *seeds* are implanted directly into the tumor.

Radioisotope injections. The effectiveness of radioactive solutions injected into the body is based on their affinity for certain body tissues. Radioactive iodine, for instance, is effective in treating malignant thyroid tissue because it concentrates in thyroid tissue. Similarly, radioactive phosphorus has an affinity for bone tissue. The tissue in which a radioactive substance accumulates is called a *target*.

SURGERY

Surgery is the treatment of a disease or disorder through an operation in which diseased tissue is removed, a damaged structure is repaired, symptoms are relieved, or any combination of the preceding is performed. So although surgical procedures vary according to the area of the body, the tissue or organ involved, and the nature of the disorder, all surgery has one or more of the following purposes:

1. To repair a damaged or defective organ.
2. To remove a diseased organ or tissue (called *extirpative surgery*, eks-tir'pa-tiv, EXTIRP/O uprooting;
   debridement, day-breed-mon', is the removal of foreign substances and dead tissue from a wound).
3. To relieve the symptoms of a disease or disorder (called *palliative surgery*).
4. To transplant tissues or organs.

The *surgeon* is the individual who specializes in performing operations. The *general surgeon* is familiar with surgery in all areas of the body. Today the general surgeon deals with those areas of the body not treated by the special surgeon. The gastrointestinal tract, tumors, especially breast tumors, and amputations are some of the types of surgery performed by the general surgeon. Surgeons are usually specialists in a specific area of medicine. Here are some examples.

Orthopedic surgery

Orthopedic surgery deals with the treatment of *fractures* (broken bones). Congenital defects, such as scoliosis and clubfoot, are also treated by orthopedic surgeons.

Plastic surgery

Plastic surgery deals with the repair of external acquired and congenital defects. *Skin grafting* is the application of skin from one area of the body to a damaged area (e.g., a burned area). The *dermatome*, a special instrument for cutting skin, is used to remove skin for grafts. Plastic surgeons also perform cosmetic surgery to reduce signs of aging, such as wrinkles and sagging cheeks.

Ophthalmic surgery

The two most common disorders treated by ophthalmic surgeons are the removal of cataracts and the relief of intraocular pressure caused by glaucoma.

Otolaryngolic surgery

This branch of surgery is concerned with diseases of the ears and the throat, especially the larynx. Surgery to restore hearing and the removal of a cancerous larynx (laryngectomy) are performed by otolaryngologists.

Neurosurgery

Operations on the brain are usually performed to remove tumors or to repair damage caused by skull fractures.

Thoracic surgery

Generally the term thoracic surgery indicates surgery of any organ in the thoracic cavity. The heart and lungs are the most important organs treated by thoracic surgeons. Acquired and congenital heart disease and both lung and esophageal cancer are the disorders commonly treated by thoracic surgeons. Subdivisions of this branch of surgery are also common—for example, cardiovascular surgeons.

Surgery of the urinary tract and reproductive organs

Surgery of the urinary tract and male reproductive organs is performed by a *urological surgeon*. Prostatectomy, a partial or total removal of the prostate gland, is a common operation performed by urosurgeons. *Gynecologists* specialize in treating disorders and diseases of the female reproductive organs. The two most common operations performed by gynecologists are the removal of cancerous growths of the female reproductive organs and the removal of all or a portion of the reproductive organs (hysterectomy). The care of a woman throughout pregnancy and immediately after childbirth is handled by an *obstetrician*. Two operations performed by an obstetrician are an *episiotomy*, the cutting of the perineum for easier delivery, and a *cesarean section*, delivery through the uterus. Obstetricians also treat complications that arise during delivery.

Asepsis

Because surgery involves cutting the skin to enter the body, strict precautions must be taken to prevent harmful microorganisms from entering the body. The prevention of microorganisms from entering the body and causing an infection is called *asepsis*. Before the operation, all objects that will come in contact with the area to be operated must be made *sterile*. Linens, pans, jars, and similar items are placed in a chamber called an *autoclave* (aw'to-klayv) where they are sterilized by pressurized steam at temperatures of 115°C and higher. Pressurized-steam sterilization destroys both microorganisms and their spores. Surgical instruments are placed in a chamber similar to the autoclave. Instruments and rubber parts that are damaged by steam can be sterilized with gas and disinfectants. *Disinfectants* are chemicals that destroy microorganisms or limit their growth. The operating room is thoroughly cleansed with disinfectants, and the surgical team apply a disinfectant to their hands and arms after scrubbing. Here is a list of some of disinfectants commonly used.

Type	*Example*	*Comments*
Alcohols	Ethyl, isopropyl	Widely used to disinfect skin
Phenols and their derivatives (cresols)	Hexachlorophine	Now thought to be carcinogenic
Oxidants	Hydrogen peroxide potassium permanganate	"Foaming" substances, kill germs by freeing oxygen
Halogens	Iodine, betadine	Used as surface germicides

Anesthesia

The loss of sensation in all or part of the body can be artificially induced in the operating room by the use of an anesthesia-producing drug. Unconsciousness may also accompany the loss of sensation. The *anesthesiologist* administers the anesthesia and is responsible for monitoring the patient's *vital signs*—pulse, blood pressure, and respiration—and for keeping any other records used in that operation (e.g., electrocardiogram, electroencephalogram).

A *general anesthetic* produces a loss of sensation in the entire body and unconsciousness. The effects of a general anesthetic occur in three stages.

Stage I. Blood pressure is normal. Pupils react normally to light and the pulse is irregular.

Stage II. Blood pressure is high. Pupils are dilated and the pulse is rapid.

Stage III. This is usually referred to as the operative stage. Blood pressure is normal and the pupils are small. The pulse is regular but slow.

General anesthetics are administered by having the patient breathe a gas or inhale a vapor given off by a liquid. Both types of administration are called *inhalation anesthesia.* Such liquids as ethyl ether, halothane, methoxyflurane, divinyl ether, ethyl chloride, and trichlorethane are examples of vaporized anesthetics. Examples of gases are nitrous oxide, ethylene, and cyclopropane. Most general anesthetics have several drawbacks, making their use in certain operations undesirable or even hazardous. The disadvantages range from explosibility to mucous accumulation and nausea.

Besides inhalation anesthetics, certain general anesthetics can be administered intravenously. The most widely used *intravenous general anesthetic* is sodium pentothal (thiopental, a barbiturate). Anesthesia is quick and postoperative complications, such as nausea and vomiting, are not common. Sodium pentothal is frequently administered in a mild form to relax patients given a spinal anesthetic.

Unlike general anesthetics, *area anesthetics* desensitize only a certain area of the body. There are three types of area anesthetics: spinal, regional, and local. A *spinal anesthetic* is injected into the subarachnoid space of the spinal column. Spinal anesthesia is commonly used in operations of the lower extremities and abdomen. Procaine (Novocaine, -caine is a derivative of cocaine), tetracaine (Pontocaine), and dibucaine (Nupercaine) are widely used spinal anesthetics. *Regional anesthetics* are injected into nerves supplying a particular region of the body. As a result, nerve impulses are blocked. Here are some examples of nerve *blocks.*

Brachial plexus block.   Entire area is anesthetized.

Paravertebral block.   Viscera and abdominal wall are anesthetized.

Transsacral or caudal block.   The perineum and portions of the lower abdomen are anesthetized.

Local anesthetics are injected into a certain area of tissue and produce anesthesia only in that area. The application of an anesthetic directly into the tissue to be cut is also called *infiltration anesthesia*. Local anesthetics are effectively used in operations that are short and require only a simple procedure. Dentists frequently use a local anesthetic before drilling into a tooth, and superficial wounds are normally sutured under a local anesthetic. Procaine, tetracaine, and lidocaine (Xylocaine) are examples of local anesthetics.

Operating positions

In positioning the patient on the operating table, the primary concern is the type of operation to be performed. Normally the patient is lying on his back until the anesthesia is administered. Here is a list of the common operating positions.

Supine (sou'pine, SUPIN/O lying on the back, also called dorsal recumbent)
The patient is flat on his back. This position is used for operations on the anterior surface of the body and many of the major body organs.

Trendelenburg position
This position provides for the clear exposure and separation of the abdominal organs. Both the patient's head and legs are lowered so that the body is curved. In the reverse Tredelenburg position, the patient's entire body is slanted in the direction of his feet. This position if used for gallbladder operations.

Sim's position
The patient is lying on her left side, chest partially prone, with her right thigh and knee drawn up. This position is used in operations on the cervix, for uterine curretage, and irrigation of the uterus after labor.

Fowler's position
The patient is in a partially sitting position. This position is used to facilitate breathing by improving lung expansion; it also prevents the pooling of blood in the pulmonary vessels.

Lithotomy position
This is the same as the supine position except that the patient's legs are raised and held in stirrups. This position is used in operations involving the pelvic organs and genitals.

Lateral position
The patient is placed on his side. This position is used in kidney operations.

Prone position (PRON/O lying face forward)
The patient is on his chest. This position is common in back and spine operations. The

jackknife is a prone position in which the patient's buttocks are raised. This position is used in surgery of the prostate.

Surgical Instruments

Today the surgeon makes use of a variety of instruments ranging from the simple knife (scalpel) used for centuries to complex devices, such as the heart–lung machine. Each surgical procedure involves the use of instruments made specifically for that procedure or a particular structure of the body. The instruments most commonly used in making and closing an incision are called a *simple instrument setup*. In the operating room the *Mayo instrument stand* holds the simple instrument setup, and special instruments needed for the operation are placed on another instrument stand. A basic instrument setup contains the following items.

    Scalpel.   Scalpels are surgical knives used to cut tissue. They may have permanent or removable blades.

    Scissors.   A scissors is a two-edged cutting instrument. Scissors come in all sizes and shapes—straight, curved, angular.

    Forceps.   Forceps are used for holding or removing objects. They come in a variety of shapes, sizes, and type of teeth.

    Hemostats.   Hemostats are special forceps that are used to block blood vessels to keep blood loss to a minimum. Their shapes and sizes vary according to the blood vessels and tissues where they are used.

    Retractors.   These instruments hold back tissues and muscles so that the operative site is clearly exposed.

    Probe.   Probes are used for the in-depth examination of tissue.

    Suture needles and suture materials.   These devices are used to close an incision.

    The names for most surgical instruments, such as scissors, clamps, saws, and drills, indicate both their function and their general shapes. Many instruments are named after the individuals who developed them.

    Below is a list of surgical instruments and procedures with which you should be familiar.

       amputation.   The surgical removal of a body part

       anastomosis.   The surgical formation of a passageway between two structures

       apposition.   The adding or placing of several layers of tissue and properly fitting them

       approximation.   The nearness or closeness to a structure

       avulsion.   The tearing away of a body part, e.g. the fingers. Through surgery the part can sometimes be reattached.

       bougie (boo'zhee).   A cylindrical device used to dilate and examine canals

cannula (kan′ou-la).   A hollow metal tube containing a trocar

catheter (kath′e-ter).   A tube inserted into vessels or canals to introduce or to remove fluids, or to keep the passageway open

clamp.   A surgical device used to hold in place tissue, veins, etc.

clips.   Devices for holding or fastening

coaptation.   The process of fitting or matching the parts of a structure, e.g. the pieces of a fractured bone

crushing.   The reduction of a large object(s) into smaller objects, e.g. the crushing of a stone in the bladder

curet, currette (ku′ret).   A scraper that is shaped like a spoon. It is used for removing substances from a cavity. For example, in a D and C (dilatation and curettage) the uterine wall is scraped.

debridement (day-breed-mon′).   The removal of infected or damaged tissue or foreign substances from a wound

decompression.   The release of pressure, e.g. gas or fluid, from a cavity or sack. The bladder can be decompressed with a catheter.

decortication.   The removal of the covering or outer portion of a structure

dehiscence (de-hiss′sense).   The splitting open of a wound

desiccation (des-i-kay′shun).   The process of drying up

destruction.   The death of tissue or of an organ

dilation.   The expansion of a structure by means of an instrument

disarticulation.   Amputation at a joint

dissection.   Cutting into parts

drainage.   The drawing off of fluid from a cavity. For example, after a choledochotomy, a T tube can be placed in the duct to keep it open and to allow for the drainage of bile.

drapes.   Plastic or cloth coverings used during surgery

dressing.   The covering applied to a wound, diseased area, or incision. Sometimes dressings are impregnated with antibacterial agents (e.g. nitrofurazone) or substances (e.g. scarlet red) that stimulate the growth of epithelial tissue (epithelization).

drill and burr.   The boring of a hole into a structure such as the cranium with a rotary type cutter

electrocoagulation.   The use of electrical current to promote coagulation

elevator.   An instrument used to raise a structure

endoscopes.   Tube-shaped devices equipped with a small light for viewing a hollow or cavity. Examples of endoscopes are the anoscope, proctoscope, and sigmoidoscope.

endoscopy.   The use of a tubelike device to examine a canal, passageway, or cavity

enucleation (e-new-klee-ay'shun).   The removal of a mass (e.g. a tumor) in its entirety

evacuation.   The removal of a substance from a cavity, e.g. stones from the bladder

evisceration.   The process of taking out the organs (viscera) from a cavity

exploratory surgery.   Surgery performed to find the origin of an ailment, for example, exploratory laparotomy

extirpation (eks-tir-pay'shun).   The surgical removal of a structure

fistulization (fis-tue-lie-zay'shun).   The process of making tubelike opening into a structure. This tubelike opening leads to the outside of the body or to another structure. For example, thoracic duct fistulas are used to drain off lymph.

fusion.   The joining of two parts or structures

gauze.   A loosely woven fabric

gouge.   An instrument for cutting bone tissue

graft.   The attaching of healthy skin or tissue to a damaged area of the body; *autograft:* tissue is taken from another area of the patient's body; *homograft:* tissue is taken from a donor (e.g., a cadaver); *heterograft* (also called xenograft): tissue is taken from an animal such as a pig (porcine xenograft).

hook.   A curved instrument used for holding, grabbing, or pulling

incision and drainage.   Cutting into a body cavity to withdraw fluid

insertion.   The process of implanting

introduction.   The insertion of an object or substance into the body or body structure

intubation.   The placement of a tube into a hollow structure, for example, the insertion of a tube into the larynx to facilitate breathing

implantation.   The insertion of a foreign substance into a body structure, for example, the placement of radioactive seeds into a tumor *irrigation.*   The process of cleansing a cavity/canal or wound with water or a specially prepared solution, for example, the irrigation of the external auditory canal with an irrigation syringe. An *irrigator* is a suction device used to introduce fluid into the cavity or wound.

ligation.   The tying of a blood vessel. A *ligature* is a piece of suture material used to tie a blood vessel.

manipulation.   The movement, by the hands, of body structures. For example, in rheumatoid arthritis, joint manipulations in which the joints are stretched are performed to provide relief from the adhesions.

marsupialization (mar-sou-pe-al-eye-zay'shun).   Surgically making a pouch from the sac left by a tumor that has been removed

needles.   Slender steel devices for puncturing, stitching, etc.

perfusion.   The passage of gasses or fluids through tissues, e.g. the perfusion of oxygen

prostheses.   Artificial devices or structures used to replace natural structures, for example, breast prosthesis used for mastectomy patients

reconstruction.   The surgical repair of functional or cosmetic deformities, for example, surgery to correct damage caused by burns

reduction.   The placement of a structure into its normal position, for example, properly aligning a fractured bone

repair.   To restore, through surgery, damaged tissue by replacement or by fixing the damage

resection.   The removal of a portion of a structure

rongeur (ron'zhur).   An instrument for removing pieces of bone

simple and radical excision.   Simple excision is the surgical removal of only the affected tissue or structure; radical excision is the removal of the affected tissue and a portion of the surrounding healthy tissue, for example, a simple and radical mastectomy.

shunt (by-pass).   A passage used to divert the flow of fluid, for example, the external shunt used in hemodialysis

snare.   An instrument having a wire loop that is used for removing growths such as polyps

speculum (SPECUL/O, mirror).   An instrument for dilating a canal so that it can be examined. For example, the vagina and cervix can be viewed by means of a speculum.

sponges.   Absorbent pads used in surgery to soak up fluids or to apply medication

stripping.   The use of pressure to remove the contents of a vessel, e.g. a blood vessel

suction.   The withdrawal from a cavity of a substance, especially a fluid or secretion, by means of a vacuum device, for example, the suctioning of respiratory secretions

tenaculum (ten-ak'ou-lum).   A hook-shaped instrument used to grasp and hold tissue (e.g. a blood vessel)

transplantation.   The removal of living tissue from one area of the body to another area, or from one individual to another

trephination (tref-in-ay'shun).   The removal of a portion of a bone with a cylindrical saw called a *trephine* (tree-fine')

trocar (tro'kar).   An instrument with a very sharp point that is used to puncture a cavity and to drain fluids. A trocar can be used to drain a blocked bladder.

The surgical incision is closed by suturing. A *suture* is a material substance used to close a wound so that healing may occur. There are basically two types of suture material: suture made from absorbable material and suture made from nonabsorbable material. Absorbable suture material, called surgical gut, is made from the collagenous tissues of animals (e.g., sheep's intestines) or from the fibrous tissues of beef cattle (called *fascia lata*, fa'she-a la'ta). The suture material is processed so that it can be packaged according to a specific gauge and tensile strength. The greatest advantage of natural suture material is that it is absorbed by the surrounding tissue. Since absorption rate is important, surgical gut may be treated to resist absorption for a longer period of time. *Type C* suture is surgical gut that has been chemically treated to resist absorption for a longer period. *Type A* suture has not been treated.

Nonabsorbable suture materials are not absorbed by the surrounding tissues during healing. Several nonabsorbable suture materials are available. Silk is a commonly used suture material. Other substances range from cotton and nylon to wire and Teflon. Their high tensile strength and nonirritating qualities make nonabsorbable materials excellent for suturing.

Suture needles are used to fasten the suture material to the tissue. There are three methods of classifying suture needles.

1. According to the eye of the needle
   (a) Ordinary round or square eye
   (b) Split-eye (French)—split at the end of the needle to facilitate threading
   (c) Atraumatic needle—suture is attached to the needle during manufacturing.

2. According to the tip of the needle
   (a) Cutting point—used to suture dense tissue
   (b) Tapered point—used for delicate tissue

3. According to the shape of the needle
   (a) Straight
   (b) Curved, semicurved, or any variation

Special Surgical Techniques

Astonishing progress has been made in surgical techniques and instruments so that today surgeons can work on the small, delicate structures of the eye, ear, and brain.

Stereotactic surgery

Stereotactic surgery has become an important area of neurosurgery in recent years. The brain is mapped out by the use of a special form of x ray called a *CAT scan* (*C*omputerized *A*xial *T*omography), which gives a three-dimensional x ray. The center of the disorder or the diseased tissue is located and a probe inserted into that site. The disorder is subjected to electrical, chemical, or cold treatment. Stereotactic surgery has made it possible to treat disorders centered in the brain that previously could not be accurately reached or that required extensive surgery. The use of the probe or electrode in stereotactic surgery requires only that a small hole be made in the skull.

Cryosurgery

In *cryosurgery* diseased tissue is destroyed by the application of an extremely cold substance. Hollow probes containing liquid nitrogen are used to freeze and remove the diseased tissue. The moist tissue quickly adheres to the probe and is then removed. Cataracts can be frozen and removed in this manner.

Microsurgery

The use of the *surgical microscope* has enabled surgeons to operate on structures that are difficult to see with normal vision. The repair of small blood vessels and nerves and operations on the eye, bile ducts, and reproductive organs can now be performed without harming surrounding structures by using the surgical microscope. *Microinstruments* and microsurgical procedures have been developed for use with the surgical microscope.

Ultrasonic and laser surgery

The application of ultrasonic and laser devices to surgery is still in its early stages. Ultrasonic units produce sound waves that are too high to be heard by the human ear. When directed at an area of the body, the sound waves bound back and their *echoes* or reflections are recorded by an instrument called an *oscilloscope*. The "echo" differs, depending on the depth and density of the tissue. The record produced by an oscilloscope is called an *echogram*. The echogram is especially helpful in locating structures deep within the brain. Surgically, ultrasonic devices can be used to dissolve cataracts or to destroy diseased nerve tissue in previously inaccessible areas of the brain.

The application of laser (*L*ight *A*mplification by *S*timulated *E*mission of *R*adiation) technology to surgery is still in its infancy. These beams of light can be used to *cauterize* (destroy by burning) diseased tissues, such as tumors.

EXERCISES

I. Give the meaning for each of the following medical words. Divide each word into base(s), prefix, and suffix; underscore the letter(s) that has the primary stress. *Example:*

IONIC   pertaining to ions   <u>ion</u>/ic

1. ISOMETRIC (METR/O measure) ....

2. TERATISM ....

3. TRANSECTION ....

4. ASTEREOGNOSIS ....

5. CRYOGEN ....

6. MULTISONOUS ....

7. RADIOTOXEMIA ....

8. LUCOTHERAPY ....

9. PHOTOKINETIC ....

10. CINECYSTOURETHROGRAM ....

11. ISOTONIA ....

12. TELALGIA ....

13. RADICIFORM ....

14. DISSECT ....

15. SEPTICEMIA ....

16. VITAMIN ....

17. CAUTERIZE ....

18. PALLIATE ....

19. SECTION ....

20. ISOMORPHOUS ....

21. ATAXIA ....

22. ELECTROCAUTERY ....

23. HALOID ....

24. ROENTGENOGRAPHY ....

25. PHOTOLYTIC ....

    II. Make medical words from the following phrases. Indicate the primary stress by underlining the stressed letter(s). *Example:*

instrument for measuring extremely cold temperatures

    cry<u>om</u>eter
....

1. out of place

....

2. to cut into two (parts)

....

3. the prevention of putrefaction

....

4. surgery using the surgical microscope

....

5. pertaining to a substance that absorbs radiation

....

6. the branch of medicine that deals with treating women during pregnancy and childbirth

....

7. using cold to treat a disease

....

8. cauterizing by using heat

....

9. image produced by ultra sound waves

....

10. production of severe deformities in a fetus

....

11. the treatment of a disease with x rays

....

12. allowing light to pass through

....

13. a writing or description of a particular area of the body

....

14. instrument for examining the depth of an object

....

15. abnormal fear of light

....

III.   Match the following descriptions with their medical words.

1. x rays ....   a. fluoroscope

2. negative pole of an x-ray machine ....   b. teletherapy

3. positive pole of an x-ray machine ....   c. target

4. produced by a high-voltage emission of electrons ....   d. contrast medium

5. allow x rays to pass   ....   e. cineradiography

6. absorb x rays   ....   f. roentgens

7. substance that is used to obtain better differentiation of

    x-rayed tissue   ....   g. radioisotope

8. instrument that projects the x-rayed image onto a

    screen   ....   h. cathode

9. a procedure for taking x rays in which everything but the

    tissue under examination is blurred out   ....   i. hard radiation

    j. seeds

10. a motion-picture or serial-type radiography   ....   k. anode

11. exposure of living tissue to radiation   ....   l. radiopaque

12. atomic alteration of a cell exposed to radiation   ....   m. irradiation

13. a radioactive substance used to treat malignancies   ....   n. translucent

14. a form of treatment in which the radioactive substance is   o. tomography

    kept at a distance from the patient   ....   p. ionization

15. radioactive needle implanted directly into malignant

    tissue   ....

16. the tissue for which a radioactive substance has an

    affinity   ....

     IV. Give the name of the surgical specialist who would perform the following operations.

1. surgery of the major organs of the chest   ....

2. cataracts   ....

3. fracture   ....

4. hysterectomy   ....

5. amputation   ....

6. skin grafting   . . . .

7. laryngectomy   . . . .

8. episiotomy   . . . .

9. brain tumor   . . . .

10. prostatectomy   . . . .

V. Fill in the blanks for the following statements.

1. Preventing microorganisms from entering the body and causing an infection is called

. . . .

2. An . . . . is a chamber in which lines, pan, etc. are sterilized.

3. Chemicals that are used to destroy microorganisms or inhibit their growth are called

. . . .

4. An . . . . administers anesthesia and monitors the . . . .

. . . .

5. Anesthetics that produce anesthesia in the entire body are called . . . .
anesthetics.

6. . . . . anesthetics are those anesthetics that are administered in the form of
a gas or vapor.

7. Sodium pentothal is a . . . . anesthetic that is administered . . . .

. . . .

8. A . . . . anesthetic is administered by injection into the subarachnoid space

of the . . . .

9. Regional anesthetics produce a . . . . in a particular area
of the body.

10. Another name for local anesthesia is . . . . anesthesia.

VI.   Multiple choice: Underline the correct letter.

1.   The operating position in which the patient is flat on his back
     (a) prone
     (b) Trendelenburg
     (c) supine
     (d) lithotomy

2.   A position that permits good exposure of the abdominal organs
     (a) lateral
     (b) supine
     (c) prone
     (d) Trendelenburg

3.   The position in which the patient is on his chest
     (a) prone
     (b) supine
     (c) lithotomy
     (d) lateral

4.   A spoon-shaped scraper
     (a) trocar
     (b) curette
     (c) tenaculum
     (d) endoscope

5.   An instrument for removing pieces of bone
     (a) gouge
     (b) rongeur
     (c) cannula
     (d) curette

6.   An instrument for dilatating a canal
     (a) cannula
     (b) irrigator
     (c) gouge
     (d) speculum

7.   Suture material made from collagenous tissue of animals
     (a) surgical gut
     (b) absorbable material
     (c) can be treated to resist absorption longer
     (d) all of the above

8.   Suture material used to tie off a blood vessel
     (a) ligature
     (b) tenaculum
     (c) curette
     (d) none of the above

9. An example of a nonabsorbable suture material
    (a) silk
    (b) gut
    (c) wire
    (d) fascia lata
    (e) both (a) and (c)

10. A suture needle that is manufactured with the suture material directly attached to it
    (a) split-eye needle
    (b) square-eye needle
    (c) atraumatic needle
    (d) French needle

11. The removal of a mass such as a tumor in its entirety
    (a) desiccation
    (b) reduction
    (c) approximation
    (d) enucleation

12. A cylindrical saw used to remove a portion of bone
    (a) rongeur
    (b) bougie
    (c) trephine
    (d) curet

13. The removal of organs from their body cavity
    (a) enucleation
    (b) fistulization
    (c) resection
    (d) evisceration

14. The use of pressure to remove the contents of a vessel
    (a) reduction
    (b) irrigation
    (c) stripping
    (d) manipulation

15. Absorbent pads used in surgery to soak up fluids or to apply medication
    (a) dressings
    (b) sponges
    (c) prostheses
    (d) shunts

16. The surgical formation of a passageway between two structures
    (a) anastomosis
    (b) trephination
    (c) perfusion
    (d) intubation

17. Surgically making a pouch from the sac left by a tumor that has been removed
    (a) marsupialization
    (b) avulsion
    (c) coaptation
    (d) dehiscence

18. The removal of the covering or outer portion of a structure
    (a) extirpation
    (b) avulsion
    (c) decortication
    (d) resection

19. The splitting open of a wound
    (a) desiccation
    (b) dehiscence
    (c) debridement
    (d) decompression

20. Tissue for grafting taken from the body of a donor
    (a) autograft
    (b) homograft
    (c) xenograft

VII.   Match the following descriptions with their medical names.

1. surgical use of three-dimensional x rays ....   a. ultrasonic surgery

2. x-ray procedure for producing three-dimensional
                                                              b. laser surgery
   x rays ....
                                                              c. microsurgery
3. surgical use of cold to destroy diseased tissue ....
                                                              d. CAT scan
4. form of surgery that deals with structures too small for

   ordinary surgery ....   e. echogram

5. use of high-frequency sound waves to dissolve   f. stereotactic surgery

   cataracts ....   g. cryosurgery

6. instrument to record sound waves ....   h. oscilloscope

7. record produced by sound waves ....

8. use of a beam of light to cauterize diseased tissues ....

ANSWERS TO EXERCISES

I.

1. having equal measure, is/o/metr/ic
2. a severe congenital malformation, terat/ism
3. a cutting across, trans/(s)ec/tion
4. inability to recognize solid objects, a/stere/o/gnosis
5. substance that produces cold temperatures, cry/o/gen
6. producing many sounds, mult/i/son/ous
7. blood poisoning caused by a radioactive substance, radi/o/tox/emia
8. treatment with light, luc/o/therapy
9. pertaining to substance that moves under light, phot/o/kine/tic
10. serial x ray of the bladder and urethra, cine/cyst/o/urethr/o/gram
11. having equal tension, is/o/ton/ia
12. pain locate far from its stimulus, tel/algia
13. root shaped, radic/i/form
14. to cut apart, dis/sec/t
15. blood poisoning, sept/ic/emia
16. substance essential for life, vit/amin
17. to burn with a special instrument, cauter/ize
18. to relieve, alleviate, palli/ate
19. a cutting, sec/tion
20. having an equal form or shape, is/o/morph/ous
21. lack of regulation, a/tax/ia
22. burning with an electronic device, electr/o/cauter/y
23. resembling salt, hal/oid
24. process of making an x ray, roentgen/o/graphy
25. destroyed by light, phot/o/ly/tic

II.

1. extopic;   2. bisect;   3. antisepsis;   4. microsurgery;   5. radiopaque;
6. obstetrics;   7. cryotherapy;   8. thermocautery;   9. ultrasonogram;
10. teratogenesis;   11. roentgenotherapy;   12. translucent;   13. topography;
14. stereoscope;   15. photophobia.

III.

1. f;   2. h;   3. k;   4. i;   5. n;   6. l;   7. d;   8. a;   9. o;
10. e;   11. m;   12. p;   13. g;   14. b;   15. j;   16. c.

IV.

1. thoracic surgeon;   2. ophthalmic surgeon;   3. orthopedic surgeon;
4. gynecologist;   5. general surgeon;   6. plastic surgeon;
7. otolaryngeal surgeon;   8. obstetrician;   9. neurosurgeon;   10. urosurgeon.

V.

1. asepsis; 2. autoclave; 3. disinfectants; 4. anesthesiologist, vital signs;
5. general; 6. inhalation; 7. general, intravenously; 8. spinal, spinal column;
9. nerve block; 10. infiltration.

VI.

1. (c); 2. (d); 3. (a); 4. (b); 5. (b); 6. (d); 7. (d); 8. (a);
9. (e); 10. (c); 11. (d); 12. (c); 13. (d); 14. (c); 15. (b);
16. (a); 17. (a); 18. (c); 19. (b); 20. (b).

VII.

1. f; 2. d; 3. g; 4. c; 5. a; 6. h; 7. e; 8. b.

20 Mental Illness

COMBINING FORMS

	Meaning	Example
PSYCH/O (sy′ko)	mind	PSYCHOPHYSIOLOGIC (sy-ko-fiz-e-o-log′ik), a combination of emotional and physical illness
MENT/O (men′to)	mind	DEMENTIA (de-men′she-a), a mental deterioriation and loss of intellectual functioning occurring after age 18
-PHRENIA (free′ne-a)	mind	BRADYPHRENIA (bra-de-free′ne-a), mental slowness
SCHIZ/O (skiz′o)	split	SCHIZOPHRENIA (skiz-o-free′ne-a), a severe psychosis affecting young adults and characterized by a loss of contact with reality
HEBE- (he′be)	youth	HEBEPHRENIC (he-be-free′nik), pertaining to a type of schizophrenia characterized by childish behavior
-MANIA (may′ne-a)	extreme compulsion or preoccupation	PYROMANIA (pie-ro-may′ne-a), a compulsion to set fires
KLEPT/O (klep′to)	stealing	KLEPTOMANIA (klep-toe-may′ne-a), a compulsion to steal
EGO- (e′go)	I, self	EGOCENTRIC (e-go-sen′trik), an extreme emphasis on the self
CATA- (ka′ta)	down	CATATONIA (ka-ta-toe′ne-a), a subdivision of schizophrenia characterized by a rigid body position and a trance-like state
-PHOBIA (foe′be-a)	fear	XENOPHOBIA (zen-o-foe′be-a), an extreme fear of strangers

Mental illness refers to those mind-altering conditions that affect an individual's behavior so that the individual cannot function positively in society. A person is judged mentally ill by those health care specialists who are experienced in treating mental disorders and who would consider that individual's behavior abnormal. The two primary health care specialists who deal with mental disorders are *psychologists* and *psychiatrists* (IATR/O, physician). Psychologists are specialists in behaviorial sciences and theories about mental illness. Mental tests are frequently administered by psychologists. Psychiatrists are physicians who have specialized in the treatment of mental disorders. The use of medications and other forms of therapy to treat the mentally ill is the responsibility of the psychiatrist.

Mental disorders can be classified into four major categories: *organic psychoses, schizophrenia, affective psychoses,* and *neuroses.*

Organic psychoses (also called *organic mental disorders*) is the term used to refer to those forms of mental illness that have been caused by an injury to the brain or by some interference with normal brain function. One form of organic psychosis is *acute organic brain syndrome.* This form of mental disorder can be described as a drug-induced mental disorder (*toxic psychosis*). Such a disorder is characterized by general disorientation accompanied by disturbances of perception (e.g., hallucinations, illusions) and of sensation (e.g., depression, euphoria). Alcohol and narcotics are examples of substances that can produce this form of mental disorder. *Chronic brain syndrome*, another form of organic psychosis, is caused by brain injury, brain tumors, or old age. *Senile dementia* is the most commonly occurring form of chronic brain syndrome. In this disorder the brain atrophies, resulting in the loss of memory and intellectual functions, altered personality, and sometimes hallucinations and illusions.

Schizophrenia is a severe *psychosis* (a mental disorder of sufficient severity to warrant treatment) characterized by a withdrawal from reality, delusions, hallucinations, and changes in both behavior and mood. There are several types of schizophrenia. The table shows examples of this disorder.

Type	*Major Characteristics*
Catatonic	Rigid and/or awkward posture, trancelike state, excessive activity or paralyzed motor function
Paranoid	Delusions of persecution, greatness, and jealousy
Hebephrenic	Childish behavior, incoherence
Schizo-affective	Combination of schizophrenia and manic-depressive behavior

Usually schizophrenia occurs in individuals between the ages 16 to 25. Although environment may have some influence on the development of schizophrenia, genetic make-up is the major causative factor.

Affective disorders are those forms of mental illness that are accompanied by a change in mood. There are basically two forms of affective disorders: *mania* and *depression. Manic psychosis* is characterized by a heightened mood, increased level of activity, and feelings of greatness and power. *Depression,* on the other hand, is characterized by a general feeling of melancholy and sadness. Poor sleep, poor appetite, a lack of interest in normal activities, and the inability to concentrate frequently accompany depression.

Neuroses are extreme or exaggerated feelings of obsession, compulsion, phobia, or anxiety. Many of us possess some aspects of neurotic behavior; however, neuroses usually do not become serious unless they interfere with normal activities. Two common forms of neurotic behavior are *phobias* and *compulsive behavior* (the urge to perform certain acts). Examples of phobias are a fear of high places (acrophobia) and a fear of closed places (claustrophobia). Compulsive behavior can be described as the engaging in an act while, at the same time, trying to avoid that very act. Senseless habits are examples of compulsive neuroses.

Here is a select list of terms commonly used in psychology and psychiatry.

aggression.   Forcefulness, the intent to use or the use of force in action and/or speech. The object of the aggression may be an individual, a group, or oneself.

anxiety.   A feeling of apprehension or tension resulting from something that is feared or anticipated. Anxiety is frequently manifested by sweating, headache, increased pulse, and tenseness.

compulsion.   An irresistible urge to act in a manner that is irrational and against one's will. The need to perform a compulsive act and the unwillingness to perform that act frequently give rise to anxiety.

defense mechanism.   A misperception that brings about a reduction or relief of mental conflicts or anxiety. Rationalization is an example of a defense mechanism.

delusion.   A persistent false belief about oneself, another, an object, etc., that won't yield to logic. Delusions of persecution, the belief that everyone is against the individual, are examples of delusion.

depression (retarded depression).   A feeling of sadness or melancholy in which the individual becomes inactive, unable to concentrate, and dejected. Agitated depression is characterized by restlessness and loquaciousness.

drive.   A deep-seated urge.

ego.   One of the three Freudian divisions of the psyche (ego, id, superego). The ego is the repository of perceptions and concepts. It aids the psyche in adapting to reality by mediating between the primitive instincts of the id and the acquired prohibitions of the superego.

emotion.   A mental state or feeling. Examples of emotions are fear, love, surprise, anger, etc.

fantasy. The use of the imagination (e.g., daydreaming) to resolve conflicts or to seek gratification.

hallucination. The perception of objects that do not exist in external reality. A *hallucinogen* is a substance that induces hallucinations.

id. A Freudian concept that refers to the aspect of the psyche that houses primitive instincts.

illusion. The misinterpretation of the objects of sensory perception.

mania. An excessive or unreasonable preoccupation with something. For example, megalomania is an excessive preoccupation with feelings of greatness, power, wealth.

masochism. A condition or state in which one derives pleasure (frequently sexual) by being physically or mentally abused.

mental retardation. An abnormal lack of intelligence as determined by IQ testing. Adjustment to normal social activities is difficult. The levels of retardation are

> Mild   (50–70 IQ)
> Moderate   (35–49 IQ)
> Severe   (20–34 IQ)
> Profound   (below 20 IQ)

narcissism. An abnormal, obsessive love for one's self, frequently accompanied by a sexual desire for one's own body.

obsession. A persistent preoccupation with a feeling or impulse.

organic psychosis. A mental disorder resulting from some physical cause, such as a tumor, trauma, or infection.

paranoia. A chronic mental disorder characterized by somewhat organized feelings of persecution and/or grandeur.

phobia. An exaggerated, usually unreasonable, fear of someone or something. For example, claustrophobia is a morbid fear of closed places.

psychopathic personality. An emotional and behavioral state in which the individual is aware of reality but engages in amoral or antisocial activities for self-gratification. These acts are carried out with little feelings of anxiety or guilt.

psychosis. A severe mental disorder characterized by a loss of contact with reality or a distortion of reality. *Neurosis,* on the other hand, is an excessive feeling of anxiety, an obsession or compulsion, or phobia in which there is no loss of contact with reality.

psychotherapy. The treatment of a mental disorder.

repression.   A form of defense mechanism by which unacceptable impulses or feelings are kept from entering the consciousness, resulting in the production of tension. The repressed thought also becomes more powerful in its interactions with other thoughts.

sadism.   Pleasure, especially sexual, is derived from inflicting physical or mental pain on someone.

schizophrenia.   A form of psychosis in which the individual loses contact with reality and engages in delusions, hallucinations, and regressive behavior.

sublimation.   The diversion of unacceptable drives into socially and personally acceptable outlets.

superego.   A Freudian concept that refers to that part of the psyche that is the repository of social rules and morality.

suppression.   A conscious effort to exclude or conceal unacceptable thoughts, feelings, impulses, etc.

withdrawal.   A pathological retreat from reality.

EXERCISES

I.   Give the meaning for each of the following medical words. Divide each word into base(s), prefix, and suffix; underline the letter that has the primary stress. *Example:*

PSYCHOTHERAPY   the treatment of a mental illness   psych/o/<u>the</u>rapy

1. DIPSOMANIA

2. PSYCHIATRIST

3. PANPHOBIA

4. PSYCHOSIS

5. HYPERPHRENIA

6. NYMPHOMANIA

7. HEBEPHRENIA

8. DEMENTED

9. PHOTOPHOBIA

10. CATATONIA ....

11. MYSOPHOBIA (MYS/O, dirt) ....

12. HEBETIC ....

13. IDIOPHRENIC ....

14. NECROMANIA ....

15. PSYCHODIAGNOSTIC ....

> **II.** Make medical words from the following phrases. Indicate the primary stress by underlining the stressed letter(s). *Example:*

pertaining to behavior characterized by an excessive preoccupation with something

<u>ma</u>nic
....

1. a term used to describe a physical condition produced by a mental condition or state

....

2. pertaining to a type of schizophrenia characterized by a rigid body position and a trance-like state

....

3. a compulsion or desire to set fires

....

4. a major form of psychosis affecting young adults and characterized by a loss of contact with reality

....

5. excessive preoccupation with one's self

....

6. pertaining to a person who has a severe mental disorder that causes him to lose contact with reality

....

7. characterized by or resembling schizophrenic behavior

....

8. pertaining to the mind

....

9. abnormal fear of closed places

....

10. referring to an individual who has a compulsion for stealing

....

    III. Fill in the blanks for each statement.

1. A physician who specializes in the treatment of mental disorders is called a ....

....

2. A .... is a specialist in the theories about mental illness and in the administration of diagnostic tests.

3. .... refers to those forms of mental illness that are the result of brain injury or altered function.

4. Drug-induced mental disorders are called ....

5. .... is a form of chronic brain syndrome that occurs in old age.

6. .... is a severe psychosis characterized by a withdrawal from reality, delusions, hallucinations, and altered mood and behavior.

7. The two forms of affective mental disorders are .... and ....

....

8. .... is characterized by a heightened mood, excessive activity, and feelings of grandeur.

9. .... is characterized by a general melancholy, sadness, and reduced activity.

10. A compulsive, obsessive form of behavior that frequently results in anxiety or phobias

is called a ....

IV.   Match the following descriptions with their medical words.

1. an irresistible urge to act in a manner that is irrational and

   contrary to one's will ....

2. an illogical false belief about oneself, another, objects,

   etc. ....

3. a form of schizophrenia characterized by childish

   behavior ....

4. a conscious effort to exclude unacceptable thoughts, feelings,

   impulses from the mind ....

5. an exaggerated, usually unreasonable fear of someone or

   something ....

6. an abnormal self-love ....

7. an obsessive preoccupation with something ....

8. rationalization ....

9. a form of psychosis in which the individual loses contact

   with reality ....

10. a division of the psyche that mediates between the other

    two divisions ....

11. the subconscious removal from the memory of unacceptable

    thoughts or impulses ....

12. daydreaming ....

13. an abnormal lack of intelligence as determined by IQ

    testing ....

14. the externalization of a feeling ....

15. the division of the psyche that is the repository for primitive

    instincts ....

a. fantasy

b. depression

c. masochism

d. hallucination

e. compulsion

f. supression

g. drive

h. id

i. mental
    retardation

j. defense
    mechanism

k. hebephrenia

l. paranoid
    schizophrenia

m. mania

n. delusion

o. schizophrenia

p. catatonic
    schizophrenia

q. psychopathic
    personality

r. phobia

16. a feeling of sadness or melancholy ....

17. a form of schizophrenia characterized by a rigid posture and a

    trancelike state ....

18. the division of the psyche that is the repository of societal

    rules and morality ....

19. used to describe the emotional and behavioral state of an
    individual who knowingly engages in antisocial activities

    ....

20. the treatment of a mental disorder ....

21. a feeling of apprehension or tension resulting from something

    that is feared or anticipated ....

22. the derivation of pleasure, frequently sexual, from physical

    or mental abuse ....

23. a form of schizophrenia characterized by delusions of

    persecution, and/or greatness, and jealousy ....

24. a deep-seated urge ....

25. the perception of objects that do not exist outside the

    mind ....

s. anxiety

t. superego

u. narcissism

v. psychotherapy

w. ego

x. repression

y. emotion

ANSWERS TO EXERCISES

I.

1. an abnormal compulsion to drink (especially alcohol), dips/o/<u>ma</u>nia
2. a physician who treats mental disorders, ps<u>ych</u>/iatr/ist
3. an abnormal fear of everything, pan/<u>phob</u>ia
4. a severe mental disorder in which the individual loses contact with reality, ps<u>ych</u>/osis
5. excessive mental activity, hyper/<u>phren</u>ia
6. an excessive desire (in the female) for sexual intercourse, nymph/o/<u>ma</u>nia
7. a type of schizophrenia characterized by childish behavior, hebe/<u>phren</u>ia
8. used to describe an individual who has lost his mental functions, de/<u>ment</u>/ed
9. a severe intolerance to light, phot/o/<u>phob</u>ia
10. a type of schizophrenia characterized by a rigid body position and a trancelike state, cata/<u>ton</u>/ia

11. an abnormal fear of dirt, mys/o/<u>pho</u>bia
12. occurring at puberty, he<u>be</u>/tic
13. originating in the mind, idi/o/<u>phren</u>/ic
14. an abnormal preoccupation with dead bodies, necr/o/<u>ma</u>nia
15. pertaining to the use of psychological testing to determine an individual's mental condition, psych/o/dia<u>gnos</u>/tic

II.

1. psychoso<u>ma</u>tic;   2. cata<u>ton</u>ic;   3. pyro<u>ma</u>nia;   4. schizophrenia;
5. ego<u>ma</u>nia;   6. psy<u>cho</u>tic;   7. <u>schiz</u>oid;   8. <u>men</u>tal;   9. claustro<u>pho</u>bia;
10. klepto<u>ma</u>niac.

III.

1. psychiatrist;   2. psychologist;   3. organic mental disorders/organic psychosis;
4. toxic psychoses;   5. senile dementia;   6. schizophrenia;
7. mania and depression;   8. mania;   9. depression;   10. neurosis.

IV.

1. e;   2. n;   3. k;   4. f;   5. r;   6. u;   7. m;   8. j;   9. o;
10. w;   11. x;   12. a;   13. i;   14. y;   15. h;   16. b;   17. p;
18. t;   19. q;   20. v;   21. s;   22. c;   23. l;   24. g;   25. d.

Combining form	Meaning	Examples*
DACTYL/O (dak'til-o)	finger, toe	DACTYLITIS (dak-til-eye'tis), inflammation of the bones or the fingers and toes in young children DACTYLOMEGALY (give meaning) . . . .
IN/O (in'o)	fiber	INOCYST (in'o-cyst), a fibrous capsule INONEUROMA . . . .
-AGRA (ag'ra)	severe pain	PODAGRA (pod-ag'ra), severe pain in the foot joints, gout ARTHRAGRA . . . .
-KINESIA	movement, motion	DYSKINESIA (dis-ki-nee'ze-a), poor, defective movement AUTOKINESIS . . . .
HYAL/O (hi'a-lo)	glass, glasslike transparent	HYALINE (hi'a-line), glassy transparent HYALOENCHONDROMA . . . .

*Give the meaning of the word preceding the blanks in the space provided.

Combining form	Meaning	Examples
POD/O (po'do)	foot	PODALGIA (po-dal'ge-a), pain in the foot MACROPODIA
AXI/O (aks'e-o)	axis	SUBAXIAL (sub-aks'e-al), located below the axis of a structure EPAXIAL
VAG/O (va'go)	vagus nerve 10 cranial nerve	VAGOTOMY (va-got'o-me), incision of the vagus nerve VAGOMIMETIC
VERRUC/O (ver-rou'ko)	wart	VERRUCIFORM (ver-rou'se-form), shaped like a wart VERRUCOSE
-LALIA (lay'le-a)	speech	DYSLALIA (dis-lay'le-a), a speech impairment **RHINOLALIA**
CULD/O (kul'do)	pouch, the peritoneal pouch behind the uterus	CULDOSCOPY (kul-dos'ko-pe), examining the pelvic organs of a female by means of an endoscope that is sent through the posterior vaginal wall **CULDOCENTESIS**
SPLANCHN/O (splank-no)	viscera, internal organs	SPLANCHNEMPHRAXIS (splank-nem-fraks'is), obstruction of an internal organ **SPLANCHNODYNIA**

Combining form	Meaning	Examples
TRACHEL/O (tray′kel-o)	neck of the uterus	TRACHELECTOMOPEXY (tray-kel-ek-to-mo′peks-e), partial removal of the neck of the uterus and fixing in place of the remainder TRACHELITIS
FISTUL/O (fis′tou-lo)	a fistula, an abnormal tube or pipe-like structure	FISTULECTOMY (fis-tou-lek′toe-me), excision of a fistula FISTULOTOME
SYRING/O (sir-in′go)	any tubelike structure, a fistula	SYRINGOTOMY (sir-in-got′o-me), incision of a fistula SYRINGE
-CLEISIS (kly′sis) -KLEISIS (kly′sis)	closure, blockage	OTOCLEISIS (ot-o-kly′sis), closure of the ear ENTEROAPOKLEISIS
EME/O (em′e-o)	vomiting	EMETIC (e-met′ik), a substance that induces vomiting HYPEREMESIS
SCHIZ/O (skiz′o)	split, division fissure	SCHIZOPHRENIA (skiz-o-free′ne-a), a group of mental disorders characterized by a split personality THORACOSCHISIS
MYX/O (mik′so)	mucus	MYXADENITIS (miks-ad-en-eye′tis), inflammation of a mucous gland MYXIOSIS

Combining form	Meaning	Examples
BLENN/O (blen/o)	mucus	BLENNORRHAGIA (blen-o-ray'je-a), discharge of mucus BLENNEMESIS
APIC/O (ap'i-ko)	tip	APICECTOMY (ap-i-sek'toe-me), excision of the root of a tooth APICITIS
FEBR/I (feb're)	fever	FEBRILE (feb'ril), pertaining to a fever FEBRIFACIENT
UVUL/O (ou-vou'lo)	the uvula, a lobe-like structure hanging from the soft palate	UVULOPTOSIS (ou-vou-lop-toe'sis), prolapse of the uvula UVULOTOME
VENTR/O (ven'tro)	belly	VENTRAD (ven'trad), toward the belly DORSIVENTRAL
GALACT/O milk	milk	GALACTEMIA (ga-lak-tee'me-a), milky condition of the blood AGALACTIA
THI/O (thy'o)	sulfur	THIOGENIC (thy-o-gen'ik), sulfur producing THIOPEXY
AUR/O (or'o)	gold	AUROTHERAPY (or-o-ther'a-pe), treatment using gold AURIC

Combining form	*Meaning*	*Examples*
FERR/O (fer'o)	iron	FERROUS (fer'us), pertaining/containing iron FERROPEXIA
		. . . .
SILIC/O (sil'i-ko)	flint, dust	SILICOSIS (sil-i-ko'sis), pneumonicosis caused by the inhalation of silicon dust SILICOTUBERCULOSIS
		. . . .
AER/O (air'o)	air, gas	AEROGRAM (air'o-gram), x ray of an organ that has been filled with air AEROSINUSITIS
		. . . .
BARY- (bar'e)	weight, pressure	BARYPHONIA (bar-e-fon'e-a), heavy/difficult speech BAROREFLEXES
		. . . .
-SCHESIS (skey'sis)	a holding back, suppression of a discharge	UROSCHESIS (your-o-skey'sis), suppression of urine ISCHEMIA
		. . . .
GER/O (jer'o) GERONT/O (je-ron'to)	age, the aged	GERONTOLOGY (je-ron-tol'o-ge), the study of aging GEROMORPHISM
		. . . .
-GEUSIA (gou'ze-a)	taste	AGEUSIA (a-gou'ze-a), absence of the sense of taste DYSGEUSIA
		. . . .

Medical Abbreviations

abd	abdomen
AC	axiocervical, alternating current
ACG	apex cardiogram
acG	accelerator globulin (factor V)
ACTH	adrenocorticotropic hormone
AD	right ear (auris dextra)
ADC	anodic duration contraction, axiodistocervical
ADH	antidiuretic hormone
ADP	adensoine diphosphate
ADPase	adenosine diphosphatase
AGA	accelerated growth area
A/G ratio	albumin-globulin ratio
ah	hypermetropic astigmatism
AHF	antihemophilic factor (factor VIII)
AHG	antihemophilic factor (factor VIII)
AI	aortic insufficiency
AJ	ankle jerk
alb	albumin
am	ametropia, myopic astigmatism
AMI	acute myocardial infarction
AML	acute myoblastic leukemia
AMP	adenosine monophosphate
amp	amperage, ampule
An	anisometropia, anodal, anode
anat	anatomic
ANS	autonomic nervous system
A-P	anterioposterior
A + P	auscultation and percussion
APC	aspirin, phenacetin, and caffeine (read as one)
A-P&Lat	anterioposterior and lateral
APF	animal protein factor (vitamin B_{12})
ARD	acute respiratory disease
AS	left ear (auris sinistra)
ASCVD	arteriosclerotic cardiovascular disease
Ast	astigmatism
AT	mean manifest magnitude of repolarization of the myocardium
ATCC	American Type Culture Collection
ATN	acute tubular necrosis
ATP	adenosine triphosphate
ATPase	adenosine triphosphatase
ATS	equine antitetanus serum
at vol	atomic volume
at wt	atomic weight
AV	arteriovenous, atrioventricular
Av	avoirdupois weight

B bacillus

BBB bundle branch block

B cells lymphocytes produced in bone marrow

BBT basal body temperature

BE barium enema

BFP biologic false positive reaction

BM bowel movement

BMR basal metabolic rate

BS blood sugar

BSA body surface area

BSR blood sedimentation rate

BT bleeding time

BTU British thermal unit

BUN blood, urea, nitrogen (used to test kidney function)

C Celsius, centigrade

Ca calcium

Ca cancer

Cal large calorie

cal small calorie

CAT Scan computerized axial tomography

CBC complete blood count

CBG corticosteroid-binding globulin

CBS chronic brain syndrome

cc cubic centimeter

CEA carcinoembryonic antigen

CCU coronary care unit

CDC Center for Disease Control

cg centigram

CHD congenital heart disease

CHF congestive heart failure

CHINA chronic infectious neuropathic agent

CID cytomegalic inclusion disease

Cl chlorine

CLSH corpus-luteum-stimulating hormone

cm centimeter

CMR cerebral metabolic rate

CMV cytomegalic virus

CNS central nervous system

Co cobalt

CO_2 carbon dioxide

CoA coenzyme A

COPD chronic obstructive pulmonary disease

CPD cephalopelvic disproportion

CR conditioned reflex

Cr chromium

Cs cesium

CS conditioned stimulus

CSF cerebrospinal fluid

CSM cerebrospinal meningitis

CSR corrected sedimentation rate

CST convulsive shock therapy

CTR cardiothoracic ratio

CV cardiovascular

CVA cardiovascular accident, cerebrovascular accident

CVD cardiovascular disease

Cx cervix

DC direct current

D&C dilatation and curettage

dB decibel

DJD degenerative joint disease

DOA dead on arrival

DOE dyspnea on exertion

DT delirium tremens

DTR deep tendon reflex

dx diagnosis

ECG   electrocardiogram

ECS   electroconvulsive shock

ECT   electroconvulsive therapy

EEG   electroencephalogram

EHBF   estimated hepatic blood flow

EKG   electrocardiogram

EMC   encephalomyocarditis

EMF   erythrocyte maturation factor

EMG   electromyogram

EMI   *E*lectronics *M*usic *I*nstruments, Ltd., abbreviation for the computerized axial tomography scanner (named after its manufacturer)

ENT   ear, nose, and throat

EOM   extraocular movement

ERBF   effective renal blood flow

ERG   electroretinogram

ERPF   effective renal plasma flow

ERV   expiratory reserve volume

ESR   erythrocyte sedimentation rate

EST   electroshock therapy

EVB   Epstein-Barr virus

FB   foreign body

FBS   fasting blood sugar

FD   focal distance

FDA   Food and Drug Administration

Fe   iron

FFA   free fatty acids

FH   family history

fl   fluid

FRF   follicle-stimulating hormone releasing factor

FSF   fibrin-stabilizing factor

FSH   follicle-stimulating hormone

FUO   fever of undetermined origin

fx   fracture

GBS   gallbladder series

GFR   glomerular filtration rate

GI   gastrointestinal

GOT   glutamic-oxaloacetic transaminase

GP   general practitioner

GTH   gonadotropic hormone

GTT   glucose tolerance test

GU   genitourinary

GYN   gynecology

H   hydrogen

HAA   hepatitis-associated antigen

hb   hemoglobin

HCl   hydrochloric acid

HCG   human chorionic gonadotropin

HCT   hematocrit

HE   helium

H&E   hematoxylin and eosin stains

HEENT   head, eye, ear, nose, and throat

HF   Hageman factor (factor XII)

HGB   hemoglobin

H_2O water

Hg   mercury

HSV   herpes simplex virus

HVD   hypertensive vascular disease

IC   inspiratory capacity

ICU   intensive care unit

ICT   insulin coma therapy

I&D   incision and drainage

ID   intradermal

Ig   immunoglobulin

IH   infectious hepatitis

IHSS   idiopathic hypertrophic subaortic stenosis

IM   intramuscular (injection)

IOP   intraocular pressure

IST	insulin shock therapy		mm Hg	millimeters of mercury
IU	international unit		mono	monocyte
IUD	intrauterine device		MS	multiple sclerosis
IV (iv)	intravenous		MSL	midsternal line
IVCD	intraventricular conduction delay		myel	myelocyte
IVP	intravenous pyelogram			
			N	nitrogen
K	potassium		Na	sodium
kg	kilogram		NAD	no appreciable disease
			NF	National Formulary
LATS	long-acting thyroid stimulator		NG	nasogastric
LD	lethal dose		ng	nanogram
LDH	lactic dehydrogenase		NPO	nothing by mouth
LE	lupus erythematosus			
LLL	left lower lobe		O	oculus (eye)
LLQ	left lower quadrant		O_2	Oxygen
LMP	last menstrual period		O_2 cap	oxygen capacity
LP	lumbar puncture		O_2 sat	oxygen saturation
LPN	licensed practical nurse		OB	obstetrics
LUL	left upper lobe		OD	oculus dexter (right eye)
LUQ	left upper quadrant		OFC	occipitofrontal circumference
LV	left ventricle		OR	operating room
LVH	left ventricular hypertrophy		OS	oculus sinister (left eye)
lymphs	lymphocytes			
			P	phosphorus
MBC	maximum breathing capacity		P	position, pulse, pupil
MCH	mean corpuscular hemoglobin		P_2	pulmonic second heart sound
MCHC	mean corpuscular hemoglobin concentration		P&A	percussion and auscultation
MCV	mean corpuscular volume		PAC	premature atrial contraction
MD	Doctor of Medicine		PAT	paroxysmal atrial tachycardia
mg	milligram		PBI	protein bound iodine
mHg	millimeters of mercury		PCG	phonocardiogram
MI	myocardial infarction		PD	doctor of pharmacy, interpupillary distance
ml	milliliter		PDA	patent ductus arteriosus
MM	mucous membrane		PDR	Physicians' Desk Reference
mm	millimeter		PE	physical examination

PEG	pneumoencephalogram
PH	past history
pH	hydrogen ion concentration
PID	pelvic inflammatory disease
PKU	phenylketonuria
PMB	polymorphonuclear basophil leukocytes
PME	polymorphonuclear eosinophil leukocytes
PMI	point of maximal impulse
PMN	polymorphonuclear neutrophil leukocytes
PNH	paroxysmal nocturnal hemoglobinuria
polys	polymorphonuclear leukocytes
PPD	purified protein derivative
Pr	presbyopia
psi	pounds per square inch
PSP	Phenylsulfonthalein (dye for kidney test)
PT	physical therapy, prothrombin time
PTT	partial thromboplastin time
PVC	premature ventricular contraction
PZI	protamine zinc insulin
R	respiration
Ra	radium
rad	radiation absorbed dose
RAI	radioactive iodine
RBC	red blood cell
rbc	red blood count
Rh	Rhesus blood factor
RLL	right lower lobe
RLQ	right lower quadrant
RM	respiratory movement
RN	registered nurse
R/O	rule out
RP	retrograde pyelogram
RUL	right upper lobe
RUQ	right upper quadrant
RV	residual volume
RVH	right ventricular hypertrophy
SA	sinoatrial
sat	saturated
sc	subcutaneously
SD	skin dose, standard deviation
SE	standard error
sed rate	erythrocyte sedimentation rate
SGOT	serum glutamic oxaloacetic transaminase
SGPT	serum glutamic pyruvic transaminase
SOB	shortness of breath
sp gr	specific gravity
SQ	subcutaneous
SR	review of systems, sedimentation rate
STAPH	Staphylococcus
STREP	streptoccus
STS	serologic test for syphillis
T	temperature, thoracic
tab	tablet
T&A	tonsillectomy and adenoidectomy
T cells	lymphocytes produced in the thymus gland
TAT	Thematic Apperception Test, toxin-antitoxin
TB	tuberculosis
TBI	total body irradiation
TLC	total lung capacity
TNI	total nodal irradiation
TPR	temperature, pulse, and respiration

tr	tincture		VD	veneral disease
TS	test solution		VDH	valvular disease of the heart
TSH	thyroid-stimulating hormone		VDRL	Veneral Disease Research Laboratories
tus	tussis (cough)		vf	field of vision
U	unit		VPB	ventricular premature beat
UGI	upper gastrointestinal		VR	vocal resonance
UP	uteropelvic		WBC	white blood cell
URI	upper respiratory infection		wbc	white blood count
USP	United States Pharmacopoeia		WD	well developed
VC	vital capacity		wt	weight
VCG	vector cardiogram			

APPENDIX 3   Drugs

This list of drugs serves two purposes: to familiarize you with the names, both generic and proprietary, of several drugs and to help you gain a knowledge of their uses. Consider this list an introduction, a sampling. Some drugs are listed with their generic or proprietary names. Although only one or two proprietary names may be listed for a generic name, there may be several brand names available. *Combination drug* indicates the several drugs that make up a proprietary drug. For an extensive listing of drugs and their uses, consult the most recent edition of the *Physician's Desk Reference.*

acetaminophen (a-see-ta-min'o-fen).   A non-narcotic analgesic that does not contain aspirin.

acetohexamide (a-see-toe-heks'a-mide).   A sulfonylurea used to increase the release of insulin from the pancreas.
Brand name: Dymelor

Achromycin-V (a-kro-my'sin).   A broad spectrum antibiotic.
Generic name: tetracycline HCl

Actifed (ak'ti-fed).   An antihistamine and decongestant.
Combination drug: triprolidine
      hydrochloride
      pseudoephedrine
      hydrochloride

actinomycin D (ak-tin-o-my'sin).   An antibiotic used in the treatment of several forms of cancer; for example, leukemia, sarcomas, and certain types of tumors that occur in children.

ADRENERGIC AGENTS (sympathomimetic).   Act similarly to epinephrine. They produce constrictions of the peripheral blood vessels, increased heart rate and output, stimulation of the CNS, and relaxation of the visceral muscles.

ADRENERGIC BLOCKING AGENTS.   Sympatholytic drugs that have an effect opposite to that of epinephrine. These drugs produce vasodilation, hypotension, increased gastrointestinal activity, and decreased heart rate and output.

Adria (ay'dre-a).   An antibiotic used in cancer therapy.
Generic name: adriamycin

adriamycin (ay-dre-a-my'sin).   An antibiotic used in cancer therapy.
Brand names: Adria, Doxorubicin

Aldactazide (al-dak'ta-zide).   A diuretic used to treat hypertension.
Combination drug: spironolactone
      hydrocholorthiazide

Aldactone (al-dak'tone). A diuretic taken orally; does not deplete potassium.
Generic name: spironolactone

Aldomet esther (al'doe-met). A sympathetic inhibitor used in the management of hypertension, especially hypertensive emergencies.
Generic name: methyldopa

Aldoril (al'dor-il). An antihypertensive.
Combination drug: methyldopa
hydrochlorothiazide

ALKALOIDS, (plant). Substances derived from plants and used to treat tumors because of their ability to block mitosis.

ALKYLATING AGENTS. Drugs used to treat tumors because of their ability to affect DNA structure.

alpha-methyldopa (al'fa-me-thil-doe'pa). A vasodilator used in the treatment of diseases of the blood vessels such as hypertension.

aminophylline (am-i-no-fil'in or am-i-nof'i-lin). A bronchodilator used to treat asthma.

amitriptyline (am'i-trip'ti-lin). An antidepressant effective in controlling psychoses.
Brand name: Elavil

ammonium chloride.
1. An expectorant that increases bronchial secretions.
Brand names: Dextrotussin Syrup, Triamicol Decongestant Cough Syrup
2. Also used to treat metabolic alkalosis.
Brand name: Zypam Tablets

amoxicillin (a-moks-i-sil'in). A form of penicillin.
Brand name: Amoxil

Amoxil (a-moks'il). A form of penicillin.
Generic name: amoxicillin

amphetamine (am-fet'a-mean/am-fet'a-min). A central nervous system stimulant.
Brand name: Benzedrine

Amphojel (am'foe-jel). A non-systemic antacid containing aluminum.

ampicillin (am-pe-sil'in). A form of penicillin

used to treat diseases caused by gram positive and gram negative bacteria.

amyl nitrate. An antianginal agent administered by inhalation.

ANALGESICS. Drugs that relieve pain.

ansolysen (an-so-lie'sin). An antihypertensive agent that acts on the sympathetic division of the autonomic nervous system.
Generic name: pentolinium

ANTACID. A substance that reduces or neutralizes acidity.

ANTIANGINAL AGENTS. Decrease arterial and ventricular pressure, produce coronary vasodilation, and reduce cardiac output.

ANTIARRHYTHMIC AGENTS. Reduce/control irregular heart actions.

ANTIBIOTICS. Drugs that destroy microorganisms or halt their growth. Several antibiotics are effective antitumor drugs; they block DNA and RNA synthesis.

ANTICOAGULANTS. Substances that affect the clotting properties of the blood.

ANTICONVULSANTS. Drugs that are used to control *convulsions* (involuntary activity of voluntary muscles) *and seizures* (convulsions along with other disturbances e.g. unconsciousness).

ANTIDIABETIC AGENTS. Substances that act on the level of blood sugar by promoting the release of insulin from the pancreas, or by increasing the body's utilization of glucose.

ANTIEMETIC AGENTS. Drugs that are effective in controlling vomiting and nausea.

ANTIHISTAMINES. Drugs that block allergic responses.

ANTIHYPERTENSIVE AGENTS. Drugs that reduce blood pressure chiefly through vasodilation.

ANTIHYPOTENSIVE AGENTS. Drugs that elevate arterial blood pressure.

ANTILIPEMICS. Drugs that reduce serum

lipid concentration (hyperlipidemia); used to prevent or reduce arterial occlusion.

antilymphocytic globulin. An immunosuppressive agent.

ANTIMETABOLITES. Antitumor drugs that affect DNA and RNA synthesis.

ANTITHYROID AGENTS. Drugs that cause the production of thyroid hormones to decrease; they are used to control hyperthyroidism.

ANTITUMOR DRUGS. A general term used to describe several types of drugs that are effective in the treatment of cancer because of their ability to interfere with, or block cellular processes. Antitumor drugs are alkylating agents, antimetabolites, alkaloids (plant), antibiotics, nitrosourea compounds, immune stimulants, and hormones.

Antivert (an'ti-vert). An antihistamine.
Generic name: meclizine HCl

Apresoline (a-pres'o-leen). A vasodilator used in the treatment of hypertension.
Generic name: hydralazine

Ara-C. An anti-metabolite used to treat leukemia.
Generic name: arabinosyl cytosine

Aramine (a'ra-min). An anti-hypotensive agent (vasoconstrictor) that elevates arterial blood pressure.
Generic name: metaraminol

Asbron (az'bron). An expectorant.

Atarax (a'ta-raks). An antihistamine; it is also used to relieve tension and anxiety.
Generic name: hydroxyzine hydrochloride

azathioprine (az-a-thy'o-prin). An antipurine used as an immunosuppressive agent.
Brand name: Imuran

BCG—bacillus Calmette-Guerin. Used as an immunity stimulant.
Brand names: Glaxo, TKE

BCNU. An abbreviation for a nitrosourea compound used in cancer treatment (lymph cancers, Hodgkins disease, brain tumors).
Generic name: bischloroethylnitrosourea

belladona (bel-a-don'a). An antispasmodic agent that produces muscle relaxation in the GI tract; it also has a sedative effect.

Benadryl (ben'a-dril). An antihistamine.
Generic name: diphenhydramine

Bendectin (ben-dek'tin). An anti-emetic used to control vomiting and nausea, especially during pregnancy.
Combination drug:
doxylamine succinate
pyridoxine hydrochloride

Benzedrine (ben'ze-dreen). Brand name for amphetamine.

bethanechol (be-thane'kol). A cholinergic drug frequently used after surgery to stimulate urination.
Brand name: Urecholine

biquanides (by'qwa-nides). A type of antidiabetic agent that reduces intestinal glucose absorption, reduces liver gluconeogenesis, and increases body utilization of glucose.

bisacodyl (bis-a-ko'dil). A cathartic.
Brand name: Dulcolax

bischloroethylnitrosurea (abbreviation: BCNU) (bis-klor-o-ethil-ny-tros-you-ree'a). A nitrosourea compound used in cancer treatment (lymph cancers, Hodgkin's disease, brain tumors).

bishydroxycoumarin (bis-hy-droks-ee-kou'marin). An anticoagulant.
Brand names: Coumadin, Dicumarol

Bleo (blee'o). An antibiotic used in cancer therapy.
Generic name: Bleomycin

bleomycin (blee-o-my'sin). An antibiotic used in cancer therapy.
Brand names: Blenoxane, Bleo

Bonamine (bo'na-meen). An antihistamine.
Generic name: Meclizine

busulfan (bou-sul'fan). An alkylating agent used in cancer therapy.

Butazolidin (bu-ta-zol′i-din), also Butazolidin Alka. An anti-inflammatory and analgesic agent used in the treatment of arthritis.
Combination drug:
phenylbutazone
aluminum hydroxide gel
magnesium trisilicate

Cafergot (ka′fer-got). A drug used in the management of migraine headaches.
Generic name: ergotamine tartrate

carbamazepine (kar-ba-maz′e-peen). An anticonvulsant.

Cardilate (kar′di-late). An antianginal agent.
Generic name: erythrityl tetranitrate

carmustine (kar-mus′teen). A nitrosourea compound used in cancer therapy.

cathartic (ka-thar′tik). A substance that induces bowel movement; a strong purgative.

CCNU. A nitrosourea compound used in cancer therapy.
Brand name: Lomustine

chloestyramine (ko-le-sty′ra-min). An antilipemic.
Brand name: Questran

chloral hydrate. A sedative.

chlorambucil (klor-am′bue-sil). An alkylating agent used in the treatment of chronic leukemia and myeloma.
Brand name: Leukeran

chlordiazepoxide (klor-di-az-e-poks′ide). A tranquilizer used in the treatment of depression and anxiety.
Brand name: Librium

chlorothiazide (klor-o-thy′a-zide). A diuretic, administered orally.
Brand name: Diuril

chlorpheniramine (klor-fen-ire′a-min). An antihistamine.
Brand name: Chlor-Trimeton

chlorpropamide (klor-pro′pa-mide). A sufonyl-urea used in the management of diabetes.
Brand name: Diabinase

chlorthalidone (klor-thal′i-done). A diuretic.
Brand name: Hygroton

Chlor-Trimeton (klor-try′me′ton). An antihistamine.
Generic name: chlorpheniramine

CHOLINERGIC AGENTS. Drugs that affect the parasympathetic nerve fibers. They increase gastrointestinal activity, contraction of the urinary bladder, vasodilatation of the peripheral blood vessels, skeletal muscle tone, and reduce heart rate. Cholinergic agents are frequently referred to as parasympathomimetic drugs.

choloxin (kol-oks′in). An antilipemic used to reduce blood cholesterol levels.
Generic name: sodium dextrothyroxine

clofibrate (klo-fy′brate). An antilipemic that reduces triglyceride and cholesterol levels in the blood.
Brand name: Atromid S

Compazine (kom′pa-zeen). An antiemetic
Generic name: prochlorperazine

Cortef (kor′tef). An adrenal cortical steroid used in the treatment of cancers (lymphomas, Hodgkin's disease, and multiple myeloma).
Generic name: hydrocortisone

CORTICOSTEROID (kor-tee-ko-ster′oyd). A steroid derived from the cortex of the adrenal gland; because corticosteroids increase blood flow and decrease arterial resistance, they are effective antihypotensive agents; several are used in cancer therapy (e.g. treatment of leukemia).

Cosmegen (koz′me-jen). An antibiotic used in cancer therapy.
Generic name: actinomycin D

Coumadin (kou′ma-din). An anticoagulant.
Generic name: bishydroxycoumarin

coumarin (kou′ma-rin). An anticoagulant that is administered orally and has a prothrombin depressing effect.

cyclandelate (sy-klan'de-late).   An antilipemic that relaxes the arterial wall causing increased blood flow.
Brand name: Cyclospasmol

cyclophosphamide (sy-klo-fos'fa-mide).   An alkylating agent used in cancer therapy.
Brand names: Cytoxan, CYT

Cyclospasmol (sy-klo-spaz'mol).   An antilipemic agent that relaxes the arterial wall causing increased blood flow.
Generic name: cyclandelate

CYT.   An alkylating agent used in cancer therapy.
Generic name: cyclophosphamide

Cytellin (sy-tell'in).   An antilipemic that reduces the cholesterol level of the blood.
Generic name: sitosteral(s)

Cytomel (sy'toe-mel).   A thyroid replacement drug.
Generic name: liothyronine sodium

cytosine arabinoside (sy'toe-sin ar-a-bin'a-side).   An antimetabolite used in the treatment of leukemia.
Brand name: Ara-C

Cytoxan (sy'toks-an).   An alkylating agent used in cancer therapy.
Generic name: cyclophosphamide

Dalmane (dal'main).   Used to treat insomnia.
Generic name: flurazepam hydrochloride

Darvon (dar'von).   An analgesic.
Generic name: propoxyphene

Daunomycin (dawn-o-my'sin).   An antibiotic used in cancer therapy.
Generic name: daunorubicin

daunorubicin (dawn-o-rou'bi-sin).   An antibiotic used in cancer therapy.
Brand names: Daunomycin, Rubidomycin

Decadron (dec'a-dron).   A corticosteroid used in cancer therapy, especially in the treatment of lymphomas, Hodgkin's disease, and multiple myeloma.
Generic name: dexamethasone

Delalutin (de-lay'lou-tin).   A progestin used in the treatment of endometrial adenocarcinoma.

Delta Cortef (del'ta Cor'tef).   A corticosteroid used in cancer therapy, especially lymphomas, Hodgkin's disease, multiple myeloma.
Generic name: prednisolone

Deltasone (del'ta-sone).   A corticosteroid used in cancer therapy, especially in the treatment of lymphomas, Hodgkin's disease, multiple myeloma.
Generic name: prednisone

Demerol (dem'er-ol).   A narcotic analgesic.
Generic name: meperidine

Depo-Provera (de'po-pro'ver-a).   A progestin used to treat ovarian and endometrial cancers.
Generic name: medroxyprogesterone acetate

dexamethasone (dex-a-meth'a-sone).   A corticosteroid used to treat lymphomas, Hodgkin's disease, and multiple myeloma.
Brand name: Decadron

Diabinese (di-a'bin-e-se).   A sulfonylurea used in the management of diabetes.
Generic name: chlorpropamide

diazepam (di-az'e-pam).   A tranquilizer used to control depression and anxiety.
Brand name: Valium

diazoxide (di-az-oks'ide).   A vasodilator.
Brand name: Hyperstat

Dibenzyline (di-ben'zi-line).   A sympathetic inhibitor used in the treatment of hypertension.
Generic name: phenoxybenzamine

Dicumarol (di-kou'ma-rol).   An anticoagulant.
Generic name: bishydroxycoumarin

diethylstilbestrol (di-eth-yl-stil-bes'trol).   An estrogen used to treat prostatic cancer.

digitalis (dig-i-tal'is).   Used to control arrhythmia and weak heart beat. The most common forms of digitalis are the digitalis glycosides. Digitalis, digoxin, and digitoxin are examples of digitalis glycosides.

digitoxin (di-ji-toks'in). A digitalis glycoside used to treat arrhythmia and weak heart beat.

digoxin (di-goks'in). A digitalis glycoside used to treat arrhythmia and weak heart beat.

Dilantin (dy-lan'tin). Used to control convulsive disorders; it is also an antiarrhythmic agent.
Generic name: diphenylhydantoin sodium

dimenhydrinate (di-men-hy'dri-nate). Used to treat feelings of nausea and vomiting that occur in motion sickness.
Brand name: Dramamine

Dimetapp (dim'e-tapp). Elixir or Extentabs—a decongestant and antihistamine.
Combination drug:
　brompheniramine maleate
　phenylephine hydrochloride
　phenylpropanolamine hydrochloride

diphenylhydantoin sodium (di-fee-nil hy-dan'-toe-in). Used to control convulsive disorders; it is also an antiarrhythmic.
Brand name: Dilantin

diuretics. Drugs that increase the output of urine. Diuretics are frequently used to treat mild hypertension because they decrease sodium levels in the blood which in turn reduces plasma and extracellular fluids.

Diuril (di-your'il). A thiazide that acts as a diuretic.
Generic name: chlorothiazide

Donnatal (don'a-tal). An anticholinergic used to treat motion sickness and spasms of the gastrointestinal tract.
Combination drug:
　phenobarbital
　hyoscyamine sulfate
　atropine sulfate
　hyoscine hydrobromide

Doxorubicin (doks-o-rou'bi-sin). An antibiotic used in cancer therapy.
Generic name: adriamycin

Dramamine (dra'ma-meen). Used to treat motion sickness by relieving feelings of nausea and vomiting.
Generic name: dimenhydrinate

Drixoral (driks'or-al). An antihistamine and decongestant.
Combination drug:
　dexbrompheniramine maleate
　pseudoephedrine sulfate

Dulcolax (dul'ko-laks). A strong cathartic.
Generic name: bisacodyl

Dyazide (die'a-zide). A diuretic used in the treatment of hypertension.
Combination drug: triamterene
　　　　　　　　hydrochlorothiazide

Dymelor (dy-mel'or). A sulfonylurea used to manage diabetes.
Generic name: acetohexamide

Dyrenium (dy-ren'i-um). A diuretic that does not deplete potassium.
Generic name: triamterence

Edecrin (E'de-krin). A strong diuretic.
Generic name: ethacrynic acid

E.E.S. An antibiotic.
Generic name: erythromycin (ethylsuccinate)

Elavil (el'a-vil). A tranquilizer used in the control of severe mental illnesses.
Generic name: amitriptyline

EMETIC (e-met'ik). A drug used to induce vomiting and nausea.

Empirin with codeine (Em'pir-in, ko'deen). A narcotic analgesic.
Combination drug: aspirin and codeine

E-Mycin (E-my'sin). Erythromycin in a special tablet form that prevents the drug from being deactivated by gastric secretions.

Enduron (en'dur-on). A thiazide diuretic.
Generic name: methychlothiazide

ephedrine (e-fed'rin). An antihistamine.

epinephrine (ep-i-nef'rin). A vasoconstrictor.
Brand name: Adrenalin

Epsom salts. A laxative that induces defecation through water retention in the intestine.
Generic name: magnesium sulfate

Equagesic (ek-wa-gee'zik). An analgesic.
Combination drug: meprobamate
ethoheptazine citrate
aspirin

ergotamine tartrate (er-got'a-min tar'trait). Used in the treatment of migraine headaches.
Brand name: Cafergot

erythrityl tetranitrate (e-rith'ri-til te-tra-ny'trait). An antianginal agent.
Brand name: Cardilate

erythromycin (e-rith-roe-my'sin). An antibiotic used to treat bacterial infections, e.g. infections of the respiratory tract.
Brand names: E.E.S., E-Mycin, Ilosone

Esidrix (es'i-driks). A thiazide used as a diuretic.
Generic name: hydrochlorothiazide

Estinyl (es'tin-il). An estrogen used to treat breast cancer.
Generic name: ethinyl estradiol

ethacrynic acid (eth-a-cry'nik). A strong diuretic.
Brand name: Edecrin

ethinyl estradiol (e-thy'nil es-tra'di-ol). An estrogen used to treat breast cancer.
Brand name: Estinyl

ethosuximide (eth-o-suks'i-mide). An anticonvulsant.

Eutonyl. A sympathetic inhibitor used to treat hypertension.
Generic name: pargyline

expectorant (eks-pek'tor-ant). A drug that aids in the removal of mucus by loosening secretions.

Fiorinal (fyour'in-al). An analgesic used to relieve tension headaches.
Combination drug: butalbital
aspirin
phenacetin
caffeine

5-fluorouracil (5-FU) (flew-o-roe-ou'ra-sil). An antimetabolite used in cancer therapy.

fluoxymesterone (flew-oks-i-mez'ter-own). An androgen used to treat breast cancer.

furosemide (fyour-o-sem'ide). A strong diuretic.
Brand name: Lasix

Gantrisin (gan'tri-sin). A sulfonamide used to treat infections of the urinary tract.
Generic name: sulfisoxazole

Gelusil (jel'you-sil). An antacid.
Generic name: magnesium trisilicate combined with aluminum hydroxide

Glaxo (glaks'o). An immune stimulant used in cancer therapy.
Generic name: Bacillus Calmette-Guerin

glyceryl guaiacolate (glis'er-il gwai-a-col'ate). An expectorant.

guanethidine (gwan-eth'i-dine). A sympatholytic drug used to reduce blood pressure and block the hypersecretion of epinephrine.

heparin (hep'a-rin). An anticoagulant.

heroin (her'o-in). A narcotic used as an analgesic.

hydralazine (hi-dral'a-zine). A vasodilator.

Hydrea (hi-dree'a). A drug used in cancer therapy.
Generic name: hydroxyurea

hydrochlorothiazide (hi-dro-klo-ro-thy'a-zide). A thiazide used as a diuretic.
Brand name: Hydrodiuril, Esidrix

hydrocortisone (hi-dro-kor'ti-sone). An anti-inflammation, antipruritic agent that produces vasoconstriction; also used to treat cancerous tissue that respond to hormone stimulation.
Brand names: Cortef, Solu-Cortef

Hydrodiuril (hi-dro-di-your'il). A thiazide used as a diuretic.
Generic name: hydrochlorothiazide

hydroxyprogesterone (hi-droks-e-pro-jes'ter-own). A progestin used in cancer therapy.

hydroxyurea (hi-droks-e-you-ree′a). Used in cancer therapy.
Brand name: Hydrea

Hygroton (hi-gro′ton). A thiazide used as a diuretic.
Generic name: chlorthalidone

Hyperstat (hi′per-stat). A vasodilator used to treat hypertension.
Generic name: diazoxide

Ilosone (il′o-sone). An antibiotic.
Generic name: erythromycin (estolate)

imidazole carboxamide (im-i-daz′ole car-boks′-a-mide). A drug used in cancer therapy.
Brand name: DTIC

IMMUNE STIMULANTS. Used to stimulate the body's immune defense system, or in some cases antibodies are directly administered to the patient. Immune stimulants are used in cancer therapy.
Example:
Generic name: BCG (bacillus Calmette-Guerin)
Brand names: GLAXO, TKE

Imuran (im′you-ran). An immunosuppressive agent.
Generic name: azathioprine

Inderal (in′der-al). A sympathetic inhibitor used in the treatment of hypertension and arrhythmia.
Generic name: propranolol

Indocin (in′doe-sin). Anti-inflammatory agent used in the treatment of arthritis; it also has analgesic and antipyretic effects.
Generic name: indomethacin

I-PAM. An alkylating agent used in cancer therapy.
Generic name: L-Phenylalanine mustard

ipecac, syrup of (ip′e-kak). An emetic.

Ismelin (iz′mel-in). A sympathetic inhibitor used in the treatment of hypertension.
Generic name: guanethidine.

isoproterenol (eye-so-pro-te′re-nol). A bron-chodilator used to treat bronchial asthma, bronchitis, and certain allergies.
Brand name: Isuprel

Isordil (eye-sor′dil). An antianginal agent.
Generic name: isosorbide dinitrate

isosorbide dinetrate (i-so-sor′bide). An anti-anginal agent.
Brand name: Isordil

isoxsuprine hydrochloride (i-soks′su-prine). An antilipemic that increases blood flow and reduces blood cholesterol level.
Brand name: Vasodilan

Isuprel (eye-sup′rel). A bronchodilator used to treat bronchial asthma, bronchitis, and certain allergies.
Generic name: isoproterenol

Keflex (kef′leks). Antibiotic used to treat several types of infections, e.g. infections of the respiratory and urinary tracts.
Generic name: cephalexin

Lanoxin (lan-oks′in). A digitalis glycoside used to treat arrhythmia and weak heart beat.
Generic name: digoxin

Lasix (la′siks). A strong diuretic.
Generic name: furosemide

L-Asparaginase (az-par′a-jin-ase). Used in cancer therapy.

LAXATIVE. A substance used to induce defecation.

L-dopa (do′pa). Used to treat Parkinson's disease by strengthening neurotransmission.
Generic name: levodopa

Leukeran (lew′ker-an). An alkylating agent used in cancer therapy.
Generic name: Chlorambucil

levodopa (le-vo-do′pa). Used to treat Parkinson's disease by strengthening neurotransmission.
Brand name: L-dopa

Levoid (le′void). A thyroid replacement drug.
Generic name: levothyroxine sodium

Levophed (lev'o-fed).   A vasoconstrictor used to treat hypotension.
Generic name: norepinephrine

levothyroxine sodium (lev-o-thy-roks'in).   A thyroid replacement drug.
Brand name: Levoid

Librax (lib'raks).   An anticholingeric used to treat tension, anxiety, and spasms of the gastrointestinal tract.
Combination drug:
chlordiazepoxide hydrochloride
clidinium bromide

Librium (lib're-um).   A tranquilizer used to control depression and anxiety.
Generic name: chlordiazepoxide

lidocaine (lie'doe-kane).   A local anesthetic, also an antiarrhythmic.
Brand name: Xylocaine

liothyronine sodium (lie-o-thy'roe-nine).   A thyroid replacement drug.
Brand name: Cytomel

Lomotil (lo'mo-til).   An antidiarrheal agent.
Generic name: diphenoxylate hydrochloride with atropine sulfate

Lomustine (lo-mus'teen).   A nitrosourea compound used in cancer therapy.
Generic name: CCNU

Maalox (may'loks).   A non-systemic antacid containing magnesium.
Generic name: magnesium hydroxide and aluminum hydroxide

Macrodantin (mak-ro-dan'tin).   An antibacterial used to treat infections of the urinary tract.
Generic name:
nitrofurantoin macrocrystals

magnesium sulfate (epsom salts).   A laxative that induces defecation by causing water retention in the intestine.

magnesium trisilicate.   Combined with aluminum hydroxide, used as an antacid.
Brand name: Gelusil

mechlorethamine (me-klor-eth'a-mine).   An alkylating agent used in cancer therapy.
Brand name: Mustargen

Medrol (med'rol).   An adrenocortical steroid used in cancer therapy.
Generic name: methyl prednisone

medroxyprogesterone acetate (me-droks-e-pro-jes'ter-own).   A progestin used in cancer therapy.
Brand names: Provera, Depo-Provera

Mellaril (mel'a-ril).   A tranquilizer used for severe mental disorders.
Generic name: thioridazine

melphalan (mel'fa-lan).   An alkylating agent used in the treatment of breast cancer.

meprobamate (me-pro-ba'mate).   A tranquilizer.

MER.   An immune stimulant extracted from the bacillus Calmette-Guerin and used in cancer therapy.

mercaptopurine (6-MP) (mer-cap-toe-pu'reen).   An antimetabolite used in the treatment of acute leukemia.

merperidine (mer-per'i-dine).   A narcotic analgesic.
Brand name: Demerol

metaraminol (met-a-ram'i-nol).   A vasoconstrictor used to treat hypotension.
Brand name: Aramine

methimazale (meth-im'a-zale).   An antithyroid agent used in the treatment of hyperthyroidism.
Brand name: Tapazole

methotrexate (MTX) (meth-o-treks'ate).   An antimetabolite used in the treatment of acute leukemia and choriocarcinoma.

methychlothiazide (meth-i-klo-thy'a-zide).   A thiazide used as a diuretic.
Brand name: Enduron

methyl CCNU.   A nitrosourea compound used in cancer therapy.
Brand name: Semustine

methyldopa (meth-il-do'pa). A sympathetic inhibitor used to treat hypertension.
Brand name: Aldomet

methylprednisolone (meth-il-pred-nis'o-lone). A corticosteroid used to treat hypotension.
Brand name: Solumedrol

methyl prednisone (meth-il pred-ne'zone). A corticosteroid used to treat lymphomas, Hodgkin's disease, and multiple myeloma.

methylxanthines (meth-il-zan'thines). Bronchodilators used to treat asthma.
Brand name: Aminophylline

Milk of Magnesia. A laxative; causes water to be retained in the intestine.

mithramycin (mith-ra-my'sin). An antibiotic used in the treatment of cancer, especially leukemia.

morphine (mor'feen). A narcotic analgesic.

Motrin (mo'trin). An anti-inflammatory agent used in the treatment of arthritis; it also has analgesic and antipyretic effects.
Generic name: ibuprofen

MTX. An antimetabolite used to treat cancer.
Generic name: methotrexate

Mustargen (mus'tar-jen). An alkylating agent used in the treatment of cancer.
Generic name: mechlorethamine

Mutulane (mu'tul-lane). Used in cancer therapy.
Generic name: procarbazine

myleran. An alkylating agent used in cancer therapy. See also busulfan.

Naprosyn (na'pro-sin). An anti-inflammatory agent used to treat arthritis.
Generic name: naproxen

Naqua (na'qua). A thiazide used as a diuretic.
Generic name: trichlormethiazide

Neo-synephrine (nee-o-sin-ef'rin). A vassopressor.
Generic name: phenylephrine

nitroglycerin (ni-tro-glis'er-in). A vasodilator

to which the coronary blood vessels are especially sensitive. Nitroglycerin is especially useful in relieving angina pectoris.

nitrol ointment. An antianginal agent topically applied.

nitroprusside (ny-tro-prus'ide). A vasodilator used to treat hypertension.

NITROSOUREA COMPOUNDS. Antitumor drugs which block protein synthesis.

norepinephrine (nor-ep-e-nef'rin). A vasoconstrictor used to treat hypotension.
Brand name: Levophed

Novacain (no'vo-kane). A local anesthetic.
Generic name: procaine

nystatin (nys'ta-tin). An antifungal agent.

Oncovin (on'co-vin). A plant alkaloid used to treat cancer.
Generic name: vincristine

Orinase (or'in-ase). A sulfonylurea used to treat diabetes.
Generic name: tolbutamide

Ortho-Novum (or'tho no'vum). An oral contraceptive.
Combination drug: norethindrone
mestranol

Ovral (ov'ral). An oral contraceptive.
Combination drug: synthetic progestogen
ethinyl estradiol

Parafone Forte (par'a-fown for'te). A muscle relaxant.
Combination drug: chlorzoxazone
acetaminophen

pargyline (par'gi-line). A sympathetic inhibitor used to treat hypertension.
Brand name: Eutonyl

Pavabid (pa'va-bid). A vasodilator.
Generic name: pavaverine hydrochloride

penicillin VK. A potassium salt of penicillin V.
Brand name: Robicillin VK, Pen-Vee-K

pentaerythrityl tetranitrate (pen-ta-e-rith'ri-til tet-ra-ny'trate). An antianginal agent.
Brand name: Peritrate

pentobarbital (pen-to-bar'bi-tal). A barbiturate used as a sedative or hypnotic.

pentolinium (pen-to-lin'i-um). A sympathetic inhibitor used to treat hypertension.
Brand name: Ansolysen

Pen-Vee-K. A potassium salt of penicillin V.
Generic name: penicillin V potassium

Percodan (per'ko-dan). A narcotic analgesic used to relieve severe pain.
Combination drug:
oxycodone hydrochloride
oxycodone terephthalate
aspirin
phenacetin
caffeine

Peritrate (per'i-trate). An antianginal agent.
Generic name: pentaerythrityl tetranitrate

Phenaphen with codeine (fen'a-fen). A narcotic analgesic.
Generic name:
acetaminophen with codeine

Phenergan (fen'er-gan). An antiemetic.
Generic name: a phenothiazine

phenobarbital (fe-no-bar'bi-tal). Used as a sedative and hypnotic.

phenothiazine(s) (fe-no-thy'a-zine). An antiemetic.
Brand names: Phenergan, Thorazine

phentolamine (fen-tol'a-mine). A sympatholytic drug used as a vasodilator; it is also used to prevent excess epinephrine secretion caused by a hyperfunction of the adrenal gland.

L-Phenylalanine mustard (fen-yl-al'a-nine). An alkylating agent used in cancer therapy.
Brand name: I-PAM

phenylephrine (fen-il-ef'rin). A vasoconstrictor.
Brand name: Neo-synephrine

phenytoin (fen-i-toe'in). An anticonvulsant.

polythiazide (pol-e-thy'a-zide). A thiazide used as a diuretic.
Brand name: Renese

Pontocaine (pon'toe-kane). A local anesthetic.
Generic name: tetracaine

prednisolone (pred-nis'o-lone). A corticosteroid used in cancer therapy.
Brand name: Delta Cortef

prednisone (pred'ni-sone). A corticosteroid used in cancer therapy, especially in the treatment of acute lymphocytic leukemia.
Brand name: Deltasone

Premarin (prem'ar-in). A vaginal cream used to treat conditions resulting from menopause, e.g. atrophic vaginitis.
Generic name: conjugated estrogens

primidone (pri'mi-done). An anticonvulsant.

procainamide (pro-kane-am'ide). An antiarrhythmic.
Brand name: Pronestyl

procaine (pro-kane). A local anesthetic.
Brand name: Novacain

procarbazine (pro-kar'ba-zeen). Used in cancer therapy.
Brand name: Mutulane

prochlorperazine (pro-klor-per'a-zeen). Antiemetic.
Brand name: Compazine

Proloid (pro-loyd). A thyroid replacement drug.
Generic name: thyroglobulin

Pronestyl (pro-nes'til). An antiarrhythmic agent.
Generic name: procainamide

propoxyphene (pro-poks'i-feen). An analgesic.
Brand name: Darvon

propranolol (pro-pran'o-lol). An antiarrhythmic agent.
Brand name: Inderal

propylthiouracil (pro-pil-thy-our'a-sil). An antithyroid drug.

Provera. A progestin used to treat ovarian and endometrial cancers.

Generic name:
medroxyprogesterone acetate

Pyribenzamine (pie-re-ben′za-meen).   An antihistamine.
Generic name: tripelennamine

Questran (ques′tran).   An antilipemic agent that increases the production of bile from cholesterol.
Generic name: cholestyramine

Quibron (quib′ron).   An expectorant.

quinidine sulfate (quin-i-dine).   An antiarrhythmic.

Regitine (rej′i-teen).   An anti-ischemic agent.

Renese (ren′ez).   A thiazide used as a diuretic.
Generic name: polythiazide

reserpine (re-ser′peen).   A sympathetic inhibitor used to treat hypertension.
Brand names: Reserpoid, Sandril, Serpasil

Robitussin (ro′bi-tuss-in).   An expectorant.

Rubidomycin (ru-bid′o-my-sin).   An antibiotic used in cancer therapy.
Generic name: daunorubicin

Sandril (san′dril).   A sympathetic inhibitor used to treat hypertension.
Generic name: reserpine

secobarbital (sek-o-bar′bi-tal).   A barbiturate used as a sedative or hypnotic.

Semustine (se-mus′teen).   A nitrosourea compound used in cancer therapy.
Generic name: methyl-CCNU

Ser-Ap-Es.   An antihypertensive agent.
Combination drug:
reserpine
hydralazine hydrochloride
hydrochlorothiazide

Serpasil (ser′pa-sil).   A sympathetic inhibitor used to treat hypertension.
Generic name: reserpine

Sinequan (sin′-e-qwan).   An antidepressant.
Generic name: doxepin HCl

sitosteral (s).   An antilipemic that reduces blood cholesterol level.
Brand name: Cytellin

Slow-K.   A potassium chloride supplement in slow release tablet form, used to treat hypokalemia.

Solucortef (so-lou-kor′tef).   A corticosteroid used in cancer therapy, also used as a vasodilator.
Generic name: hydrocortisone

Solumedral (so-lou-med′ral).   A corticosteroid used as a vasodilator.
Generic name: methylprednisolone

spironolactone (spi-ro-no-lak′tone).   A diuretic that does not deplete potassium.
Brand name: Aldactone

Stelazine (stel′a-zeen).   A tranquilizer used to control severe mental disturbances.
Generic name: phenothiazine

streptomycin (strep-toe-my′sin).   An antibiotic used to treat illnesses produced by many gram-positive and gram-negative bacteria.

streptozoticin (strep-toz-o-tie′sin).   A nitrosourea compound used in cancer therapy.

SULFONYLUREAS (sul-fo-nil-you-re′az).   A group of drugs used to treat diabetes. These drugs cause the pancreas to release insulin.

Sumycin (sou-my′sin).   An antibiotic.
Generic name: tetracycline (hydrochloride)

SYMPATHETIC INHIBITORS.   These drugs affect the sympathetic division of the autonomic nervous system. They reduce vasomotor tone. These drugs are especially useful in the treatment of hypertension.

Synthroid (sin′throyd).   A thyroid replacement drug.
Generic name: levothyroxine sodium

Tagamet (tag′a-met).   A histamine H_2 antagonist used in the treatment of stomach ulcers.
Generic name: cimetidine

Talwin (tal'win).   A potent analgesic.
Generic name: pentazocine hydrochloride

Tapazole (tap'a-zole).   An antithyroid drug.
Generic name: methimazole

testosterone propionate (tes-tos'ter-own pro'pe-o-nate).   An androgen, used to treat breast cancer.

tetracaine (tet'ra-kane).   A local anesthetic.
Brand name: Pontocaine

tetracycline (tet-ra-sy'klin).   An antibiotic used to treat various streptococcal and staphyloccal infections in addition to gram-negative bacteria.
Brand names: Achromycin-V, Sumycin

THIAZIDES (thy'a-zides).   A group of diuretics which are administered orally.

thioquanine (6-TG) (thy-o-gua'nine).   An antimetabolite used in cancer therapy.

Thiotepa (thy-o'te-pa).   An alkylating agent used in cancer therapy.
Generic name:
triethylene thiophosphoramide

Thorazine (thor'a-zeen).   A tranquilizer used to control severe mental disturbances.
Generic name: phenothiazine

thyroglobulin (thy-ro-glob'you-lin).   A thyroid replacement drug.
Brand name: Proloid

THYROID REPLACEMENT DRUGS.   Used to treat hypothyroidism.

TKE.   An immune stimulant used in cancer therapy.
Generic name: bacillus Calmette-Guerin

tolazamide (toe-la'za-mide).   A sulfonylurea used in the treatment of diabetes.
Brand name: Tolinase

tolbutamide (tol-bu'ta-mide).   A sulfonylurea used to treat diabetes.
Brand name: Orinase

Tolinase (tol'in-ase).   A sulfonylurea used to treat diabetes.
Generic name: tolazamide

Tranxene (tranks'een).   A tranquilizer.
Generic name: clorazepate dipotassium

triameterence (tree-a-me'ter-ence).   A diuretic that does not deplete potassium.
Brand name: Dyrenium

Triavil (try'a-vil).   An antidepressant and tranquilizer.
Combination drug: perphenazine amitriptyline

trichlormethiazide (tri-klor-me-thy'a-zide).   A thiazide used as a diuretic.
Brand name: Naqua

triethylene thiophosphoramide (tri-eth'il-ene thy-o-fos-for'a-mide).   An alkylating agent used in cancer therapy.
Brand names: TSPA, Thiotepa

tripelennamine (tri-pel-en'na-meen).   An antihistamine.
Brand name: Pyribenzamine

TSPA.   An alkylating agent used in cancer therapy.
Generic name:
triethylene thiophosphoramide

Tylenol with codeine (tie'le-nol).   A narcotic analgesic.
Generic name: acetaminophen and codeine

Urecholine (you-re-ko'leen).   A cholinergic drug used after surgery to stimulate urination.
Generic name: bethanechol

Valium (val'i-um).   A tranquilizer used to treat depression and anxiety.
Generic name: diazepam

Vasodilan (va-so-die'lan).   An antilipemic that increases blood flow.
Generic name: isoxsuprine hydrochloride

VASODILATORS.   Drugs that cause the blood vessels to dilate.

V-Cillin K.   An antibiotic.
Generic name: penicillin V potassium

Velban (vel'ban).   A plant alkaloid used in the treatment of various cancers such as Hodg-

kin's disease, breast cancer, and choriocarcinoma.
Generic name: vinblastine

Vibramycin (vib-ra-my'sin).   A broad spectrum antibiotic.
Generic name: doxycycline

vinblastine (VLB) (vin-blas'teen). A plant alkaloid used in the treatment of various cancers such as Hodgkin's disease, breast cancer, and choriocarcinoma.
Brand name: Velban

vincristine (VCR) (vin-cris'teen).   A plant alkaloid used in cancer therapy.
Brand name: Oncovin

Xylocaine (zy'lo-kane).   A local anesthetic which also has an antiarrhythmic effect.
Generic name: lidocaine

Zyloprim (zy'lo-prim).   An anti-uric acid agent used to reduce the level of uric acid in the blood, for the treatment of gout.
Generic name: allopurinol

APPENDIX 4 Review Exercises

REVIEW UNIT I

The following exercises will help you review the basic elements of medical terminology presented in the first five chapters. If you have any difficulty with an exercise, don't hesitate to refer to the text.

I. For each of the following medical words underline the base(s), give the meaning of the base(s), and give the meaning of the entire word. *Example:*

HYSTERECTOMY   uterus   removal of the uterus
....

1. HYDROTHERAPY ....

2. VENOUS ....

3. DYSTROPHY ....

4. HEMOPOIESIS ....

5. DENTAL ....

6. TOXICOLOGY ....

7. NEURALAGIA ....

8. APPENDECTOMY ....

9. GASTRITIS ....

10. IATROGENIC ....

11. CARDIOLOGY ....

12. THERMAL ....

13. UROGENITAL ....

14. LINGUAL ....

15. HEPATITIS ....

II. For each pair of medical words indicate the type of duplication and give the meaning of the base. *Example:*

HEMATOLOGIST   HEMOLYTIC

two forms of the same base   blood
....

1. BRONCHIECTASIS   BRONCHOPULMONARY

....

2. POSTGANGLIONIC   GANGLIAL

....

3. ABORAL   STOMATOPATHY

....

4. PELVIPERITONITIS   PELVOSCOPY

....

5. SPERMOBLAST   SPERMATOZOA

....

6. LABIODENTAL   CHEILOPLASTY

....

7. OCULAR   OPHTHAMOLOGIST

....

8. HYPODERMIC   DERMATITIS

....

9. DENTIST   PERIODONTICS

. . . .

10. OVIFORM   OVOGENESIS

. . . .

11. PNEUMOHYDROTHORAX   PNEUMONIA

. . . .

12. LINGUAL   GLOSSODYNIA

. . . .

13. VENOUS   PHLEBITIS

. . . .

14. MEGACARDIA   MEGALOGASTRIA

. . . .

III.   For the following lists of medical words give the suffix of each word and the meaning of the suffix only. Do not be concerned about the meaning of the entire word.

List 1: Simple Suffixes

1. PSYCHOSIS . . . .

2. GASTRIC . . . .

3. SARCOID . . . .

4. CARDIOMEGALY . . . .

5. ILIAC . . . .

6. UREMIA . . . .

7. HYPERTHYROIDISM . . . .

8. FIBROSIS . . . .

9. EPIGASTRIUM . . . .

10. RETRACTOR ....

11. PROCTOSCOPE ....

12. LYMPHOMA ....

13. SPINAL ....

14. PAPILLARY ....

15. NEPHRITIS ....

16. SCAPULAR ....

17. PHARMACIST ....

18. PHARYNGEAL ....

List 2: Compound Suffixes

1. RECTOSCOPY ....

2. THORACENTESIS ....

3. VENOSTASIS ....

4. HEMATOLOGY ....

5. MUCORRHAGIA ....

6. HEPATODYNIA ....

7. OSTEOTOME ....

8. RECTOCLYSIS ....

9. COLOSTOMY ....

10. HEPATOPATHY ....

11. DYSMENORRHEA ....

12. DENTALGIA ....

13. ALBUMINURIA ....

14. ERYTHROPENIA ....

15. SEPTICEMIA ....

16. GASTROPTOSIS ....

17. PHAGOCYTE ....

18. NEPHROTOMY ....

19. ANGIOGRAM ....

20. PARAPLEGIA ....

21. URINALYSIS ....

22. ENCEPHALOGRAPHY ....

23. LARYNGOSCOPE ....

24. CHEILOSTOMATOPLASTY ....

25. ORCHIOCELE ....

26. CEREBROMALACIA ....

27. ELECTROCARDIOGRAPH ....

28. ENTERORRHEXIS ....

29. TONSILLECTOMY ....

30. NEPHROSCLEROSIS ....

31. PHLEBECTASIA ....

32. SPLENOMEGALY ....

33. GASTRORRHAPHY ....

34. PEDIATRICS ....

35. RHINOSTENOSIS ....

36. SALPINGOPEXY ....

      IV. For the following list of medical words give the prefix and the meaning of the prefix. Do not be concerned about knowing the meaning of the entire word.

1. EPIGLOTTIS ....

2. INTRATHORACIC ....

3. CIRCUMCISION ....

4. SUPRALUMBAR ....

5. POSTHYPNOTIC ....

6. ANTENATAL ....

7. DYSPEPSIA ....

8. HEMIAMBLYOPIA ....

9. ANAEROBIC ....

10. SUBDERMAL ....

11. PERICARDIUM ....

12. EXCORIATION ....

13. ADDUCTION ....

14. DICHROMIC ....

15. ENDODERM ....

16. TRANSDUCTION ....

17. CONGLUTINATION ....

18. ABAXIAL ....

19. SEMINORMAL ....

20. DISINFECTANT ....

21. HYPOTONIC ....

22. PERFUSION ....

23. BIFOCAL ....

24. SYNTHESIS ....

25. ANTIBIOTIC ....

26. DECALCIFICATION ....

27. PRESPINAL ....

28. ENARTHRITIS ....

29. INSPIRATION ....

30. ANALYSIS ....

31. INFRARED ....

32. DIATHERMY ....

33. SUPEROXIDE ....

34. PROSTHESIS ....

35. ECTOGENOUS ....

36. AUTONOMIC ....

37. INTERFEMORAL ....

38. PARASYMPATHETIC ....

39. EUPNEA ....

40. CONTRAVOLITIONAL ....

41. EXTRAVASCULAR ....

42. HYPERTONIC ....

43. INSOMNIA ....

    V. For the following list of words cover the pronunciation guide, pronounce each word aloud, and mark the primary stress. Check your answers with the pronunciation guide.

1.	CIRRHOSIS	si-roe'sis
2.	OSTEOPSATHYROSIS	os-tee-op-sa-thy-roe'sis
3.	GANGLIA	gang'le-a
4.	TENDOSYNOVITIS	ten-doe-sin-o-vie'tis
5.	CARDIOTACHOMETER	kar-de-o-tak-om'e-ter
6.	CHONDROCYTE	kon'dro-syt
7.	PSEUDOMEMBRANOUS	sou-do-mem'bra-nus
8.	EUPNEA	up-nee'a
9.	XANTHODERMA	zan-tho-der'ma
10.	PHLEGM	flem'
11.	JEJUNOSTOMY	jee-jou-nos'toe-me
12.	ABAXIAL	ab-ak'se-al
13.	PSYCHOSIS	sy-koe'sis
14.	COCCI	kok'eye
15.	XIPHOID	zif'oid
16.	PHLEBOMYOMASTOSIS	fleb-o-my-o-ma-toe'sis
17.	NEUROGLIAL	new-rog'le-al
18.	OMPHALOCELE	om-fal'o-seel
19.	OSTEOMALACIA	os-tee-o-ma-lay'she-a
20.	PNEUMOTHORAX	new-mo-tho'raks
21.	CILIARY	sil'e-er-e
22.	NEPHROPTOSIS	nef-rop-toe'sis
23.	GENITOURINARY	jen-i-toe-your'i-nar-e

24. PTYALISM tie'a-lizm

25. AUTOGENIC aw-toe-jen'ik

    VI. This exercise will help you to pronounce medical words as whole words instead of groups of little words that have been combined. For each medical word underline the letter(s) that has the primary stress.

1. OSTEOPATHY

2. GASTRECTOMY

3. CYTOLOGY

4. PHARYNGEMPHRAXIS

5. NEPHROTOMY

6. PERIMENINGITIS

7. UROGRAPHY

8. TENDOLYSIS

9. OPHTHALMATROPHY

10. STOMATOPATHY

11. HYPOPHYSECTOMY

12. HEMOLYSIS

13. HYPERPNEA

14. LYMPHADENOPATHY

15. RHINOMETER

    VII. Each word below presents a possible spelling problem. After studying the word, briefly describe the problem. *Example:*

INTERVENOUS   for   INTRAVENOUS

.........Confusion between prefixes has led to a misspelling of intravenous.............

1. *P*SEUDARTHROSIS

....

2. THYMECTOMY   for   THYMUSECTOMY

....

3. HYPERCAPNIA   for   HYPOCAPNIA

....

4. PTILOSIS and TYLOSIS

....

5. R*H*EUMATISM

....

6. DITHERMY for DIATHERMY

....

7. C*H*ONDROBLAST

....

8. APPERCEPTION for ADPERCEPTION

....

9. APEX and APICAL

....

10. THORACENTESIS for THORACOCENTESIS

....

11. SYMPATHECTOMY for SYNPATHECTOMY

....

12. SINUITIS for SINUSITIS

....

13. DIABETES for DIABETES MELLITUS

....

14. PEROSTEUM for PERIOSTEUM

....

15. SYCOSIS for PSYCHOSIS

....

16. *P*NEUMONIA

....

17. COCCYDYNIA   for   COCCYGODYNIA

....

18. LARYNX   and   LARYNGOLOGIST

....

19. IMPERFORATE   for   INPERFORATE

....

20. ERYTHREMIA   for   ERYTHROCYTHEMIA

....

21. DISURIA   for   DYSURIA

....

22. SALPINX   and   SALPINGOSTOMY

....

VIII.   In the following list give the plural form for each word.

Singular   *Plural*

1. BULBUS   ....

2. APEX   ....

3. EDEMA   ....

4. ANALYSIS   ....

5. ARTHRON   ....

6. FOSSA   ....

7. LOBUS   ....

8. AXIS   ....

9. CICATRIX   ....

10. TEMPUS   ....

11. SOMA ....

12. BACTERIUM ....

13. COCHLEA ....

14. CORTEX ....

15. NEUROSIS ....

16. STROMA ....

17. PHALANX ....

18. NEURON ....

19. GUTTA ....

20. MYCOSIS ....

21. GYRUS ....

22. LAMINA ....

23. MATRIX ....

24. VARIX ....

25. MYRINX ....

26. RUGA ....

27. COLUMNA ....

28. SULCUS ....

29. MUSCULUS ....

30. NEMA ....

31. OVUM ....

32. ANTRUM ....

33. SERUM ....

34. CHORDA ....

35. PILUS ....

IX. Answer the following multiple choice, true or false, and fill-in-the-blank questions.

1. Refers to a condition present at birth
(a) neonatal
(b) congenital
(c) acquired
(d) none of the above

2. An .... is the blockage of a passageway.

3. A complication is a secondary disease or disorder that follows a disease or disorder.

T / F   ....

4. A pattern of signs and symptoms that indicate a specific disease is called a ....

....

5. The invasion of the body or part of it by disease-causing microorganisms
(a) complication
(b) inflammation
(c) suppuration
(d) infection

6. The slipping downward of an organ
(a) prolapse
(b) displacement
(c) edema
(d) occlusion

7. A term meaning observable, capable of being examined, and treatable
(a) congenital
(b) clinical
(c) diagnosis
(d) prognosis

8. Edema is the stretching of an organ. T / F   ....

9. An illness that has a long duration is described as ....

10. Another word for suppurative is ....

11. Blood pressure, body temperature, respiration, and heart rate are
    (a) vital signs
    (b) objectives of pathology
    (c) etiology of diseases
    (d) symptoms of diseases

12. A disease is a disorder of the body (or mind) in which body structures and functions are

    affected. T / F ....

13. A disease that occurs without any observable signs is called
    (a) trauma
    (b) anomaly
    (c) asymptomatic
    (d) purulent

14. To look for the causes of a disease is to be concerned with its ....

15. .... is the result of body tissues reacting to injury.

16. The prediction of the course and outcome of a disease
    (a) treatment
    (b) syndrome
    (c) prognosis
    (d) diagnosis

17. .... refers to an illness that occurs suddenly and is accompanied by severe
    symptoms.

18. .... are the signs of a disease and are based on careful observation and
    examination of a patient.

19. A wound to the body caused by an external agent is called a trauma.

    T / F ....

20. .... is the application of a form of therapy.

Review Unit I
Answers to Exercises

I.

1. hydrotherapy, water, treatment, treatment by means of water
2. venous, vein, pertaining to a vein
3. dystrophy, nourishment, poor nourishment
4. hemopoiesis, blood, produce, production of blood

5. <u>dental</u>, tooth, pertaining to the teeth
6. <u>toxic</u>ology, poison, area of medicine that deals with poisons, their effects on the body, and their antidotes
7. <u>neur</u>algia, nerve, pain in a nerve
8. <u>appendec</u>tomy, appendix, excision of the appendix
9. <u>gastri</u>tis, stomach, inflammation of the stomach
10. <u>iatro</u>genic, doctor, produce, produced or caused by a doctor
11. <u>cardi</u>ology, heart, study of the heart and its diseases
12. <u>therma</u>l, heat, pertaining to heat
13. <u>uro</u>genital, urinary tract, reproductive organs, pertaining to the urinary tract and reproductive organs
14. <u>lingua</u>l, tongue, pertaining to the tongue
15. <u>hepa</u>titis, liver, inflammation of the liver

II.

1. different combining vowels, bronchus, windpipe
2. two forms of the same base, mass of nerve cell tissues (mainly nerve cell bodies) outside the brain or spinal cord
3. different bases, mouth
4. different combining vowels, pelvis
5. two forms of the same base, sperm
6. different bases, lip
7. different bases, eye
8. two forms of the same base, skin
9. different bases, tooth
10. different combining vowels, egg
11. two forms of the same base, air
12. different bases, tongue
13. different bases, vein
14. two forms of the same base, enlargement

III.

List 1

1. -osis, abnormal condition
2. -ic, pertaining to
3. -oid, resembling
4. -y, condition, process
5. -ac, pertaining to
6. -a, condition
7. -ism, condition (frequently resulting from a prior condition)
8. -ous, pertaining to, containing
9. -ium, a part (in relation to the whole), region
10. -or, a doer of a specific task
11. -e, instrument
12. -oma, tumor
13. -al, pertaining to

14. -ary, pertaining to
15. -itis, inflammation
16. -ar, pertaining to
17. -ist, one who specializes in
18. -eal, pertaining to

List 2

1. -scopy, examination (visual)
2. -centesis, surgical puncture to withdraw fluid
3. -stasis, halting
4. -logy, study of
5. -orrhagia, excessive flow
6. -odynia, pain
7. -tome, instrument for cutting
8. -clysis, washing, irrigation
9. -ostomy, process of making an opening
10. -pathy, disease, diseased condition
11. -orrhea, flow, discharge
12. -algia, pain
13. -uria, urine condition
14. -penia, deficiency
15. -emia, blood condition
16. -ptosis, falling, prolapse
17. -cyte, a cell
18. -tomy, incision
19. -gram, record
20. -plegia, stroke
21. -lysis, breakdown
22. -graphy, process of recording
23. -scope, instrument for examining (visually)
24. -plasty, surgical repair
25. -cele, hernia
26. -malacia, softening
27. -graph, instrument for recording
28. -orrhexis, rupture
29. -ectomy, excision
30. -sclerosis, hardening
31. -ectasia, dilatation
32. -megaly, enlargement
33. -orrhaphy, process of suturing
34. -iatrics, healing
35. -stenosis, narrowing, stricture
36. -pexy, fixing in place

IV.

1. epi-, over, upon, on; 2. intra-, within; 3. circum-, around;
4. supra-, above, over; 5. post-, after; 6. ante-, before;

7. dys-, difficult, painful;   **8.** hemi-, half;   **9.** an-, without;   **10.** sub-, under;
11. peri-, around;   **12.** ex-, out of, from;   **13.** ad-, toward;   **14.** di-, two;
15. endo, inner, inside;   **16.** trans-, across, through, over;   **17.** con-, with, together;
18. ab-, from, away from;   **19.** semi-, half;   **20.** dis-, apart, free from;
21. hypo-, under, less than normal;   **22.** per-, through;   **23.** bi-, two;
24. syn-, with, together;   **25.** anti-, against;   **26.** de-, from;
27. pre-, before, in front of;   **28.** en-, in, within;   **29.** in-, in, into;
30. ana-, up, back again;   **31.** infra-, below;   **32.** dia-, through;
33. super-, above, over;   **34.** pros-, to, in addition to, near;   **35.** ecto-, outside, outer;
36. auto-, self;   **37.** inter-, between;   **38.** para-, beside, alongside, abnormal;
39. eu-, good, well;   **40.** contra-, against;   **41.** extra-, outside of, beyond;
42. hyper-, above, excessive;   **43.** in-, not.

VI.

1. osteopathy, os-tee-op'a-the;   **2.** gastrectomy, gas-trek'toe-me;
3. cytology, sy-tol'o-je;   **4.** pharyngemphraxis, far-in-jem-frak'sis;
5. nephrotomy, ne-frot'o-me;   **6.** perimenigitis, per-e-men-in-jy'tis;
7. urography, you-rog'ra-fe;   **8.** tendolysis, ten-dol'i-sis;
9. ophthalmatrophy, of-thal-mat'roe-fe;   **10.** stomatopathy, sto-ma-top'a-the;
11. hypophysectomy, hi-pof-i-sek'toe-me;   **12.** hemolysis, he-mol'i-sis;
13. hyperpnea, hi-perp-nee'a;   **14.** lymphadenopathy, lim-fad-e-nop'a-the;
15. rhinometer, ry-nom'et-er.

VII.

1. Avoid omitting the silent letter.
2. Shortened form is competing with full form.
3. Prefixes are confused.
4. Homophones are confused.
5. Avoid omitting the silent letter.
6. misspelling resulting from confusion of prefixes
7. Avoid omitting the silent letter.
8. assimilation of sounds
9. Name and combining form differ.
10. shortened form competing with full form
11. assimilation of sounds
12. shortened form competing with full form
13. shortened form competing with full form
14. misspelling resulting from prefix confusion
15. homophones confused
16. Avoid omitting silent letter.
17. shortened form competing with full form
18. Name and combining form differ.
19. assimilation of sounds
20. shortened form competing with full form

21. misspelling resulting from prefix confusion
22. Name and combining form differ.

VIII.

1. bulbi;   2. apices;   3. edemata;   4. analyses;   5. arthra;   6. fossae;
7. lobi;   8. axes;   9. cicatrices;   10. tempora;   11. somata;
12. bacteria;   13. cochleae;   14. cortices;   15. neuroses;   16. stromata;
17. phalanges;   18. neura;   19. guttae;   20. mycoses;   21. gyri;
22. laminae;   23. matrices;   24. varices;   25. myringes;   26. rugae;
27. columnae;   28. sulci;   29. musculi;   30. nemata;   31. ova;
32. antra;   33. sera;   34. chordae;   35. pili.

IX.

1. (b);   2. occlusion;   3. T;   4. syndrome;   5. (d);   6. (a);   7. (b);
8. F, a swelling;   9. chronic;   10. purulent;   11. (a);   12. T;   13. (c);
14. etiology;   15. inflammation;   16. (c);   17. acute;   18. symptoms;
19. T;   20. treatment.

REVIEW UNIT II

I. The Body Regions: For each set of body regions put the medical words into correct order.

1.	thoracic cervical pubic	neck	chest	groin
		. . . .		
2.	deltoid orbital perineal	eye	base of trunk	shoulder
		. . . .		
3.	gluteal frontal buccal	buttocks	forehead	cheek
		. . . .		
4.	scapular umbilical mammary	shoulderblade	breast	navel
		. . . .		
5.	femoral brachial plantar	arm	thigh	sole of the foot
		. . . .		
6.	occipital cubital lumbar	base of skull	lower back	front of elbow
		. . . .		

7. patellar   palm   wrist   knee   back of knee
    popliteal
    volar   ....
    carpal

II.   Match each body cavity with its medical name.

1. houses the brain ....   a. nasal cavity

2. contains the spinal cord ....   b. abdominal cavity

3. eye socket ....   c. alimentary canal

4. nose cavity ....   d. spinal cavity

5. mouth cavity ....   e. thoracic cavity

6. chest cavity ....   f. celomic cavity

7. different portions of the same cavity (use two
                                                   g. cranial cavity
    letters) ....
                                                   h. buccal cavity
8. general name for the three cavities that house the

    viscera ....   i. orbital cavity

                                                   j. pelvic cavity
9. digestive tract ....

III.   Arrange the following list of directional terms into pairs of antonyms.

1. ....   superior
                                                                    superficial
2. ....   medial
                                                                    deep
3. ....   distal
                                                                    posterior
4. ....   inferior
                                                                    lateral
                                                                    proximal
5. ....   anterior

IV. Match the following descriptions with their medical words.

1. circular, cone-shaped movement ....

2. a movement that separates two portions of an

    extremity ....

3. a hand in a backward position ....

4. the lowering of a body part ....

5. the movement of an extremity away from the median plane

    of the body ....

6. a bending action that brings two portions of an extremity

    together ....

7. a hand in a face-forward position ....

8. the drawing backward of a body part ....

9. the movement of an extremity toward the median plane of

    the body ....

10. the turning of a structure on its axis ....

11. the feet turned inward ....

12. the feet turned outward ....

13. forward movement/protrusion of a body part ....

14. the raising of a body part ....

a. eversion

b. supination

c. inversion

d. protraction

e. elevation

f. adduction

g. circumduction

h. depression

i. extension

j. pronation

k. retraction

l. abduction

m. rotation

n. flexion

V. Fill in the blanks for the following statements.

1. The .... plane cuts the body horizontally.

2. The .... plane divides the body into front and rear sections.

3. The .... or .... plane cuts the body into right and left
    halves.

4. Surface examination of the body by feeling is called ....

VI. Numbers and Colors: Match the combining forms with their meanings. You may use some letters several times.

1. di		a.	one, single
2. centi		b.	two, double
3. multi		c.	three
4. melano		d.	four
5. nigro		e.	one hundredth
6. chloro		f.	many
7. glauco		g.	white
8. mono		h.	black
9. tri		i.	red
10. polio		j.	green
11. erythro		k.	blue
12. cyano		l.	yellow
13. haplo		m.	gray
14. kilo		n.	one thousandth
15. albo			
16. diplo			
17. quadri			
18. uni			
19. milli			
20. tetra			
21. xantho			

22. rubo . . . .

23. poly . . . .

24. leuko . . . .

VII. The Skin: For each medical word underline the letter(s) with the primary stress, give the meaning for the word, and write the combining form with its meaning. *Example:*

<u>DER</u>MAL   pertaining to the skin   derm/o, skin
. . . .

1. TRICHORRHEA . . . .

2. SEBORRHAGIA . . . .

3. UNGUAL . . . .

4. HOLISTIC . . . .

5. EXOCRINE . . . .

6. INTRACUTANEOUS . . . .

7. ACANTHOID . . . .

8. FOLLICULAR . . . .

9. ADIPECTOMY . . . .

10. DIAPHORETIC . . . .

11. DERMATITIS . . . .

12. MEROGENESIS . . . .

13. SUDORIFIC . . . .

14. KERATOSIS . . . .

15. DERMALGIA . . . .

16. HIDRADENITIS . . . .

17. ONYCHOTOMY ....

18. DEPILATE ....

      VIII.   The Musculoskeletal System: Match the following combining forms with their meanings. Some letters may be used twice.

List 1

1. CERVIC/O	a.	palate
2. LAMIN/O	b.	spinal cord, bone marrow
2. SACR/O	c.	bent
4. STERN/O	d.	bone
5. TARS/O	e.	upper jawbone
6. PUB/O	f.	wrist
7. PELV/O	g.	upper arm
8. ULN/O	h.	collarbone
9. SCAPUL/O	i.	hand bones
10. MANDIBUL/O	j.	outer bone of the forearm
11. OSTE/O	k.	kneecap
12. LUMB/O	l.	heel bone
13. FIBUL/O	m.	neck
14. COST/O	n.	lower back
15. TIBI/O	o.	humped
16. METATARS/O	p.	vertebra
17. ACETABUL/O	q.	flat bone of the neural arch of a vertebra
18. FEMOR/O	r.	breastbone

19. CARP/O ....

20. HUMER/O ....

21. CHONDR/O ....

22. PALAT/O ....

23. SPONDYL/O ....

24. MYEL/O ....

25. KYPH/O ....

26. PATELL/O ....

27. ISCHI/O ....

28. RADI/O ....

29. CALCANE/O ....

30. ILI/O ....

31. METACARP/O ....

32. MAXILL/O ....

33. SUBMAXILL/O ....

34. CRANI/O ....

35. THORAC/O ....

36. VERTEBR/O ....

37. LORD/O ....

38. RACHI/O ....

39. SCOLI/O ....

40. COCCYG/O ....

s.   cartilage

t.   finger or toe bones

u.   lower portion of the hipbone

v.   calf bone

w.   foot bones

x.   ankle

y.   pelvis

z.   shoulder bone

aa. lower jawbone

bb. cranium

cc. sacrum

dd. rib

ee. spinal column

ff. curved

gg. tailbone

hh. thighbone

ii. saucerlike cavity of the hipbone

jj. elbow

kk. portion of the scapula that articulates with the clavicle

ll. inner bone of the forearm

mm. shinbone

nn. superior part of the hipbone

41. CLAVICUL/O ....   oo. pubic bone

42. OLECRAN/O ....   pp. chest

43. ACROMI/O ....

44. PHALANG/O ....

List 2

1. ARTHR/O ....   a. bundle of muscle fibers

2. FIBR/O ....   b. ligament

3. MYOS/O ....   c. away

4. FASCI/O ....   d. flesh

5. TEN/O ....   e. joint

6. ARTICUL/O ....   f. muscle

7. BURS/O ....   g. both

8. SYNDESM/O ....   h. fibrous membrane that covers and
                                         separates muscles

9. MUSCUL/O ....   i. lubricating fluid of the joints

10. TENDIN/O ....   j. sac containing synovial fluid

11. SYNOVI/O ....   k. fiber

12. APO- ....   l. tendon

13. FASCICUL/O ....

14. TEND/O ....

15. SARC/O ....

16. AMPHI- ....

17. MY/O ....

IX.   The Nervous System: Match the combining forms with their meanings.

<table>
<tr><td>

1. GANGLI/O or

   GANGLION/O ....

2. ENCEPHAL/O ....

3. FER/O ....

4. PARASYMPATH/O,

   PARASYMPATHIC/O, or

   PARASYMPATHETIC/O ....

5. MENING/O or MENINGI/O ....

6. AUT/O ....

7. VENTRICUL/O ....

8. NEUR/O ....

9. MYEL/O ....

10. ASTR/O ....

11. CEREBR/O ....

12. GLI/O ....

13. MYELIN/O ....

14. OLIG/O ....

15. SPIN/O ....

16. MES/O ....

17. SYMPATH/O, SYMPATHIC/O,

    or SYMPATHETIC/O ....

18. CEREBELL/O ....
</td><td>

a. nerve

b. membranes covering the brain and spinal cord

c. cerebellum

d. few, deficient in

e. glue, adhesive

f. cerebrum

g. ganglion

h. branch

i. sympathetic division of the ANS

j. carry, conduct

k. self

l. brain

m. thalamus

n. spinal cord

o. parasympathetic division of the ANS

p. star shaped

q. small cavity, ventricle

r. myelin

s. small

t. spinal cord

u. middle
</td></tr>
</table>

19. MICR/O ....

20. THALAM/O ....

21. RAM/O ....

      X. Synonymous bases: Match the combining forms that have the same meaning.

         Synonyms   *Meaning*

1. .... SUBMAXILL/O

   .... ARTICUL/O

2. .... TENDIN/O

   .... DERMAT/O

3. .... ONYCH/O

   .... SUDOR/O

   .... TEN/O

4. .... VERTEBR/O

   .... MY/O

5. .... MANDIBUL/O

   .... CUT/I

6. .... PIL/L

   .... TEND/O

7. .... MUSCUL/O

   .... HIDR/O

8. .... UNGU/O

   .... SPONDYL/O

   .... ARTHR/O

9. .... DIAPHOR/O

.... MYOS/O

.... TRICH/O

XI. Give the meaning for each of the following medical words. Divide each word into base(s), prefixes, and suffix; underline the letter(s) with the primary stress. *Example:*

AUTOGENIC   self-producing   auto/gen/ic

1. TENODESIS ....

2. CHONDROGENESIS ....

3. RAMIFICATION ....

4. CORTICOSPINAL ....

5. ARTHROTOME ....

6. STERNOCOSTAL ....

7. DERMATOMYCOSIS ....

8. ONYCHOPHAGY ....

9. ARTHROSYNOVITIS ....

10. OLIGEMIA ....

11. MYELOPOIESIS ....

12. GLIOMA ....

13. DERMATOMYOSITIS ....

14. SPONDYLALGIA ....

15. MYOMA ....

16. OSTEOCLAST ....

17. OLECRANOID ....

18. EFFERENT ....

19. VENTRICULOGRAPHY ....

20. COSTECTOMY ....

21. ADIPOGENOUS ....

22. SCOLIOSOMETRY ....

23. SYNDESMOPEXY ....

24. MAXILLITIS ....

25. NEURASTHENIA ....

26. CEREBROMALACIA ....

27. ADIAPHORESIS ....

28. UNGUAL ....

29. MYITIS ....

30. BURSITIS ....

31. ILIOGEMORAL ....

32. MENIGOMYELOCELE ....

33. HIDROADENITIS ....

34. KERATOSIS ....

35. GANGLIONECTOMY ....

XII. For each group of words underline the misspelled word and write the correct spelling in the space provided.

1. ENDOCRINE   TRICOLOGIST   KERATOSIS

....

2. UMBILICAL   GLUTEAL   PATELAR

....

3. MILIMETER   LEUKODERMA   MELANOCYTE

. . . .

4. DIAFORETIC   ONYCHITIS   PACHYDERMA

. . . .

5. RACHITIS   SPONDILOSYNDESIS   CLACANEAL

. . . .

6. EFERENT   MENINGITIS   ASTROGLIAL

. . . .

7. LORDOSCOLIOSIS   SYNDESMOPEXY   APONUROSIS

. . . .

8. PILLOSIS   ORBITAL   CYNANODERMA

. . . .

9. THORACOCENTESIS   RABDOMYOSARCOMA   CHONDROGENESIS

. . . .

10. NEUROSTHENIA   GLIOMATA   RAMOSE

. . . .

Review Unit II
Answers to Exercises

I.

1. cervical, thoracic, pubic; 2. orbital, perineal, deltoid; 3. gluteal, frontal, buccal;
4. scapular, mammary, umbilical; 5. brachial, femoral, plantar;
6. occipital, lumbar, cubital; 7. volar, carpal, patellar, popliteal.

II.

1. g; 2. d; 3. i; 4. a; 5. h; 6. e; 7. b and j; 8. f;
9. c.

III.

superior, inferior; superficial, deep; medial, lateral;
distal, proximal; posterior, anterior.

IV.

1. g;   2. i;   3. j;   4. h;   5. l;   6. n;   7. b;   8. k;   9. f;
10. m;   11. c;   12. a;   13. d;   14. e.

V.

1. transverse;   2. coronal;   3. median, midsagittal;   4. palpation.

VI.

1. b;   2. e;   3. f;   4. h;   5. h;   6. j;   7. m;   8. a;   9. c;
10. m;   11. i;   12. k;   13. a;   14. n;   15. g;   16. b;   17. d;
18. a;   19. n;   20. d;   21. l;   22. i;   23. f;   24. g.

VII.

1. trichorrhea, excessive loss of hair, trich/o, hair
2. seborrhagia, excessive secretion of sebum, seb/o, sebum
3. ungual, pertaining to the nails, ungu/o, nail
4. holistic, pertaining to the whole, hol/o, whole
5. exocrine, externally secreting, -crine, to secrete
6. intracutaneous, within the skin, cut/i, skin
7. acanthoid, spiny, thorny, acanth/o, spine or thorn
8. follicular, pertaining to follicles, follicul/o, small cavity
9. adipectomy, excision of fatty tissue, adip/o, fat
10. diaphoretic, sweat-producing, diaphor/o, sweat
11. dermatitis, inflammation of the skin, dermat/o, skin
12. merogenesis, reproduction by segmentation, mer/o, part, gen/o, produce
13. sudorific, sweat-producing, sudor/o, sweat
14. keratosis, abnormal horny growth, kerat/o, horny
15. dermalgia, pain in the skin, derm/o, skin
16. hidradenitis, inflammation of sweat glands, hidr/o, sweat, aden/o, gland
17. onychotomy, incision of a finger/toe nail, onych/o, nail
18. depilate, to remove hair, pil/o, hair

VIII.

List 1

1. m;   2. q;   3. cc;   4. r;   5. x;   6. oo;   7. y;   8. ll;
9. z;   10. aa;   11. d;   12. n;   13. v;   14. dd;   15. mm;
16. w;   17. ii;   18. hh;   19. f;   20. g;   21. s;   22. a;   23. p;
24. b;   25. o;   26. k;   27. u;   28. j;   29. l;   30. nn;   31. i;
32. e;   33. aa;   34. bb;   35. pp;   36. p;   37. c;   38. ee;
39. ff;   40. gg;   41. h;   42. jj;   43. kk;   44. t.

List 2

1. e;   2. k;   3. f;   4. h;   5. l;   6. e;   7. j;   8. b;   9. f;
10. l;   11. i;   12. c;   13. a;   14. l;   15. d;   16. g;   17. f.

IX.

1. g;   **2.** l;   **3.** j;   **4.** o;   **5.** b;   **6.** k;   **7.** q;   **8.** a;   **9.** t;
10. p;   **11.** f;   **12.** e;   **13.** r;   **14.** d;   **15.** n;   **16.** u;   **17.** i;
18. c;   **19.** s;   **20.** m;   **21.** h.

X.

cut/i, dermat/o, skin;   trich/o, pil/o, hair;
sudor/o, diaphor/o, hidr/o, sweat;   ungu/o, onych/o, nail;
mandibul/o, submaxill/o, lower jawbone;   spondyl/o, vertebr/o, vertebra;
arthr/o, articul/o, joint;   ten/o, tend/o, tendin/o, tendon;
my/o, myos/o, muscul/o, muscle

XI.

1. surgical fastening of a tendon, ten/o/desis
2. formation of cartilage, chondr/o/gen/esis
3. process of making branches, ram/i/fic/a/tion
4. pertaining to the cerebral cortex and spinal cord, cortic/o/spin/al
5. instrument for cutting a joint, arthr/o/tome
6. pertaining to the sternum and ribs, stern/o/cost/al
7. skin infection caused by fungus, dermat/o/myc/osis
8. nail biting, onych/o/phagy
9. inflammation of the synovial membrane of a joint, arthr/o/synov/itis
10. insufficient quantity of blood in the body, olig/emia
11. formation of bone marrow, myel/o/poie/sis
12. tumor originating in the supporting nervous tissue, gli/oma
13. inflammation of connective (muscle) tissue (skin), dermat/o/myos/itis
14. pain in a vertebra, spondyl/algia
15. tumor composed of muscle tissue, my/oma
16. a cell that breaks up and absorbs bone matter, oste/o/clast
17. elbow shaped, olecran/oid
18. conducting impulses away from the CNS, ef/fer/ent
19. x-raying of the ventricles of the brain, ventricul/o/graphy
20. excision of a rib, cost/ectomy
21. fat producing, adip/o/gen/ous
22. measurement of the degree of spinal curvature, scolios/o/metry
23. surgical fastening of a ligament, syndesm/o/pexy
24. inflammation of the upper jaw, maxill/itis
25. weakness resulting from a nervous disorder, neur/asthenia
26. softening of the cerebrum, cerebr/o/malacia
27. absence of sweat, a/diaphor/esis
28. pertaining to the nails, ungu/al
29. inflammation of a muscle, my/itis
30. inflammation of the sac containing synovial fluid, burs/itis
31. pertaining to the ilium and femur, ili/o/femor/al
32. hernia of the spinal cord and its coverings, mening/o/myel/o/cele
33. inflammation of the sweat glands, hidr/o/aden/itis

34. abnormal horny growth of the skin, kerat/osis
35. excision of a ganglion, ganglion/ectomy

     XII.

1. trichologist;   **2.** patellar;   **3.** millimeter;   **4.** diaphoretic;
5. spondylosyndesis;   **6.** efferent;   **7.** aponeurosis;   **8.** pilosis;
9. rhabdomyosarcoma;   **10.** neurasthenia.

REVIEW UNIT III

    I.   The Eye: Match each combining form with its meaning. Some letters may be used more than once.

1. PHAC/O	a. iris
2. KERAT/O	b. eyelid
3. CYCL/O	c. pupil
4. IR/O	d. eye
5. PALPEBR/O	e. sight, vision
6. EX/O	f. lens
7. OPHTHALM/O	g. eyelid
8. CORE/O	h. tear/tear duct
9. OCUL/O	i. outside
10. BLEPHAR/O	j. cornea
11. LACRIM/O	k. membrane lining the eye
12. CONJUNCTIV/O	l. white portion of the eye
13. -OPIA	m. retina
14. PUPILL/O	n. ciliary body
15. AQU/O	o. water

16. SCLER/O ....

17. CORNE/O ....

18. IRID/O ....

19. RETIN/O ....

20. DACRY/O ....

    II. The Ear: Match each combining form with its meaning. Some letters may be used more than once.

1. MALLE/O	a. baglike protrusion of a canal
2. EUSTACHI/O	b. hearing
3. UTRICUL/O	c. sac of the bony labyrinth
4. ANKYL/O	d. ear
5. AUDI/O	e. tube/eustachian tube
6. OT/O	f. wax
7. INCUD/O	g. hammer of the ear
8. TYMPAN/O	h. sac of the membranous labyrinth
9. AUR/O	i. snail-shaped portion of the middle ear
10. LABYRINTH/O	j. eardrum
11. AMPULL/O	k. stirrup
12. MYRING/O	l. eustachian tube
13. SALPING/O	m. anvil
14. STAPED/O	n. bent
15. ACOU/O	o. winding path of the inner ear
16. COCHLE/O	p. a cavity that constitutes the middle portion of the middle ear

17. VESTIBUL/O ....

18. SACCUL/O ....

19. CERUMIN/O ....

III. The Cardiovascular System: The following list of words contains several groups of synonyms. Find the synonyms and give their meaning.

	Synonym	*Meaning*	
1.	....	....	-EMIA
	....		MEGAL/O
	....		ANGI/O
2.	....	....	VEN/O
	....		NUCLE/O
3.	....	....	CORON/O
	....		MEGA-
4.	....	....	VAS/O
	....		CARDI/O
5.	....	....	OXY-
	....		HEM/O
6.	....	....	PHLEB/O
	....		OX/O
7.	....	....	HEMAT/O
	....		KARY/O

IV. The Cardiovascular System: Match each combining form with its meaning.

1. CAPILL/O ....   a. tonsil

2. IMMUN/O ....   b. small vein

3. SPLEN/O ....

4. ATHER/O ....

5. THROMB/O ....

6. AORT/O ....

7. FIBRIN/O ....

8. RETICUL/O ....

9. TON/O ....

10. ARTERI/O ....

11. SPHYGM/O ....

12. PHIL/O ....

13. FIBR/O ....

14. ANGIN/O ....

15. SER/O ....

16. BRACHY- ....

17. -IN ....

18. VALV/O ....

19. VENUL/O ....

20. STETH/O ....

21. -POIESIS ....

22. LYMPH/O ....

23. THYM/O ....

24. -STASIS ....

25. SIDER/O ....

c. network

d. abnormal widening

e. small

f. death

g. knot/node

h. affinity for

i. very small blood vessel

j. serum

k. halting

l. valve

m. cavity

n. small artery

o. round

p. safe/immune

q. artery

r. choking

s. thymus gland

t. clot

u. atrium

v. granule

w. fatty buildup

x. tension

y. short

26. ATRI/O ....   z. production

27. ANEURYSM/O ....   aa. spleen

28. PHAG/O ....   bb. fibrin

29. BAS/O ....   cc. indicates a chemical substance

30. SIN/O ....   dd. quick

31. VARIC/O ....   ee. lymph

32. -L/O ....   ff. iron

33. AGGLUTIN/O ....   gg. eat

34. GLOB/O ....   hh. pulse

35. TONSILL/O ....   ii. aorta

36. PLASM/O ....   jj. plasma

37. TACH/O ....   kk. fiber

38. NOD/O ....   ll. chest

39. GRANUL/O ....   mm. base

40. ARTERIOL/O ....   nn. clumping

41. NECR/O ....   oo. twisted vein

V. The Respiratory System: Match each combining form with its meaning. Some letters may be used more than once.

1. PHRENIC/O ....   a. the wall separating the thoracic and abdominal cavities

2. -PNEA ....   b. bronchus

3. PULM/O ....   c. carbon dioxide

4. PECTOR/O ....   d. cavity located between two parts of an organ

5. PHARYNG/O ....   e. air/lung

6. PLEUR/O ....   f. epiglottis

7. DIAPHRAGM/O ....   g. chest

8. MYC/O ....   h. nose

9. LOB/O ....   i. breathing

10. BRONCH/O ....   j. saliva

11. EPIGLOTT/O ....   k. larynx

12. RHIN/O ....   l. small bronchus

13. BRONCHI/O ....   m. lung

14. PTYAL/O ....   n. pharynx

15. DIAPHRAGMAT/O ....   o. division of an organ

16. ATEL/O ....   p. serous membrane covering the lungs and thoracic wall

17. PHREN/O ....   q. imperfect

18. MUC/O ....   r. trachea

19. NAS/O ....   s. small hollow or cavity/air cell

20. ALVEOL/O ....   t. fungus

21. SPIR/O ....   u. a thick fluid secreted by membranes

22. PNEUM/O ....   v. phrenic nerve

23. -CAPNIA ....

24. PTY/O ....

25. PNEUMON/O ....

26. PULMON/O ....

27. BRONCHIOL/O ....

28. TRACHE/O ....

29. LARYNG/O ....

30. MEDIASTIN/O ....

VI. Synonymous bases: Match the combining forms that have the same meaning.

Synonym   *Meaning*

1. .... LACRIM/O

    ....   TYMPAN/O

2. .... PNEUM/O

    ....   OCUL/O

3. .... PHREN/O

    ....   RHIN/O

4. .... AUR/O

    ....   PALPEBR/O

5. .... CORNE/O

    ....   OPHTHALM/O

6. .... PULM/O

    ....   PNEUMON/O

7. .... MYRING/O

    ....   BLEPHAR/O

8. .... KERAT/O

    ....   NAS/O

9. .... DIAPHRAGMAT/O

    ....   CORE/O

10. ....   DACRY/O

    ....   ACOU/O

11. ....   PULMON/O

    ....   OT/O

12. ....   PUPILL/O

    ....   AUDI/O

VII. Give the meaning for each of the following medical words. Divide each word into base(s), prefix, and suffix; underline the letter(s) with the primary stress.
Example:

LYMPHADENITIS   inflammation of a lymph gland   lymph/aden/<u>i</u>tis
....

1. RHINOMYCOSIS ....

2. SIDEROPENIA ....

3. IRIDECTOMY ....

4. PHARYNGEMPHRAXIS ....

5. TRACHEOSTOMY ....

6. EXOPHTHALMIA ....

7. OCULOMYCOSIS ....

8. NECROSIS ....

9. GRANULOCYTOPOIESIS ....

10. DIAPHRAGMODYNIA ....

11. ANEURYSMECTOMY ....

12. HYPOXIA ....

13. PNEUMOHYDROTHORAX ....

14. TRACHEOPYOSIS ....

15. DACRYOADENITIS ....

16. BLEPHARADENITIS ....

17. ASTHENOPIA ....

18. ANOXIA ....

19. VENOSTASIS ....

20. DYSPNEA ....

21. THROMBOLYSIS ....

22. PHAGOCYTOSIS ....

23. HEMOPTYSIS ....

24. RETINOSCOPY ....

25. KERATOID ....

26. RETICULAR ....

27. BRONCHIOLECTASIS ....

28. OPHTHALMODYNAMOMETER ....

29. PHACOMALACIA ....

30. ANGIOGRAM ....

31. TACHYARRHYTHMIA ....

32. SEPTICEMIA ....

33. HEMOTROPHIC ....

34. NEUTROPHILIA ....

35. ACAPNIA ....

VIII. For each group of words underline the misspelled word and write the correct spelling in the space provided.

1. PHLEBOPLASTY   PUPILLOSTATOMETER   HEMOTYSIS

....

2. ANKELOBLEPHARON   CYCLOPLEGIA   BASOPHIL

....

3. HEMOSIDERIN   PNEUMOHYDROTHORAX   ANEURYSMORHAPHY

....

4. CORECTOPIA   EXOPTHALMIA   PHACOMALACIA

....

5. PLASMAPHERESIS   MYKOSIS   ERYTHROPOIESIS

....

6. SFIGMOMANOMETER   BRONCHOSTENOSIS   MYRINGOSCOPE

....

7. VESTIBULAR   ARTERIOSTENOSIS   SPLENOMEGILY

....

8. CERUMINOSIS   BRACHYCARDIA   BLEPHEROPTOSIS

....

9. ATRIOVENTRICULAR   TRACHOSTOMY   CONJUNCTIVAL

....

10. LYMPHANGEOMA   CORNEOUS   DEFIBRILLATION

....

11. RETICULOENDOTHELIAL   PULMONECTOMY   STAPEDEOVESTIBULAR

....

12. EXPECTORENT   EPIGLOTTIS   POLYCYTHEMIA

....

13. STETHOMETER   MEDIASTENOPERICARDITIS   PHARYNGEMPHRAXIS

....

14. RAMIFICATION   ACAPNIA   DACROADENITIS

....

15. PROTHROMBIN   IMUNOLOGY   LYMPHOMAS

....

16. ATELLECTASIS   SCLERECTASIA   TONSILLECTOMY

....

Review Unit III
Answers to Exercises

I.

1. f;   2. j;   3. n;   4. a;   5. g;   6. i;   7. d;   8. c;   9. d;
10. b;   11. h;   12. k;   13. e;   14. c;   15. o;   16. l;   17. j;
18. a;   19. m;   20. h.

II.

1. g;   2. l;   3. h;   4. n;   5. b;   6. d;   7. m;   8. j;
9. d;   10. o;   11. a;   12. j;   13. e;   14. k;   15. b;   16. i;
17. p;   18. c;   19. f.

III.

-emia, blood, hem/o, hemat/o;   megal/o, large, mega-;
angi/o, vessel, vas/o;   ven/o, vein, phleb/o;   nucle/o, nucleus, kary/o;
coron/o, heart, cardi/o;   oxy-, oxygen, ox/o.

IV.

1. i;   2. p;   3. aa;   4. w;   5. t;   6. ii;   7. bb;   8. c;   9. x;
10. q;   11. hh;   12. h;   13. kk;   14. r;   15. j;   16. y;   17. cc;
18. l;   19. b;   20. ll;   21. z;   22. ee;   23. s;   24. k;   25. ff;
26. u;   27. d;   28. gg;   29. mm;   30. m;   31. oo;   32. e;
33. nn; 34. o;   35. a;   36. jj;   37. dd;   38. g;   39. v;
40. n;   41. f.

V.

1. v;   2. i;   3. m;   4. g;   5. n;   6. p;   7. a;   8. t;   9. o;
10. b;   11. f;   12. h;   13. b;   14. j;   15. a;   16. q;   17. a;

18. u;   **19.** h;   **20.** s;   **21.** i;   **22.** e;   **23.** c;   **24.** j;   **25.** e;
26. m;   **27.** l;   **28.** r;   **29.** k;   **30.** d.

VI.

lacrim/o, tear, dacry/o;   tympan/o, eardrum, myring/o;
pneum/o, air, pneumon/o;   ocul/o, eye, ophthalm/o;
phren/o, diaphragm, diaphragmat/o;   rhin/o, nose, nas/o;
aur/o, ear, ot/o;   palpebr/o, eyelid, blephar/o;   corne/o, cornea, kerat/o;
pulm/o, lung, pulmon/o;   acou/o, hearing, audi/o;
core/o, pupil, pupill/o.

VII.

1. fungus infection of the mucous membrane of the nose, rhin/o/myc/osis
2. deficiency of iron, sider/o/penia
3. excision of part of the iris, irid/ectomy
4. obstruction of the pharynx, pharyng/emphraxis
5. incision of the trachea to insert a tube, trache/ostomy
6. abnormal protrusion of the eyeball, ex/ophthalm/ia
7. diseased condition of the eye caused by fungus, ocul/o/myc/osis
8. death of an area of tissue, necr/osis
9. production of granulocytes, granul/o/cyt/o/poiesis
10. pain in the diaphragm, diaphragm/odynia
11. excision of an aneurysm, aneurysm/ectomy
12. deficiency of oxygen, hyp/ox/ia
13. air and fluid in the pleural cavity, pneum/o/hydr/o/thorax
14. suppurative inflammation of the trachea, trache/o/py/osis
15. inflammation of a lacrimal gland, dacry/o/aden/itis
16. inflammation of the glands of the eyelid, blephar/o/aden/itis
17. weak vision caused by fatigue, asthen/opia
18. lack of oxygen, an/ox/ia
19. pooling of blood in a vein, ven/o/stasis
20. labored breathing, dys/pnea
21. breaking up of a clot, thromb/o/lysis
22. destruction of microorganisms by phagocytes, phag/o/cyt/osis
23. spitting up blood, hem/o/ptysis
24. examination of the retina, retin/o/scopy
25. horn shaped, kerat/oid
26. pertaining to/like a net, reticul/ar
27. stretching of the bronchioles, bronchiol/ectasis
28. instrument to measure the pressure exerted by the arteries of the eye,
     ophthalm/o/dynam/o/meter
29. a softening of the lens of the eye, phac/o/malacia
30. x ray of a blood vessel, angi/o/gram
31. abnormal heartbeat accompanied by a rapid heart rate, tachy/a/rrhythm/ia
32. blood poisoning caused by pathogenic organisms and their toxins, septic/emia
33. pertaining to nutrients carried in the blood, hem/o/troph/ic
34. increase in the number of neutrophils in the blood, neutr/o/phil/ia
35. absence of carbon dioxide, a/capnia

VIII.

1. hemoptysis;   **2.** ankyloblepharon;   **3.** aneurysmorrhaphy;
4. exophthalmia;   **5.** mucosis;   **6.** sphygmomanometer; **7.** splenomegaly;
8. blepharoptosis;   **9.** tracheostomy;   **10.** lymphangioma;
11. stapediovestibular;   **12.** expectorant;   **13.** mediastinopericarditis;
14. dacryoadenitis;   **15.** immunology;   **16.** atelectasis.

REVIEW UNIT IV

I.   The Digestive System: Match each combining form with its meaning.

1. CEC/O	a.	straight
2. CHOLEDOCH/O	b.	appetite
3. AMYL/O	c.	pancreas
4. PY/O	d.	omentum
5. FEC/A	e.	gallbladder
6. POLYP/O	f.	ileum
7. BUCC/O	g.	stomach
8. GASTR/O	h.	cementum
9. DUODEN/O	i.	starch
10 MESENTER/O	j.	artificial
11. CHLORHYDR/O	k.	abdomen
12. MENT/O	l.	jaw
13. ALVEOL/O	m.	small intestine
14. PHARYNG/O	n.	pylorus
15. LAPAR/O	o.	cecum
16. RECT/O	p.	polyp
17. CHOLECYST/O	q.	pharynx

18. SUCC/O ....   r. jejunum

19. PROSTH/O ....   s. esophagus

20. -HELCOSIS ....   t. pus

21. ADEN/O ....   u. mesentery

22. ILE/O ....   v. gland

23. PEPS/I ....   w. a closing

24. PERITONE/O ....   x. dentin

25. AN/O ....   y. chin

26. COL/O ....   z. anus

27. CEMENT/O ....   aa. anus and rectum

28. HERNI/O ....   bb. liver

29. -LITHIASIS ....   cc. common bile duct

30. SIALADEN/O ....   dd. rectum

31. ENTER/O ....   ee. colon

32. HEPAT/O ....   ff. salivary gland

33. -ASE ....   gg. juice

34. ORTH/O ....   hh. duodenum

35. GNATH/O ....   ii. production of calculi

36. APPENDIC/O ....   jj. jaundice

37. OMENT/O ....   kk. appendix

38. ESOPHAG/O ....   ll. stools

39. DENTIN/O ....   mm. socket of a tooth

40. OREX/I ....   nn. formation of ulcers

41. ICTER/O ....

oo. cheek

42. SPHINCTER/O ....

pp. hernia

43. CELI/O ....

qq. S-shaped portion of the colon

44. SIGMOID/O ....

rr. enzyme indicator

45. OCCLUS/O ....

ss. hydrochloric acid

46. PROCT/O ....

tt. serous membrane of the abdominal wall and viscera

47. PANCREAT/O ....

uu. abdominal wall

48. JEJUN/O ....

vv. valvelike muscle ring

49. PYLOR/O ....

ww. digestion

II. The Urinary System: Match each combining form with its meaning.

1. URETHR/O ....

a. bunch

2. COCC/O ....

b. behind

3. -TRIPSY ....

c. water

4. TUBUL/O ....

d. urethra

5. HYDR/O ....

e. stone

6. PYEL/O ....

f. ureter

7. STAPHYL/O ....

g. spherical bacteria

8. -EMPHRAXIS ....

h. cluster/glomerulus

9. URETHER/O ....

i. small tube

10. UR/O ....

j. breaking

11. -CLASIS ....

k. renal pelvis

12. RETRO- ....

l. small nipplelike projection

13. GLOMERUL/O ....   m. urine

14. LITH/O ....   n. rubbing/crushing

15. PAPILL/O ....   o. obstruction

III. The Reproductive Systems: Match each combining form with its meaning.

1. SLAPING/O ....   a. animal life

2. EMBRY/O ....   b. hidden

3. PROSTAT/O ....   c. seminal vesicles

4. SPERMAT/O ....   d. perineum

5. PAR(T)/O ....   e. female

6. -PLASIA ....   f. fallopian tube

7. ANDR/O ....   g. bulb

8. ZO/O ....   h. pregnant

9. CERVIC/O ....   i. process of giving birth

10. SCROT/O ....   j. chorion

11. GYNEC/O ....   k. amnion

12. CYES/O ....   l. glans penis

13. EPIDIDYM/O ....   m. embryo

14. CRYPT/O ....   n. male

15. CHORI/O ....   o. vas deferens

16. PERINE/O ....   p. spermatozoa

17. BALAN/O ....   q. false

18. VAS/O ....   r. pregnancy

19. GRAVID/O ....   s.   prostate gland

20. MEN/O ....   t.   cervix

21. GAMET/O ....   u.   semen

22. VESICUL/O ....   v.   scrotum

23. TOC/O ....   w.   a fully developed reproductive cell

24. PSEUD/O ....   x.   epididymis

25. BULB/O ....   y.   formation

26. SEMIN/O ....   z.   menses

27. AMNI/O ....   aa.   birth

IV. Synonymous bases: Match the combining forms that have the same meaning.

Synonyms   *Meaning*

1. ....   SIAL/O

....   OOPHOR/O

2. ....   PHALL/O

....   REN/O

3. ....   VESIC/O

....   COLP/O

4. ....   STOMAT/O

....   LINGU/O

5. ....   CHOL/E

....   OV/O

6. ....   ORCHID/O

....   METR/O

7. .... MAMM/O

   .... PEN/O

8. .... TEST/O

   .... GLOSS/O

9. .... CHEIL/O

   .... GLYC/O

10. .... STEAT/O

    .... OO/O

11. .... HYSTER/O

    .... GENIT/O

    .... ODONT/O

12. .... OR/O

    .... BIL/I

    .... SACCHAR/O

13. .... UTER/O

    .... CYST/O

14. .... UMBILIC/O

    .... VULV/O

15. .... MAST/O

    .... ORCHI/O

    .... LABI/O

16. .... GLUC/O

    .... OVARI/O

17. .... NEPHR/O

.... SALIV/A

18. .... GON/O

.... DENT/I

19. .... LIP/O

.... EPISI/O

20. .... VAGIN/O

.... OMPHAL/O

    V. Give the meaning for each of the following medical words. Divide each word into base(s), prefix, and suffix; underline the letter(s) with the primary stress. *Example:*

MAMMOPLASTY   plastic surgery of the breast   <u>mamm</u>/o/plasty
....

1. PROSTATOVESICULITIS ....

2. CRYPTORCHIDISM ....

3. POLYPOTOME ....

4. INTRATUBULAR ....

5. CHOLECYSTOTOMY ....

6. ODONTOCLASIS ....

7. SIALOANGITIS ....

8. VASECTOMY ....

9. OOGENESIS ....

10. LIPASE ....

11. CHEILOSCHISIS ....

12. OVARIOCYESIS ....

13. CELIOTOMY ....

14. ACHLORHYDRIA ....

15. PRIMIPARA ....

16. ENDOCERVITIS ....

17. PROSTHODONTIST ....

18. INTRAPERITONEAL ....

19. ANOREXIA ....

20. NEPHREMPHRAXIS ....

21. PYELONEPHRITIS ....

22. ENURESIS ....

23. GNATHODYNAMOMETER ....

24. MASTECTOMY ....

25. PANHYSTEROCOLPECTOMY ....

26. BALANORRHEA ....

27. AMENORRHEA ....

28. HYDROPYONEPHROSIS ....

29. STAPHYLOHEMIA ....

30. GLYCOSURIA ....

31. PERIODONTAL ....

32. SUCCAGOGUE ....

33. GASTRODUODENOSTOMY ....

34. SIGMOIDOPEXY ....

35. BULBOURETHRAL ....

36. GENITALIA ....

37. PANCREATHELCOSIS ....

38. LITHOCLAST ....

39. GLOMERULAR ....

40. GAMETOGENESIS ....

41. CHORIOCARCINOMA ....

42. PARENTERAL ....

43. CEMENTOBLAST ....

44. CYSTITIS ....

45. PAPILLOMA ....

    VI. For each group of words underline the misspelled word and write the correct
spelling in the space provided.

1. GONADOTROPHIN   HYDROPHYONEPHROSIS   CECEOPTOSIS

....

2. DIVERTICULOSIS   URETHRITIS   AMMENORRHEA

....

3. PHIMOSIS   METROFIBROMA   PERETONITIS

....

4. CHOLESYSTOKININ   AMNIORRHEXIS   PROSTHESIS

....

5. MELENA   CRYPORCHIDECTOMY   GAMETOGENESIS

....

6. AURIA   NEPHROCYSTANASTOMOSIS CIRRHOSIS

....

7. AZOTEMIA   INTUSSUSCEPTION   ESOPHAGAL

....

8. CHOLEPOIESIS   CHEILITIS   URETERONYOCYSTOSTOMY

....

9. OPHORITIS   AMYLASE   OMPHALOTOMY

....

10. SPERMATOZOON   BILIRUBINEMIA   EMBRYOTOSIA

....

11. AMNIOCENTESIS   MAMOGRAPHY   ICTEROGENIC

....

12. LEUKOPLAKIA   PYELLONEPHRITIS   NOCTURIA

....

13. DYSTENTERY   DENTIBUCCAL   HEPATOLITHIASIS

....

14. LITHOCLAST   EPIDIDYMOVASOSTOMY   PAPILOCARCINOMA

....

15. HYPOSPADIA   LAPAORRHAPHY   PRIMIPARA

....

16. VASOLIGATION   GNATHODYNAMOMETER   PROSTRATECTOMY

....

17. ENDOMETREAL   HEMODIALYSIS   BALANOPREPUTIAL

....

18. SALPINGO-   OLIGUREA   PYURIA
    OOPHORECTOMY

....

Review Unit IV
Answers to Exercises

I.

1. o;	**2.** cc;	**3.** i;	**4.** t;	**5.** ll;	**6.** p;	**7.** oo;	**8.** g;
9. hh;	**10.** u;	**11.** ss;	**12.** y;	**13.** mm;	**14.** q;	**15.** uu;	
16. dd;	**17.** e;	**18.** gg;	**19.** j;	**20.** nn;	**21.** v;	**22.** f;	
23. ww;	**24.** tt;	**25.** z;	**26.** ee;	**27.** h;	**28.** pp;	**29.** ii;	
30. ff;	**31.** m;	**32.** bb;	**33.** rr;	**34.** a;	**35.** l;	**36.** kk;	
37. d;	**38.** s;	**39.** x;	**40.** b;	**41.** jj;	**42.** vv;	**43.** k;	**44.** qq;
45. w;	**46.** aa;	**47.** c;	**48.** r;	**49.** n.			

II.

1. d;	**2.** g;	**3.** n;	**4.** i;	**5.** c;	**6.** k;	**7.** a;	**8.** o;	**9.** f;
10. m;	**11.** j;	**12.** b;	**13.** h;	**14.** e;	**15.** l.			

III.

1. f;	**2.** m;	**3.** s;	**4.** p;	**5.** i;	**6.** y;	**7.** n;	**8.** a;	**9.** t;
10. v;	**11.** e;	**12.** r;	**13.** x;	**14.** b;	**15.** j;	**16.** d;	**17.** l;	
18. o;	**19.** h;	**20.** z;	**21.** w;	**22.** c;	**23.** aa;	**24.** q;	**25.** g;	
26. u;	**27.** k.							

IV.

sial/o, saliva, saliv/a; oophor/o, ovary, ovari/o; phall/o, penis, pen/o;
ren/o, kidney, nephr/o; vesic/o, bladder, cyst/o; colp/o, vagina, vagin/o;
stomat/o, mouth, or/o; lingu/o, tongue, gloss/o; chol/e, bile, bil/i;
ov/o, egg, oo/o; orchid/o, testicle/testes, orchi/o, test/o;
metr/o, uterus, hyster/o, uter/o; mamm/o, breast, mast/o;
cheil/o, lip, labi/o; glyc/o, sugar, gluc/o, sacchar/o; steat/o, fat, lip/o;
genit/o, reproductive organs, gon/o; umbilic/o, navel, omphal/o;
vulv/o, vulva, episi/o; dent/i, teeth, odont/o.

V.

1. inflammation of the prostate gland and seminal vesicles, prostat/o/vesicul/itis
2. undescended testes, crypt/orchid/ism
3. instrument to cut a polyp, polyp/o/tome
4. within a tubule, intra/tubul/ar
5. incision of the gallbladder, cholecyst/o/tomy
6. breaking of a tooth, odont/o/clasis
7. inflammation of a salivary duct(s), sial/o/ang/itis
8. cutting of the bas deferens, vas/ectomy
9. production of ova, o/o/gen/esis
10. enzyme that breaks down fat, lip/ase
11. harelip, cheil/o/schisis
12. ectopic pregnancy occurring in the ovary, ovari/o/cyes/is
13. incision of the abdomen, celi/otomy
14. absence of hydrochloric acid, a/chlor/hydr/ia

15. a woman who has given birth to her first child, prim/i/para
16. inflammation of the cervical lining, endo/cerv/itis
17. a dentist who specializes in making and fitting false teeth, prosth/odont/ist
18. inside the peritoneal cavity, intra/peritone/al
19. lack of appetite, an/orex/ia
20. renal obstruction, nephr/emphraxis
21. inflammation of the kidney and renal pelvis, pyel/o/nephr/itis
22. involuntary urination, en/ur/esis
23. instrument for measuring the pressure exerted by the closing of the jaw, gnath/o/dynam/o/meter
24. removal of the breast(s), mast/ectomy
25. removal of the entire uterus and vagina, pan/hyster/o/colp/ectomy
26. purulent discharge from the glans penis, balan/o/rrhea
27. absence of menstruation, a/men/o/rrhea
28. accumulation of urine and pus in the renal pelvis as a result of an obstruction, hydr/o/py/o/nephr/osis
29. presence of clusters of spherical bacteria in the blood, staphyl/o/hemia
30. presence of sugar in the urine, glycos/ur/ia
31. pertaining to the structures around a tooth, peri/odont/al
32. a substance that stimulates glandular secretion, succ/agogue
33. anastomosis between the stomach and duodenum, gastr/o/duoden/ostomy
34. fixation of the sigmoid colon to the abdominal wall, sigmoid/o/pexy
35. pertaining to the bulbourethral glands, bulb/o/urethral
36. the genitals, genit/al/ia
37. ulceration of the pancreas, pancreat/helcosis
38. instrument for breaking up calculi, lith/o/clast
39. pertaining to the glomerulus, glomerul/ar
40. production of gametes, gamet/o/gen/esis
41. cancer developing from the chorion, chori/o/carcinoma
42. outside/beside the intestines, par/enter/al
43. a cementum-forming cell, cement/o/blast
44. inflammation of the bladder, cyst/itis
45. a tumor with nipplelike projections, papill/oma

VI.

1. hydropyonephrosis;   2. amenorrhea;   3. peritonitis;   4. cholecystokinin;
5. cryptorchidectomy;   6. anuria;   7. esophageal;   8. ureteroneocystostomy;
9. oophoritis;   10. embryotocia;   11. amniocentesis;   12. pyelonephritis;
13. dysentery;   14. papillocarcinoma;   15. laparorrhaphy;   16. prostatectomy;
17. endometrial;   18. oliguria.

REVIEW UNIT V

I. The Endocrine System: Match each combining form with its meaning.

1. THYROID/O or THYR/O ....   a. pineal body

2. CALC/I ....   b. sodium

3. SOMAT/O ....   c. parathyroid glands

4. STER/O ....   d. top

5. PINEAL/O ....   e. growth

6. CHROM/O ....   f. glue

7. -PHYSIS ....   g. thyroid gland

8. KAL/I ....   h. solid

9. PARATHYROID/O ....   i. bad

10. -THROPIN ....   j. calcium

11. COLL/O ....   k. potassium

12. ADREN/O ....   l. adrenal glands

13. NATR/I ....   m. body

14. CAC/O ....   n. color

15. ACR/O ....   o. a substance that stimulates or activates

II. Pharmacology: Match each combining form with its meaning. Some letters may be used twice.

1. CHEM/O ....   a. sleep

2. IDI/O ....   b. convulsion

3. HYPN/O ....   c. sensitivity to pain

4. TON/O ....   d. deep sleep

5. -PHYLAXIS ....   e. cough

6. TOXIC/O ....   f. poison

7. ERG/O ....   g. perception

8. SPASM/O ....   h. chemical

9. HIST/O ....   i. protection

10. ESTHESI/O ....   j. numbness

11. PHAEMAC/O ....   k. work

12. ALGES/I ....   l. treatment

13. PYR/O ....   m. drug

14. SOMN/I ....   n. fever

15. TUSS/I ....   o. tissue

16. -THERAPY ....   p. tension

17. NARC/O ....   q. individual

18. SOPOR/I ....

19. TOX/O ....

III. Oncology: Match each combining form with its meaning.

1. CARCIN/O ....   a. tumor

2. MUT/O ....   b. beyond

3. -SARCOMA ....   c. flesh

4. ONC/O ....   d. cancer

5. -GNOSIS ....   e. malignant tumor developing from epithelial tissue

6. SARC/O ....   f. new

7. -PLASM ....   g. knowledge

8. -CAECINOMA ....   h. change

9. VIR/O ....   i. virus

10. TUM/O ....   j. malignant tumor developing from connective tissue

11. META- ....   k. swelling

12. NE/O ....   l. something formed

    IV.   Mental Illness: Match each combining form with its meaning. Some letters may be used several times.

1. SCHIZ/O ....   a. mind

2. -MANIA ....   b. youth

3. MENT/O ....   c. down

4. EGO- ....   d. split

5. HEBE- ....   e. stealing

6. -PHRENIA ....   f. self

7. PHOBIA ....   g. abnormal preoccupation

8. KLEPT/O ....   h. fear

9. CATA- ....

10. PSYCH/O ....

    V.   Radiology and Surgery: Match each combining form with its meaning. Some letters may be used twice.

1. TERAT/O ....   a. ion

2. SEC/O ....   b. arrangement

3. HAL/O ....   c. light

4. RADI/O ....   d. three dimensional

5. SON/O ....   e. extremely deformed fetus

6. IS/O ....   f. x rays

7. CAUTER/O ....   g. cold

8. STERE/O ....   h. motion

9. CINE/O ....   i. cut

10. ION/O ....   j. burn

11. SURGIC/O ....   k. root

12. OBSTERIC/O ....   l. surgery

13. LUC/O ....   m. salt

14. TOP/O ....   n. relief

15. ULTRA- ....   o. ray

16. TELE- ....   p. beyond

17. CRY/O ....   q. equal

18. PALLI/O ....   r. rotting

19. PHOB/O ....   s. sound

20. -TAXIS ....   t. place

21. RADIC/O ....   u. far

22. SEPT/O ....   v. obstetrician

23. ROENTGEN/O ....

VI. Give the meaning for each of the following medical words. Divide each word into base(s), prefix, and suffix; underline the letter(s) with the primary stress. *Example:*

ANAPHYLACTIC   pertaining to the body's overprotective reaction   ana/phylac/tic

1. CINERADIODRAPHY ....

2. ADENOCARCINOMA ....

3. RESECTION ....

4. ANTISEPSIS ....

5. SPASMOPHILIA ....

6. SOMATOTROPIN ....

7. NEUROHYPOPHYSIS ....

8. CATATONIA ....

9. PERTUSSIS ....

10. TERATOGENESIS ....

11. MULTISONOUS ....

12. CHROMODERMATOSIS ....

13. ARCROMEGALY ....

14. CRYANESTHESIA ....

15. ONCOLOGY ....

16. TELETHERAPY ....

17. CAUTERIZE ....

18. KLEPTOMANIAC ....

19. HALOGENIC ....

20. RADIOLUCENT ....

21. STEREOTACTIC ....

22. LEIOMYOMA ....

23. SARCOMPHALOCELE ....

24. PHOTOPHOBIA ....

25. TOXEMIA ....

26. POLYDIPSIA

27. DYSTONIA

28. THYROTOXICOSIS

29. PHOTOKINETIC

30. ATAXIA

31. NEOPLASM

32. MASTONCUS

33. PYROGENIC

34. IDIOPATHY

35. HYPOKALEMIA

36. CACHEXIA

37. CRYOSURGERY

38. PSYCHOTHERAPY

39. ROENTGENOTHERAPY

40. MUTAGEN

41. RHABDOMYOSARCOMA

42. CORTICOTROPIN

43. ADRENERGIC

44. CALCIPENIA

45. HEBEPHRENIA

      VII. For each group of words underline the misspelled word and write the correct spelling in the space provided.

1. RADIOISOTOPES   ANTISPAZMODIC   ANAPHYLAXIS

2. ANEPLASIA GLUCOCORTICOIDS HYPERPLASIA

....

3. HYPOCALSEMIA TOMOGRAM OXYPHILS

....

4. MITOSIS HYPERPYREXIA COLODIAL

....

5. CATHARTICS DIMENTIA SYNERGISM

....

6. HYPERADRENO- TERETOGENESIS MYXEDEMA
   CORTICALISM

....

7. EXFOLIATIVE CARCINOGENIC CINERORADIOGRAPHY

....

8. POLIDYPSIA MYCOTOXIN INTUMESCENCE

....

9. ADRENERGIC DISTONIA HYPOGLYCEMIA

....

10. CACHEXIA RADIOIMMUNOASSAY ANTITOXEN

....

11. SOPORIFIC OSTEOCARCOMMA PSYCHOPHYSIOLOGIC

....

12. DISECT OBSTETRICIAN INTERSTITIAL

....

13. SARCOPOIETIC METASTESIS STEREOTACTIC

....

14. METAMORPHOSIS SYMPATHICOMIMETIC IRIDATION

....

15. DIABETES   HYPOTHYRODISM   PHARMACOGNOSY

. . . .

16. RENTGENOGRAPHY   ONCOFETAL   PHOTOFLUOROGRAMS

. . . .

17. ALERGY   EMOLLIENTS   POLYPHAGIA

. . . .

18. NEUROSURGERY   IONIZATION   ANTITUSIVE

. . . .

19. PALLIATIVE   RADIOPHARMACEUTICALS   HYPONETREMIA

. . . .

20. PYROMANIA   LIPOSARCOMA   TELITHERAPY

. . . .

Review Unit V
Answers to Exercises

I.

1. g;   2. j;   3. m;   4. h;   5. a;   6. n;   7. e;   8. k;   9. c;
10. o;   11. f;   12. l;   13. b;   14. i;   15. d.

II.

1. h;   2. q;   3. a;   4. p;   5. i;   6. f;   7. k;   8. b;   9. o;
10. g;   11. m;   12. c;   13. n;   14. a;   15. e;   16. l;   17. j;
18. d;   19. f.

III.

1. d;   2. h;   3. j;   4. a;   5. g;   6. c;   7. l;   8. e;   9. i;
10. k;   11. b;   12. f.

IV.

1. d;   2. g;   3. a;   4. f;   5. b;   6. a;   7. h;   8. e;
9. c;   10. a.

V.

1. e;   2. i;   3. m;   4. o;   5. s;   6. q;   7. j;   8. d;   9. h;

10. a;	**11.** l;	**12.** v;	**13.** c;	**14.** t;	**15.** p;	**16.** u;	**17.** g;
18. n;	**19.** c;	**20.** b;	**21.** k;	**22.** r;	**23.** f.		

VI.

1. a series of x rays, cine/radi/o/graphy
2. malignant tumor developing from glandular tissue, aden/o/carcin/oma
3. excision of a part of a structure, re/sec/tion
4. the prevention of putrefaction, anti/seps/is
5. tendency toward convulsions, spasm/o/phil/ia
6. body-growth-stimulating hormone, somat/o/tropin
7. the posterior lobe of the hypophysis, neur/o/hypo/physis
8. a form of schizophrenia characterized by a rigid body position and a trancelike state, cata/ton/ia
9. intensive coughing, per/tuss/is
10. production of severe deformities in the fetus, terat/o/gen/esis
11. producing many sounds, mult/i/son/ous
12. skin disease accompanied by pigmentation, chrom/o/dermat/osis
13. enlargement of the bones of the extremities, acr/o/megaly
14. insensitivity to cold, cry/an/esthes/ia
15. study of tumors and their treatment, onc/o/logy
16. treatment in which the radioactive substance is kept at a distance from the patient, tele/therapy
17. to burn with a special instrument, cauter/ize
18. pertaining to a person who has a compulsion to steal, klept/o/man/iac
19. pertaining to that which produces salt, hal/o/gen/ic
20. pertaining to a substance through which x rays are able to pass, radi/o/luc/ent
21. pertaining to three-dimensional x rays, stere/o/tac/tic
22. tumor developing from smooth muscle tissue, lei/o/my/oma
23. fleshy tumor of the umbilicus, sarc/omphal/o/cele
24. an excessive intolerance to light, phot/o/phobia
25. presence of toxins in the blood, tox/emia
26. excessive thirst, poly/dips/ia
27. poor muscle tension, dys/ton/ia
28. toxicity caused by a hypofunction of the thyroid, thyr/o/toxic/osis
29. pertaining to that which is moved by light, phot/o/kine/tic
30. a lack of regulation, a/tax/ia
31. abnormal formation of new tissue, ne/o/plasm
32. tumor of the breast, mast/oncus
33. fever producing, pyr/o/gen/ic
34. disease peculiar to an individual, idi/o/pathy
35. decrease of potassium, in the blood, hypo/kal/emia
36. state of poor health, cachex/ia
37. surgically removing diseased tissue by the application of an extremely cold probe, cry/o/surgery
38. the treatment of mental illness, psych/o/therapy
39. treatment of disease with x rays, roentgen/o/therapy
40. an agent that produces change, mut/a/gen

41. cancerous tissue developing from striated muscles, rhabd/o/my/o/sar<u>c</u>oma
42. a substance that stimulates the adrenal cortex, cortic/o/<u>trop</u>in
43. pertaining to a substance that acts like adrenalin, adren/<u>erg</u>/ic
44. deficiency of calcium, calc/i/<u>pe</u>nia
45. a form of schizophrenia characterized by regressive, childish behavior, hebe/<u>phre</u>nia

VII.

1. antispasmodic;   2. anaplasia;   3. hypocalcemia;   4. colloidial;
5. dementia;   6. teratogenesis;   7. cineradiography;   8. polydipsia;
9. dystonia;   10. antitoxin;   11. osteosarcoma;   12. dissect;
13. metastasis;   14. irridation;   15. hypothyroidism;   16. roentgenography;
17. allergy;   18. antitussive;   19. hyponatremia;   20. teletherapy.

Index of Combining Forms

a-, without, 25

ab-, from, away from, 25

abdomin/o, abdomen, 61

-ac, pertaining to, 17

acanth/o, thorn, spine, 76

acetabul/o, acetabulum, cavity of the hipbone, 95

acou/o, hearing, 169

acr/o, top, extremity, 300

acromi/o, acromion—the portion of the scapula that articulates with the clavicle, 94

actin/o, ray, 325

ad-, to, toward, near, 25

aden/o, gland, 235

adip/o, fat, 76

adren/o, adrenal glands, 299

aer/o, air, gas, 389

agglutin/o, clumping, 181

-agra, severe pain, 385

-al, pertaining to, 17

alb/o, white, 67

alges/i, sensitivity to pain, 315

-algia, pain, 18

al/o, blindness, 162

aliment/o, nourish, 240

all/o, other, 326

alveol/o, alveolus—small hollow or cavity; air cell of lung; socket of a tooth, 239

ambly/o, dull, 162

ambul/o, walk, 325

amel/o, enamel, 244

amni/o, amnion, 276

amphi-, both, both sides, 97

ampull/o, ampulla—baglike protrusion of a canal or duct, 170

amyl/o, starch, 238

an-, without, 25

an/o, anus, 237

ana-, up, back again, 25

andr/o, male, masculine, 81, 273

aneurysm/o, aneurysm—abnormal widening, 182

angi/o, vessel, 179

angin/o, angina—choking 182

ankyl/o, bent, crooked, the fusion of two parts, 170

ante-, before, 25

anthrac/o, coal, 227

anti-, against, 25

aort/o, aorta, 179

apic/o, tip, 388

apo-, away, from, 97

append/o, appendic/o, appendix, 237

aqu/o, water, 156

-ar, pertaining to, 17

arteri/o, artery, 180

arteriol/o, arteriole—small artery, 180

arthr/o, joint, 96

articul/o, joint, 96

-ary, pertaining to, 18

-ase, enzyme, 238

astr/o, star-shaped, 125

atel/o, imperfect, defective, 219

ather/o, fatty buildup, 182

atri/o, cavity, atrium, 179

audi/o, hearing, 169

aur/o, ear, 169

aur/o, gold, 388

auscult/o, listen, 184

aut/o, self, 126

auto-, self, 25

axi/o, axis, 386

azot/o, nitrogen, 266

balan/o, glans penis, 74

bar/o, density, pressure, 186

bary-, weight/pressure, 389

bas/o, base, 180

bi-, bi(n)-, bi(s)-, two, double, 25, 67

bil/i, bile, 237

-blast, undifferentiated cell, primitive cell, 20

blenn/o, mucus, 388

blephar/o, eye lid, 156

bol/o, mass, lump, 237

brachi/o, arm, 61

brachy-, short, 182

bronch/o, bronchus, bronchial tube, 218

bronchi/o, bronchus, bronchial tube, 218

bronchiol/o, bronchiole—very small bronchial tube, 218

bucc/o, cheek, mouth, 61, 235

bulb/o, bulb, 274

burs/o, bursa—the sac containing synovial fluid, 96

cac/o, bad, 300
calc/i, calcium, 299
calcane/o, calcaneus—heel bone, 95
calyc/o, cup, calyces, 261
can/o, dog, 244
capill/o, capillary—very small blood vessel, 180
-capnia, carbon dioxide, 219
carcin/o, cancer, 333
-carcinoma, carcinoma—malignant tumor developing from epithelial tissue, 333
cardi/o, heart, 179
carp/o, carpus—wrist, 61, 95
cata-, down, 374
caust/o, burning, 83
cauter/o, burn, 349
cec/o, cecum, 237
-cele, hernia, herniation, 20
celi/o, abdomen, 236
cement/o, cementum, 239
-centesis, surgical puncture to withdraw fluid, 20
centi-, one hundredth, 67
cephal/o, head, 2
cerebell/o, cerebellum, 126
cerebr/o, cerebrum, 125
cerumin/o, cerumen—wax, 169
cervic/o, neck, cervix, 61, 93, 275
cheil/o, lip, 235
chem/o, chemical, drug, 315
chlor/o, green, 68
chlorhydr/o, hydrochloric acid, 238
chol/e, bile, 237
cholecyst/o, gallbladder, 237
choledoch/o, common bile duct, 237
chondr/o, cartilage, 93
chori/o, skin, membrane, 157, 276
chrom/o, color, 300
cine/o, motion, movement, 348
circum-, around, 25
cirrh/o, orange, 247
cis/o, cut, 244
-clasis, break/breaking/fracture, 260
-clast, instrument to break, 260
clavicul/o, clavicle—collarbone, 94
cleisis, closure, blockage, 387
-clysis, washing, irrigation, 20

co-, with, together, 26
cocc/o, spherical bacteria, 259
coccyg/o, coccyx—tailbone, 94
cochle/o, cochlea—snail-shaped portion of the inner ear, 170
col/o, colon, 236
coll/o, glue, 299
colp/o, vagina, 275
con-, with, together, 26
condyl/o, knuckle, 99
coni/o, dust, 227
conjunctiv/o, conjunctiva—membrane lining the eyelids, 156
contra-, against, 26
core/o, pupil, 155
cori/o, skin, 78
corne/o, horny, the cornea, 155
coron/o, crown, heart, 179
cortic/o, outer surface, cortex, 132
cost/o, rib, 94
crani/o, cranium—skull bones that enclose the brain, 93
-crine, to secrete, 76
cry/o, cold, 287, 349
crypt/o, hidden, 277
cubit/o, front of elbow, 61
culd/o, pouch, the peritoneal pouch behind the uterus, 386
cuspid/o, point, 244
cut/i, skin, 76
cyan/o, blue, 67
cycl/o, circle, ciliary body of the eye, 156
cyes/o, pregnancy, 276
cyst/o, sac, bladder, 259
cyt/o, cell, 48
-cyte, cell, 20

dacry/o, tear, 156
dactyl/o, finger, toe, 385
de-, from, 26
decidu/o, falling, 244
delt/o, shoulder, 61
dent/i, tooth, teeth, 235
dentin/o, dentin, 239
derm/o, skin, 76
dermat/o, skin, 76
di-, twice, double, 26, 67
dia-, through, 26

diaphor/o, sweat, 76
diaphragm/o, diaphragm, 218
diaphragmat/o, diaphragm, 218
diplo-, two, double, 67
dips/o, thirst, 300
dis-, apart, free from, separate, 26
dist/o, away from the trunk of the body, 63
dors/o, toward the back, 63
duoden/o, duodenum, 236
dynam/o, power, force, 164
dys-, bad, painful, difficult, 26

-e, instrument, noun marker, 17
-eal, pertaining to, 18
ec-, out, 279
-ectasia, stretching, dilation, 18
-ectasis, stretching, dilatation, 18
ecto-, outside, outer, 26
-ectomy, excision, process of cutting out, 19
-edema, swelling, 116
ego-, I, self, 374
embry/o, embryo, 276
eme/o, vomiting, 387
-emia, blood, blood condition, 18, 180
-emphraxis, obstruction, blockage, 259
emphysem/o, inflation, emphysema, 227
en-, in, within, 26
encephal/o, brain, 126
endo-, inside, inner, 26
enter/o, intestine, small intestine, 236
eosin/o, rosy red, acidic dye, 194
epi-, over, upon, on, 26
epicondyl/o, epicondyle, 99
epididym/o, epididymis, 273
epiglott/o, epiglottis, 217
episi/o, vulva, 275
-er, doer (person/thing), 17
erg/o, work, 315
erythr/o, red, 67
eschar/o, dead tissue mass, 83
esophag/o, esophagus, 236
esthesi/o, perception, feeling, 315
estr/o, sexual desire, estrogen, 279
eu-, good, well, normal, 26
eustachi/o, eustachian tube, 170

ex-, out of, from, 26
exo-, outside, 156
extra-, outside of, beyond, 26

fasci/o, fascia—fibrous membrane covering and separating muscles, 96
fassicul/o, fassiculus—bundle of muscle fibers, 97
febr/i, fever, 388
fec/a, feces, 238
femor/o, femur, 61, 95
fer/o, carry, conduct, 127
ferr/o, iron, 389
fibr/o, fiber, fibrous tissue, 96, 181
fibrin/o, fibrin, 181
fibul/o, fibula—calfbone, 95
fil/o, thread, 163
fistul/o, fistula—an abnormal tube or pipelike structure, 387
flagell/o, whip, flagellum, 277
follicul/o, follicle, 76
front/o, forehead, 61
fund/o, fundus—base of a structure, 240

galact/o, milk, 388
gamet/o, gamete—a fully developed reproductive cell, 274
gangli/o, ganglion—a collection of nerve cell bodies outside the central nervous system, 125
ganglion/o, ganglion—a collection of nerve cell bodies outside the central nervous system, 125
gastr/o, stomach, 236
gen/o, produce, 2
genit/o, reproductive organs, genitals, 274
ger/o, age, the aged, 389
geront/o, age, the aged, 389
-geusia, taste, 389
gingiv/o, gingiva, gums, 239

glauc/o, gray, greenish gray, 68
gli/o, glue, adhesive, 125
glob/o, round, globe-shaped, 181
globul/o, round body, 195
glomerul/o, cluster, glomerulus, 259
gloss/o, tongue, 235
gluc/o, sugar, 238
glute/o, buttocks, 61
glyc/o, sugar, 238
gnath/o, jaw, 239
-gnosis, knowledge, 333
-gogue, stimulant, 248
gon/o, reproductive organs, 274
gonad/o, male/female sex glands, gonads, 274
-gram, record, 19
granul/o, granule, 181
-graph, recorder, 19
-graphy, process of recording, 19
gravid/o, pregnant, 276
gust/o, taste, 163
gynec/o, woman, female, 276

hal/o, salt, 349
hapl/o, one, single, 67
hebe-, youth, 374
hect/o, one hundred, 67
-helcosis, formation of ulcers, 238
helic/o, spiral, 335
hem/o, blood, 180
hemat/o, blood, 180
hemi, half, 26
hepat/o, liver, 237
herni/o, hernia, 239
heter/o, other, 84
hidr/o, sweat, 76
hist/o, tissue, 49, 316
hol/o, whole, entire, 76
hormon/o, activate, hormone, 300
humer/o, humerus—upper arm, 94
hyal/o, glass, glasslike, transparent, 385
hydr/o, water, 260
hyper-, above, excessive, 26
hypn/o, sleep, 315
hypo-, under, less than normal, 26
hyster/o, uterus, womb, 275

i/o, violet, 160
-ia, condition, 17
iatr/o, physician, 375
-iatry, -iatrics, healing, frequently refers to a branch of medicine, 19
-ic, pertaining to, 18
icter/o, jaundice, 239
idi/o, own, individual, 315
ile/o, ileum, 236
ili/o, the illum—the superior part of the hip bone, 95
immun/o, safe, immune, 182
in-, in, into, 26
in-, not, 26
-in, sufffix indicating a chemical substance, 181
in/o, fiber, 385
incud/o, incus, anvil (second ossicle), 169
infra-, below, lower, 26
inter-, between, 26
intra-, within, 26
ion/o, ion—an atom that has given up or gained an electron, 348
iont/o, ion—an atom that has given up or gained an electron, 348
ir/o, iris, 156
irid/o, iris, 156
is/o, equal, 307, 348
isch/o, block, 142
ischi/o, the ischium—the lower portion of the hip bone, 95
-ism, a condition, usually the result of a prior condition, 17
-ist, one who specializes in, 17
-itis, inflammation, 17
-(i)um, refers to a part in relation to a whole, related to, 17

jejun/o, jejunum, 236

kal/i, potassium, 300
kary/o, nucleus, 182
kerat/o, horny, hard/horny, the cornea, 76

kilo-, one thousand, 67
-kinesia, movement, motion, 385
-kleisis, blockage, 387
klept/o, stealing, 374
kyph/o, humped, 94

-l/o, suffix indicating *small* (-le ending), 179
labi/o, lip, 235
labyrinth/o, labyrinth—intricate winding path of the inner ear, 170
lact/o, milk, 283
lacrim/o, tear, tear duct, 155
-lalia, speech, 386
lamin/o, a lamina—the flat bone of the neural arch of a vertebra, 94
lapar/o, abdominal wall, 236
laryng/o, larynx, voice box, 217
later/o, side, 63
leiomy/o, smooth muscle, 110
leuk/o, white, 67
lig/o, tie, 288
lingu/o, tongue, 235
lip/o, fat, 238
lith/o, stone, calculus, 259
-lithiasis, production of calculi, 238
lob/o, lobe, a division of an organ, 218
-logist, one who studies and treats, 19
-logy, act or process of studying, 19
lord/o, bent, 94
luc/o, light, 348
lumb/o, lower back—the loins, 61, 93
lun/o, moon, 80
lup/o, lupus, wolf, 82
lymph/o, lymph, 182
-lysis, dissolution, decomposition, destruction, 19

macul/o, spot, 81
-malacia, softening, 18
malle/o, malleus—hammer: the first of the three ossicles of the middle ear, 169

mamm/o, breast, 61, 276
man/o, thin, 191
mandibul/o, the mandible—the lower jawbone, 93
-mania, extreme compulsion or preoccupation, 374
mast/o, breast, 276
maxill/o, the maxilla—the jawbone, 93
meat/o, opening, 171
medi/o, middle, 63
mediastin/o, mediastinum—a cavity located between two parts of an organ, 217
medull/o, marrow, inner portion, 97
mega-, large, 182
megal/o, large, 182
melan/o, black, 67
men/o, menses, menstruation, 276
men/o, part, 76
mening/o, meninges—membranes of the spinal cord and brain, 126
meningi/o, meninges—membranes of the spinal cord and brain, 126
ment/o, chin, 239
ment/o, mind, 374
mes/o, middle, 126
mesenten/o, mesenteny, 237
meta-, after, beyond, 204, 333
metacarp/o, the metacarpals—the bones of the hand, 95
metatars/o, the metatarsals—the bones of the foot, 96
-meter, instrument for measuring, 18
metr/o, uterus, womb, 275
metr/o, measure, 364
-metry, measurement, 18
mi/o, less, 277
micr/o, small, 125
milli-, one thousandth, 67
mit/o, thread, 49
mol/o, grind, 244
molli/o, soften 322
mon/o, one, single, 67
morph/o, shape, form, 282, 340
muc/o, mucus—a thick fluid secreted by membranes, 218
mulc/o, soothe, 322
multi-, many, 67
muscul/o, muscle, 96

mut/o, change, 333
my/o, muscle, 96
my/o, closed, 161
myc/o, fungus, 219
myel/o, the spinal cord, bone marrow, 94, 125
myelin/o, myelin, fatty substance covering nerve fibers, 125
myos/o, muscle, 96
myring/o, eardrum, tympanic membrane, 169
mys/o, dirt, 379
myx/o, mucus, 305, 387

narc/o, numbness, narcotic, 315
nas/o, nose, 217
nat/o, birth, born, 340
natr/i, sodium, 299
ne/o, new, 333
necr/o, death, 182
nephr/o, kidney, 259
neur/o, nerve, 125
neutr/o, neither, 207
nev/o, mole, 84
nigr/o, black, 67
noct/o, night, 267
nod/o, knot, node, swelling, 182, 185
nucle/o, nucleus, 181
nyct/o, night, 162
nystagm/o, nod, 162

obstetric/o, midwife, obstetrician, obstetrics, 349
occipit/o, base of the skull, 61
occlus/o, a closing, alignment of the teeth when the jaws are closed, 239
ocul/o, eye, 155
odont/o, tooth, teeth, 235
-odynia, pain, 18
-oid, resembling, like, 18
olecran/o, the olecranon—the elbow, 95
olfact/o, smell, 164
olig/o, few, deficient in, 125
-oma, swelling, tumor, 17
oment/o, omentum, 238
omphal/o, navel, 276
onc/o, mass, tumor, 333

onych/o,   nail, nailbed, 76
oo/o,   egg, ovum, 275
oophor/o,   ovary, 275
ophthalm/o,   eye, 155
-opia,   sight, vision, 155
-or,   refers to a doer, either a
        person or thing, 17
or/o,   mouth, 235
orbit/o,   eye region, 61
orchi/o,   testis, testicle, 273
orchid/o,   testis, testicle, 273
orex/i,   appetite, 238
-(o)rrhagia,   excessive flow, 19
-(o)rrhaphy,   suturing, process of
        suturing, 19
-(o)rrhea,   flow, discharge, 18
-(o)rrhexis,   rupture, 20
orth/o,   straight, 239
-osis,   condition, usually abnormal
        or pathological, 17
oste/o,   bone, 93
-(o)stomy,   process of making an
        opening into or a connection
        between, 19
ot/o,   ear, 169
-ous,   pertaining to containing
        swelling, 18
ov/o,   egg, ovum, 275
ovari/o,   ovary, 275
ox/o,   oxygen, 180
oxy-,   oxygen, 180

pachy/o,   thick, 84
palat/o,   the palate—roof of the
        mouth, 93
palli/o,   relief, alleviation, 349
palpebr/o,   eyelid, 156
pan-,   all, entire, 289
pancreat/o,   pancreas, 237
papill/o,   nipple, a small nipple-
        like projection, 159, 259
papul/o,   pimple, 81
par(t)/o,   give birth, 276
para-,   beside, alongside,
        abnormal, 26
parasympath/o,   parasympathetic
        portion of the autonomic
        nervous system, 127
parasympathetic/o, parasympa-
        thetic portion of the
        autonomic nervous system,
        127

parasympathic/o, parasympa-
        thetic portion of the
        autonomic nervous system,
        127
parathyroid/o,   parathyroid
        glands, 299
pariet/o,   wall, 221
paroxysm/o,   sudden, sharp
        recurrence of the symptoms
        of a disease, 226
patell/o,   knee region, the
        patella—the knee cap, 61, 95
path/o,   disease, 52
-pathy,   disease, diseased
        condition, 19
pector/o,   chest, 217
pelv/o,   the pelvis, 95
pen/o,   penis, 274
-penia,   deficiency, lack, 18
pent/o,   five, 67
peps/i,   digestion, 238
pept/o,   digestion, 238
per-,   through, 26
peri-,   around, 27
perine/o,   perineum (male or
        female)—base or floor of the
        body trunk, 61, 276
peritone/o,   peritoneum—the
        serous membrane of the
        abdominal wall and viscera,
        237
-pexy,   a fixing or setting firmly in
        place by suturing, 19
phac/o,   lens, 155
phag/o,   eat, 182
phalang/o,   the phalanges—the
        finger or toe bones, 95
phall/o,   penis, 274
pharmac/o,   drug, 315
pharyng/o,   pharynx—the passage-
        way from the nasal cavity to
        the larynx, 217, 236
phe/o,   dark, 306
-pheresis,   removal, 181
phil/o,   love, affinity for
        (frequently a suffix), 180
phleb/o,   vein, 180
-phobia,   fear, 374
-phot/o,   light, 348
phren/o,   diaphragm, 218
-phrenia,   mind, 374
phrenic/o,   phrenic nerve, 218
-phylaxis,   guard, protection, 315
-physis,   growth, 299

phyt/o,   plant, fungus, 84
pil/o,   hair, 76
pin/o,   drink, 265
pineal/o,   pineal body, 300
plant/o,   sole of the foot, 61
plasm/o,   formation, growth, 181,
        191
plasm/o,   plasma—the liquid
        portion of blood, formed,
        181, 191
plas/o,   development, 203
-plasia,   formation, development,
        277
-plasm,   something formed, 333
-plasty,   surgical reshaping or
        repair, 19
-plegia,   stroke, paralysis, 18
pleur/o,   pleura—serous
        membrane covering the
        lungs and thoracic wall, 218
-pnea,   breathing, 219
pneum/o,   air, lung, 218
pneumon/o,   air, lung, 218
pod/o,   foot, 386
-poiesis,   production, 181
poli/o,   gray, whitish gray, 67
poly-,   many, 67
polyp/o,   polyp, 239
pont/o,   pons, bridge, 132
poplite/o,   back of the knee, 61
port/o,   carry, 187
post-,   after, behind, 27
pre-,   before, in front of, 27
presby/o,   old, 161
-privia,   deprived of, 308
pro-,   before, in front of, 27
proct/o,   anus and rectum, 237
pron/o,   lying face forward, 357
pros-,   to, near, in addition to, 27
prostat/o,   prostate gland, 274
prosth/o,   artificial, the
        replacement of real body
        parts with artificial ones, 239
prot/o,   first, 48
proxim/o,   located near the trunk
        of the body, 63
pseud/o,   false, 274
psych/o,   mind, 374
-ptosis,   a falling, the dropping or
        sagging of an organ, 20
pty/o,   saliva, 219
pub/o, pubi/o,   the pubis, the
        pubic bone, groin region,
        61, 95

pulmon/o, lung, 218
pulp/o, pulp, 244
pupill/o, pupil, 155
py/o, pus, 239
pyel/o, renal pelvis, 259
pylor/o, pylorus—the opening of the stomach that empties into the duodenum, 236
pyr/o, heat, fever, 315

quadri-, four, fourfold, 67
quarto-, four, fourfold, 67

rachi/o, the spinal column, 94
radi/o, the radius—the outer bone of the forearm, 95
radi/o, ray, radioactive substance, 348
radic/o, root, 349
ram/o, branch, offshoot, 126
rect/o, rectum, 237
recticul/o, network, netlike, 181
ren/o, kidney, 259
retin/o, retina, 156
retro-, backward, behind, 259
rhabdomy/o, skeletal muscle, 111
rheumat/o, discharge, 200
rhin/o, nose, 217
rhod/o, rose, visual purple, 159
roentgen/o, x-rays, 348
rub/o, red, 67
rug/o, wrinkle, 240

racchar/o, sugar, 238
saccul/o, a small bag or sac, the saccule—a small bag of the membranous, labyrinth located in the vestibule of the bony labryinth and containing maculae, 170
sacr/o, the sacrum, located between the 5th lumbar vertebra and coccyx, 94
saliv/o, saliva, 236
salping/o, tube, especially the eustachian or fallopian (uterine) tube, 170, 275

sarc/o, flesh, 96, 333
-sarcoma, sarcoma, malignant tumor developing from connective tissue, 333
scapul/o, scapula—shoulder blade, 61, 94
-schesis, a holding back, suppression of discharge, 389
schiz/o, split, split division, fissure, 374, 387
scler/o, the sclera—the white portion of the eye, 155
-sclerosis, a hardening, 20
scoli/o, curved, 94
-scope, instrument for viewing, 20
-scopy, examination, process of examining visually, 19
scot/o, dark, darkness, 159, 162
scrot/o, scrotum, 273
seb/o, sebum—fatty secretion, 76
sec/o, cut, 349
sed/o, calm, 320
semi-, half, 27
semin/o, semen—a mixture of glandular secretions and spermatozoa, 274
sept/o, rotting, putrefaction, 349
ser/o, serum, a liquid coating of serous membranes, liquid exudate of a clot, 181
sial/o, saliva, 236
sialaden/o, salivary gland, 236
sider/o, iron, 181
sigmoid/o, sigmoid colon, 237
silic/o, flint, rock dust/flint dust, 227, 389
sin/o, cavity, sinus, 179
somat/o, body, 299, 301
somn/i, sleep, 315
son/o, sound, 349
sopor/i, deep sleep, 316
spasm/o, spasm, convulsion, 316
specul/o, mirror, 361
sperm/o, spermatozoa, semen (sperm: spermatozoa and spermatic fluid), 274
spermat/o, spermatozoa, semen, 274
sphincter/o, sphincter—valve like muscle ring, 236
sphygm/o, pulse, 180

spin/o, spinal cord, 126
spir/o, breathing, 217
splanchn/o, viscera—internal organs, 386
splen/o, spleen, 182
spondyl/o, a vertebra, 93
squam/o, scaly, 378
staped/o, stapes—stirrup (third ossicle), 170
staphyl/o, bunch, 259
-stasis, arresting, halting, maintaining a constant level/suffix meaning halting, stopping, 20, 182
stat/o, stay, halting, standing still, 164
steat/o, fat, 180, 238
-stenosis, a narrowing, a stricture, 20
ster/o, solid, 299
stere/o, solid, having three dimensions, 349
stern/o, the sternum—the breast bone, 94
steth/o, chest, 180
stigmat/o, point, 159
stomat/o, mouth, 235
sub-, under, 27
submaxill/o, the lower jawbone, 93
succ/o, juice, secretion, 238
sudor/o, sweat, 76
super-, above, over, 27
supin/o, lying on the back, also called dorsal recumbent, 357
supra-, above, over, 27
-surgery, surgery, 349
surgic/o, surgery, 349
sympath/o, sympathetic portion of the autonomic nervous system, 126
sympathetic/o, sympathetic portion of the autonomic nervous system, 126
sympathic/o, sympathetic portion of the autonomic nervous system, 126
syn-, with, together, 27
syndesm/o, ligament, 96
synovi/o, synovia—the lubricating fluid of joints, 96

syring/o, any tubelike structure, a fistula, 387

tach/o, quick, 182
tal/o, the talus—the ankle bone, 95
tars/o, the tarsus—the ankle, 95
-taxis, arrangement, regulation, 349
tel-, far, distant, 349
tele-, far, distant, 349
ten/o, tendon, 96
tend/o, tendon, 96
tendin/o, tendon, 96
terat/o, extremely deformed fetus, 348
test/o, testis, testicle, 273
tetra-, four, fourfold, 67
thalam/o, the thalamus, 126
thalass/o, sea, 203
-therapy, treatment, 316
thi/o, sulfur, 388
thorac/o, the thorax, the chest, 61, 93
thromb/o, clot, 181
thym/o, thymus gland, 182
thyr/o, thyroid gland, 299
thyroid/o, thyroid gland, 299
tibi/o, the tibia—the shin bone, 95
tine/o, worm, fungus, 82
toc/o, birth, labor, 276
-tome, instrument for cutting, 20
-tomy, incision, process of cutting into, 19
ton/o, tension, stretching, osmotic pressure, 181, 316
tonsill/o, tonsil, 182
top/o, place, 279, 348
tox/o, poison, 315
toxic/o, poison, 307, 315

trache/o, trachea—windpipe, 217
trachel/o, neck of the uterus, 387
trans-, across, through, over, 27
tri, three, triple, 67
trich/o, hair, 76
triplo-, three, triple, 67
-tripsy, rubbing crushing, 260
-tropin, a substance that stimulates or activates a hormone, 299
tubercul/o, tubercle, 227
tubul/o, small tube, tubule, 259
tum/o, swelling, 333
tuss/i, cough, 316
tympan/o, tympanum—eardrum, middle ear, 169

uln/o, the ulna—the inner bone of the forearm, 95
ultra-, beyond, 349
umbilic/o, navel, 61, 276
ungu/o, nail, 76
uni-, one, single, 67
ur/o, urine, urinary tract, 260
ureter/o, ureter, 259
urethr/o, urethra, 259
-uria, urine condition, 19
uter/o, uterus, womb, 275
utricul/o, a sac, the utricle—a sac of the membranous labyrinth located in the vestibule of the bony labyrinth, 170
uvul/o, the uvula—a lobelike structure hanging from the soft palate, 388

vag/o, vagus nerve—10th cranial nerve, 386

vagin/o, vagina, 275
vallat/o, walled, 163
valv/o, valve, 179
varic/o, twisted vein—varix, 182
vas/o, a vessel, vas deferens, 179, 273
ven/o, vein, 180
venere/o, love, sexual intercourse, 284
ventr/o, belly, 63, 388
ventricul/o, a small hollow or cavity, a ventricle of the brain, 126
venul/o, small vein, venule, 180
verm/i, worm, 132, 244
verruc/o, wart, 386
vertebr/o, a vertebra, 93
vesic/o, bladder, 259
vesicul/o, small vessel, seminal vessicles, 273
vestibul/o, a cavity at the entrance of a canal, the middle portion of the middle ear, 170
vir/o, virus, 333
viscer/o, viscera, internal organs, 63
vit/o, life, 349
vitre/o, glassy, 157
vol/o, palm, 61
vulv/o, vulva, 275

xanth/o, yellow, 68
xer/o, dry, 164

-y, condition, act, process, 17
zo/o, animal life, 274

General Index

abbreviations used in prescription writing, 324–25
abdomen, anatomical divisions, 66
abdominal cavity, 63
abdominal region, 61, 66
abduction, 64
abnormal breathing, 224
abrasion, 81
abscess, 111
   pulmonary, 226
accent of medical words, 37
accessory structures of the eye, 157–59
accommodation, 160
acetabulum, 95
acidophils, 302
   adenoma of, 305
acne, 81
acquired (condition), 52
acromegaly, 305
acromion process, 94
actinic keratoses, 80
acute, 53
addiction, drug, 317
Addison's disease, 306
additive action, drug, 317
adduction, 64
adenine, 335
adenocarcinoma, 286
adenohypophysis, 300
   diseases of, 305
adenoma, 247
adipose tissue, 78
adrenal cortex, 303
   diseases of, 306
   insufficiency, 306

adrenal glands, 303
   cortex, 303
   medulla, 303
adrenal medulla, 303
   diseases of, 306
adrenergic blocking drugs, 320
adrenergic drugs, 320
adrenocorticotropic hormone, 302
adventitious breath sounds, 222
affective mental disorders, 376
afferent, 127
agglutination, 195
agglutinins, 196
aggression, 376
agnosia, 142
agranulocytes, 194
albumin, 195
alcohol, 318, 355
aldosterone, 303
   hypersecretion of, 306
aldosteronism, 306
alimentary canal, 63, 240
alkylating agents, 339
allantois, 282
alopecia, 81
alveolar sacs, 220
alveoli:
   of lungs, 220
   of mammary glands, 283
amblyopia, 162
amnion, 281
amphiarthrodial joint, 110
ampulla of ear, 172
amputation, 358
amylase, 240
anabolism, 48

analgesics, 320
anaphylactic shock, 317
anaphylaxis, 317
anaplasia, 334
anastomosis, 19, 358
anatomical position, 63
androgen, 277, 304
androgenital syndrome, 306
anemia, 202
   aplastic, 203
   hemolytic, 203
   hereditary, 203
   iron deficiency, 203
   nutritional deficiency, 203
   pernicious, 203
   sickle cell, 203
   thalassemia, 203
anesthesia, 356–57
   area, 356
   blocks, 356
   effects of, 356
   general, 356
   inhalation, 356
   local, 357
   regional, 356
   spinal, 356
anesthetics, 320
aneurysm, 201
angina pectoris, 199
angiocardiography, 201
angiography, 201
angiotensin, 304
ankle bones, 108–9
ankylosis, 172
anode, 350
antacids, 321

anterior (position), 63
anthracosis, 227
antiarrhythmic agents, 321
antibiotic, 322
antibodies, 195
anticoagulants, 321
antidiarrheal agents, 322
antidiuretic drugs, 322
antidiuretic hormone, 302
antigens, 195
antihistamines, 227
anti-infectives, 322
anti-inflammatory agents, 322
antimetabolites, 339
antipyretics, 320
antispasmodic drugs, 321
antitussives, 321
anus, 244
anxiety, 376
aorta, 183, 186
aphasia, 142
aphtha, 245
aplastic anemia, 203
apocrine glands, 80
aponeurosis, 111
apoplexy, 142
appendages of the skin, 78–80
appendicular skeleton, 108
appendix, 244
apposition, 358
approximation, 358
apraxia, 142
aqueous humor, 157
arachnoid mater, 141
    villi of, 141
area anesthetics, 356
areola, 283
arm bones, 108
arrhythmia, 199
arteries, 186
    coronary, 184
arteriogram, 352
arterioles, 186
arteriosclerosis, 201
arthritis, 113
    gouty, 113
    rheumatoid, 113
articulation, 110
asbestos, 227
asbestosis, 227
ascending colon, 244
ascites, 247
asepsis, 355

asphyxiation, 226
aspiration, 227
assimilation, of sounds, 39–40
asthma, 227
astigmatism, 161
astrocyte, 130
asymptomatic, 52
atelectasis, 226
atherosclerosis, 201
athlete's foot, 82
atrioventricular:
    node, 185
    valve, 184
atrium, 183
atrophy, 53
    glandular, 305
    muscular, 113
attraction, 39–40
atypical, 52
auditory canal, 171
auricle of the heart, 183
auscultation, 184
autoclave, 355
autonomic drugs, 320–21
autonomic nervous system, 141
AV block, 199
avulsion, 358
axon, 127
azotemia, 266

back, anatomical divisions, 59
bacterial endocarditis, 200
bacteriocidal, 322
bacteriostatic, 322
Bainbridge reflex, 186
balanitis, 285
barbiturate, 320
barium enema, 352
barium sulfate, 352
barium swallow, 352
baroreceptors, 186
Bartholin's glands, 281
basal cell carcinoma, 83
basal nuclei, 132
base of medical words, 1
basophils, 194
benign tumors, 334
beriberi, 323
betadine, 355
biconcave lens, 161
biconvex lens, 161

bile, 242, 243
bile duct, common, 243
bilirubin, 193
bilirubinemia, 247
biopsy, 337–38
blackhead, 81
bladder, urinary, 262
blastocele, 281
blastocyst, 281
blepharitis, 162
blindness, 161
blister, 81
blood, clotting, 195
blood, composition of, 191–92
blood buffers, 196
blood diseases, 202–4
blood pressure, 190–91
blood typing, 195–96
blood vessels, 186–87
    diseases of, 200–202
blue baby, 200
body, directional terms, 63
body cavities, 61
body movements, terms for, 63–64
body planes, 64
body section roentgenograms, 351
body systems, 50–51
bolus, 240
bones, cancellous, 97
bones, common features of:
    characteristics, 97
    development, 100
    markings, holes, projections, 99
    types, 99
bones, compact, 97
bones, formation and structure,
    97–100
bones, specific:
    ankle and foot, 108
    cranial, 102
    facial, 100–102
    pelvic girdle and lower
        extremity, 108
    shoulder girdle and upper
        extremity, 108
    thoracic, 107
    vertebral, 102–5
bones, tumors, 112
bougie, 358
Bowman's capsule, 264
brachial region, 61
bradycardia, 199
brain, 130–33

brain scan, 352
brainstem, 132–33
breast, 283
    tissue dysplasia, 287
    tumors, 287
breastbone, 107
breathing, 222–23
bronchi, 220
bronchioles, 220
bronchogenic carcinoma, 228
buccal cavity, 61
bulbourethral glands, 279
bundle branch block, 199
bundle of His, 185
burns, 83
bursa, 110

cachexia, 305
calcaneus, 108
calcium, 306
calculus, 266
calf bone, 108
calyces, 261
cancellous bone, 97
cancer, 333–39
    characteristics, 334
    diagnosis, 337–38
    etiology, 335–37
    treatment, 338–39
    tumor types, 334–35
cannula, 359
canthus, 159
capillary, 186
capsule, 318
carcinogens, 336–37
carcinoma, 334–35
carcinoma in situ, 286
cardiac arrest, 199
cardiac catheterization, 201–2
    left heart, 202
    right heart, 202
cardiac cycle, 185
cardiac depressants, 321
cardiac output, 186
cardiac sphincter valve, 240
cardiac tamponade, 199
cardiotonic agents, 321
cardiovascular drugs, 321
cardiovascular system, 183–204
caries, dental, 245
carpal region, 61
carpals, 108

carrier substance, 48–49
cartilage, 100
    articular, 100
    hyaline, 100
cartilaginous discs, 110
cartilaginous tumors, 112
caruncle, 159
CAT scan, 363
cataract, 162
catecholamine, 303
cathartics, 321
catheter, 359
catheterization, 201
    cardiac, 201
cathode, 350
cauda equina, 135
cauterization, 364
cecum, 244
cell:
    anatomy, 48
    division, 49
    structures, 48
celomic cavity, 63
cementum, 244
central nervous system, 130–35
    chief organs, 130
    drugs, 319–20
cerebellum, 132
    cortex, 132
cerebrospinal fluid, 141–42
cerebrovascular accident, 142
cerebrum, 130–31
    cortex, 132
    hemorrhage, 142
cerumen, 171
cervical position of vertebral
        column, 105
cervical region, 61
cervix, 280
    cancer, 286
cesarean section, 355
cesium-137, 353
chambers of the eye, 157
chancre, 284
cheeks, 240
chemical pneumonitis, 227
chemotaxis, 194
chemotherapy, 316, 338–39
    combinid, 339
Cheyne-Stokes, 224
chiasm, optic, 160
childbirth, 282
cholecystokinin, 304
cholinergic blocking agents, 321

cholinergic drugs, 320
chondrocytes, 100
chondrosarcoma, 112
choriocarcinoma, 286
chorion, 282
chorionic gonadotropin, 304
choroid layer of eye, 157
chromosomes, 49
chronic, 53
chyme, 242
cilia, 219
ciliary body, 157
ciliary muscle, 157
cineradiography, 351
circulatory system, 179–216
    diseases, 199–204
    fetal, 187
    pulmonary, 183
    systemic, 183
circumcision, 276
circumduction, 64
cirrhosis, 247
clamp, 359
clavicle, 94
cleavage furrow, 49, 281
clinical, 55
clips, 359
clitoris, 281
coagulation of blood, 195
coaptation, 359
cobalt-60, 353
coccygeal portion of vertebral
        column, 105
coccyx, 94
cochlea, 171
cold sore, 245
collarbone, 94
colloid, 302
colon, 244
color blindness, 161
colostrum, 283
coma, 142
combining form, 3
combining vowel, 3
comedo, 81
commissures, 130
common bile duct, 243
compact bone, 97
competing forms, 8–9
complication, 52
compulsion, 376
    compulsive behavior, 376
computerized axial tomography,
        363

conchae, 102
concretion, 247
condyle, 99
cones, 159, 160
congenital, 52
congenital anomaly, 52
congenital defects of the
    reproductive organs, 284
congenital heart disease, 200
conjunctiva, 159
conjunctivitis, 162
connective tissue, 49
Conn's syndrome, 306
contrast mediums, 351
    procedures using contrast
        mediums or tracer
        substances, 352
convergence, 128
corium, 78
cornea, 157, 160
coronal plane, 64
coronary thrombosis, 199
cor pulmonale, 227
corpus callosum, 130
cortex:
    adrenal, 303
    cerebellum, 132
    cerebral, 132
    kidney, 261
Corti, organ of, 171
corticoids, 303
costodiaphragmatic sinus, 221
coverings of the brain and spinal
        cord, 141
Cowper's glands, 279
cranial bones, 102
cranial cavity, 61
cranial nerves, 135
crenation, 195
crest of a bone, 99
cretinism, 305
cribriform plate, 102
cross-eye, 161
crown of tooth, 244
crushing, 359
crusts, 81
cryostat, 287
cryosurgery, 363
cryptorchidism, 285
cubital region, 61
cuboid, 108
cumulation, drug, 317
cuneiform bone, 108
curet, 359

curettage, 285
currette, 359
Cushing's syndrome, 306
cyanosis, 200
cyclopropane, 356
cystitis, 266
cytoplasm, 48
cytosine, 335

deafness, 172
debridement, 354, 359
deciduous teeth, 244
decortication, 359
deep (position), 63
defense mechanism, 376
defibrillator, 200
degeneration, 53
deglutition, 240
dehiscence, 359
deltoid region, 61
delusion, 376
demulcents, 322
dendrites, 127
dental caries, 245
dentin, 244
deoxyribonucleic acid, see DNA,
        48, 335
depressants, 319
depression, 376
dermatomes, 137
    skin grafting, 354
dermis, 78
descending colon, 244
desiccation, 359
destruction, 359
diabetes insipidus, 305
diabetes mellitus, 307
diagnosis, 52
diapedesis, 194
diaphragm, 222
diaphysis, 97
diarthrodial joints, 110
diastole, 186
diastolic pressure, 191
dibucaine, 356
diencephalon, 132
differentiation, 334
digestants, 321
digestion, 240
digestive system, 235–58
    anatomy, 240–44
    diseases, 245–47

dilatation, 53
dilation, 359
diphtheria, 226
diploid cells, 277
disarticulation, 359
disease, 52
disinfectants, 355
dislocation, joint, 112
displacement, 53
dissection, 359
distal, 63
distension, 53
diuretics, 322
divergence, 128
diverticula, 246
diverticulosis, 246
divinyl ether, 356
DNA, 48, 335
    in cancer, 335
    in template, 335
dorsal, 63
drainage, 359
drapes, 359
dressing, 359
drill and burr, 359
drive, 376
drugs, 315–32
    administration, 318–19
    effects, 317
    groups, 319–22
    nomenclature, 316
    preparations, 318
drugs for skin, 322
ductus arteriosus, 187
duodenum, 242
dura mater, 141
dwarfism, 305
dyspnea, 224

ear, 169–76
ear drum, 171
ear wax, 171
ecchymosis, 81
ectoderm, 281
ectopic pregnancy, 279
eczema, 82
edema, 53
efferent, 127
egg, see ovum
ego, 376
ejaculation, 279

electrocardiograph, 185
    electrodes, 185
    leads, 185
    tracing, 185
electrocoagulation, 360
electrolytes, 77
elevation, 64
elevator, 360
embolism, cerebrovascular, 142
embolus, 199
embryo, 281
emollients, 322
emotion, 376
emphysema, 227
empyema, 227
enamel, dental, 244
encapulated, 334
enchondroma, 112
endocarditis, bacterial, 200
endocervicitis, 286
endocrine system, 299–314
    glands, 300–304
    hormones, 300–304
    pathology, 305–7
endoderm, 282
endolymph, 171
endometritis, 286
endometrium, 280
    cancer, 286
endophthalmos, 162
endoplasmic reticulum, 48
endoscope, 360
endoscopy, 360
endosteum, 97
enlargement, 53
enterogasterone, 304
enteron, 242
enucleation, 360
enzyme, 49
eosinophils, 194
epicondyle, 99
epidermis, 78
epididymis, 279
epiglottis, 224
epilepsy, 142
epinephrine, 320
epiphysis, 97
episiotomy, 355
epithalamus, 132
epithelial tissue, 49
erythroblastosis fetalis, 203
erythrocyte, *see* red blood cells,
    192–93

esophagus, 219, 240
estrogen, 279
ether chloride, 356
ethmoid bone, 102
ethyl alcohol, 355
ethylene, 356
ethyl ether, 356
etiology, 52
eustachian tube, 171
evacuation, 360
eversion, 64
evisceration, 360
excoriation, 81
exfaliative cytology, 337
exophthalmos/exophthalmia, 162
exostosis, 112
exploratory surgery, 360
extension, 63
external auditory meatus, 171
extirpation, 354
extract, drug, 318
eye:
    anatomy, 157
    function, 159–60
    pathology, 161–62
eyebrows, 157
eyelashes, 157
eyelids, 157

facial bones, 100–102
fallopian tubes, 279
fantasy, 377
fasiculi, 111
fasting blood sugar test, 307
feces, 244
female reproductive system, 279–81
    pathology, 285–87
    structures, 279–81
femoral region, 61
femur, 108
fetus, 282
    circulation, 187
fibers, white matter of cerebrum,
    132
fibrillation, 200
fibrils, 48
fibrin, 195
fibrinogen, 195
fibroadenoma, 287
fibula, 108
filtrate, urinary, 264

finger bones, 108
fissures, brain, 131
fistulization, 360
flagellum, 277
flat bones, 99
flexion, 63
flora, intestinal, 244
fluoroscopy, 351
flutter, heart, 200
follicle:
    hair, 78
    ovarian, 280
follicle-stimulating hormone, 302
fontanels, 102
foot bones, 108
foramen:
    bone, 99
    magnum, 102
    obturator, 108
    optic, 102
    ovale, 183, 187
forceps, 358
forearm bones, 108
foreskin, 279, 285
formed elements of the blood,
    191–92
fossa, bone, 99
fossa ovale, 184
fovea centralis, 160
Fowler's position, 357
fractures, 111
    compound, 111
    simple, 111
frontal, 61
frontal bone, 102
functual residual capacity of lungs,
    223
fundus of stomach, 240
fusion, 360

gallbladder, 243
gallstones, 247
gamete, 277
gametogenesis, 277
gamma globulin, 195
ganglion, 132
gastrin, 304
gastrointestinal cancer, 247
gastrointestinal drugs, 321
gastrojejunostomy, 246
gauze, 360

gene, 321
general anesthetic, 356
genetic, 321
genetic code, 321
gestation, 281
gigantism, 305
glans penis, 279
glaucoma, 162
glioma, 143
glomerular filtrate, 264
glomerulonephritis:
    acute, 266
    chronic, 266
glomerulus, 264
glottis, 224
glucagon, 303
glucocorticoid, 303
gluconeogenesis, 243
glucose, 242, 303, 307
glucose tolerance test, 307
gluteal, 61
glycogen, 243, 303
glycosuria, 265, 307
goiter, 305
Golgi apparatus, 48
gonadal agenesis, 284
gonadal dysgenesis, 284
gonadotropin, 302
gonads, *see* ovary; testes, 277, 279
gonorrhea, 284
gouge, 360
grading of tumors, 335
grafting, skin, 354, 360
grafts, 360
granulocytes, 194
Grave's disease, 305
gray matter of brain, 132
gross anatomy, 59
growth hormone, 301
    hypersecretion, 305
    hyposecretion, 305
gyrus, 131

hair, 78
hallucination, 377
halogens, 356
halothane, 356
hand bones, 108
haploid cells, 277
haustra of colon, 244

Haversian system, 100
hearing, 170
heart:
    anatomy, 183–84
    beat, 185
    diseases, 199–200
    rate, 185
heart block, 199
heart murmur, 200
hematopoietic system, 50
hemianopia (hemianopsia), 161
hemodialysis, 266
hemoglobin, 192
hemolysis, 195
hemophilia, 203
hemorrhage, 195
hemosiderin, 193
hemostats, 195, 358
hepatic duct, 243
hepatic portal system, 187
hepatic sinusoids, 243
hepatitis, 247
hepatocarcinoma, 247
hereditary anemias, 203
heredity and cancer, 335
hermaphroditism, 284
hernia, 246
    hiatal, 246
    incarcerated, 246
herpes simplex virus, 245
hexachlorophine, 355
hilus, 220, 261
hipbone, 108
histamines, 321
histogenesis, 282
histology, 49
hives, 83
Hodgkin's disease, 204
holocrine glands, 80
hooks, 360
hormones, 300
    tropic, 301
humerus, 108
humor:
    aqueous, 157
    vitreous, 157
hyaline cartilage, 100
hyaline membrane disease, 226
hyaloid canal, 157
hyaloid fossa, 157
hydatidiform mole, 286
hydrocele, 285
hydrocephalus, 142

hydrochloric acid, 240
hydrogen peroxide, 355
hydronephrosis, 267
hydroureter, 267
hymen, 281
hyoid bone, 107
hyperadrenocorticalism, 306
hypercapnia, 191
hyperinsulinism, 307
hyperopia, 161
hyperplasia, 53, 300
    prostatic, 285
hypernea, 224
hypersensitivity, drug, 317
hypertension, 211
hyperthyroidism, 305
hypertrophy, 53
hyperuricemia, 113
hyperventilation, 224
hyphenation of medical words, 41
hypnotics, 320
hypodrenocorticalism, 306
hypoglycemia, 307
hypoglycemics, 307
hypoparathyroidism, 306
hypophysis, 300
    hormones, 301–2
    structures, 300–301
hypospadia, 284
hypothalamus, 133, 302
hypothyroidism, 305
hypoxia, 191

id, 377
idiosyncrasy, drug, 317
ileum, 242
iliac crest, 66
ilium, 108
illusion, 377
imaginary body lines, 61
immunotherapy, 339
impetigo, 82
implantation, 360
incarcerated hernia, 246
incision and drainage, 360
inclusion, 48
incus, 171
infarction, myocardial, 199
infection, 52
infectious mononucleosis, 203

inferior, 63
infertility, 284
infiltration anesthesia, 357
inflammation, 52
ingestion, 240
inhalation anesthesia, 356
inherited plasma clotting disorders,
    203
inhibitory neurons, 128
insertion, 111
insulin, 307
    shock, 307
integumentary system, 77
interatrial septum, 183
interstitial cell-stimulating
    hormone, 302
interstitial isotope therapy, 353
intracavitary isotope therapy, 353
intradermal injection, 319
intramuscular injection, 319
intravenous general anesthetic, 356
intravenous injection, 319
intrinsic factor, 203, 242
introduction, 360
intubation, 360
intussusception, 246
invagination, 246
inversion, 64
involuntary muscle, 110
iodine, 355
iris, 157
iron-deficiency anemia, 203
irregular bones, 99
irridation, 352
irrigation, 361
ischemia, 142
ischium, 108
isles of Langerhans, 303
isopropyl alcohol, 355
isotope therapy, 353

jackknife position, 358
jaundice, 247
jejunum, 242
jock itch, 82
joint capsules, 110
joints, 110
    diseases and injuries, 112–13
    types, 110

karyokinesis, 49
keloid, 81
keratin, 78
keratitis, 162
keratohyalin, 78
keratosis, 82
    seborrheic, 82
ketone bodies, 265
ketonuria, 265
kidney, 260
    anatomy, 261
Klinefelter's syndrome, 284
kneecap, 108
Krause corpuscles, 77

labia, 281
labyrinth, 172
lacrimal apparatus, 159
lacrimal bones, 102
lacteals, 197
lactiferous ducts, 283
lactogenic hormone, 302
laminae, 105
laminectomy, 94
laminograms, 351
lanugo, 78
large intestine, 244
laryngeal carcinoma, 227
larynx, 224
laser surgery, 363
lateral, 63
lateral malleolus, 66
lateral operating position, 357
laxatives, 322
leiomyoma, 334
lens of eye, 157
lentigo, 80
lesions, 81
leukemia, 203
leukocytes, *see* white blood cells,
    194–95
leukoplakia, 82, 336
Leydig, cells of, 304
lidocaine, 357
ligament, 110
ligation, 361
lipids, 243
lithotomy position, 357
litigation, 195

liver, 242–43
    neoplasms, 247
    scan, 352
lobe, 221
    cerebral, 131–32
    lung, 221
local anesthesia, 357
lower G-I series, 352
lumbar portion of vertebral
    column, 105
lumbar region, 61
lumbar vertebrae, 105
lumen, 242
lungs, 221
    cancer, 228
lunula, 80
lupus erythematosis:
    discoyd, 82
    systemic, 82
luteinizing hormone, 302
lymph, 197
lymph, disorders, 204
lymphangiography, 352
lymphatic system, 197–98
lymph capillaries, 197
lymph ducts, 197
lymphedema, 287
lymph nodes, 197
lymphocytes, 194
lymphoma, 204
lymph vessels, 197

maculae of the ear, 172
macule, 81
major body regions, 59
malaise, 173
male reproductive system, 277–79
    diseases, 283–85
    structures, 277–79
malignant tumors, 334
malignant melanoma, 84
malleus, 171
mammary glands, 283
mammary region, 61
mandible, 102
mania, 377
manic psychosis, 376
manipulation, 361
manubrium, 107

Marey's law of the heart, 186
marrow, bone, 97
marsupialization, 361
mastectomy, 287
mastication, 240
matrix, 100
maxillary bones, 102
meatus, 171
    external auditory, 171
medial, 63
medial malleolus, 66
median plane, 64
median raphe, 277
mediastinum, 219
medulla:
    brain, 132
    kidney, 261
medulla oblongata, 132
medullary canal, 97
medullary ischemic reflexes, 191
megakaryocytes, 194
Meissner's corpuscles, 77
menstruation, 280
melanin, 302
melanocyte-stimulating hormone,
    302
melatonin, 304
melena, 247
Ménière's syndrome, 173
meninges, 141
meningioma, 143
meningitis, 142
mental illness, 374–83
    definition, 375
    types, 375
mental retardation, 377
merocrine glands, 80
mesencephalon, 132
mesentery, 244
mesoderm, 282
metabolic bone disorders, 112
metabolism, 240
metacarpals, 108
metastasis, 334
metatarsals, 108
methoxyflurane, 356
microglia, 130
microsurgery, 363
micturition, 362
midsagittal plane, 64
mineralocorticoid, 303
minerals, 322

miosis, 277
miotic drugs, 162
mitochondria, 48
mitosis, 49
mitral valve, 183
    incompetency, 200
    stenosis, 200
mole, 84
monocytes, 194
mononucleosis, infectious, 203
morphogenesis, 282
morula, 281
motion sickness, 173
mouth, 240
mucus, 219
multiple myeloma, 112
multiple sclerosis, 142
mumps, 246
murmur, 200
muscular distrophy, 113
muscle attachments, 111
muscles:
    cardiac, 111
    classification, 110
    diseases, 113
    insertion, 111
    involuntary, 110
    origin, 111
    skeletal, 111
    smooth, 110
    straited, 111
    tumors, 113
    voluntary, 111
muscle tissue, 50
musculoskeletal system, 93–124
mutation, 335
myasthenia gravis, 143
mycotoxins, 337
mydriatic drugs, 162
myelogram, 352
myocardial infarction, 199
myocardium, 183
myogenic, 185
myopia, 161
myxedema, 305

nail bed, 79
nails, 78
narcissism, 377
nasal bones, 100

nasal cavity, 61
National Formulary, 317
navel, 61
navicular bone, 108
necrosis, 111
needle biopsy, 337
needles, 361
neonatal, 52
neoplasm, 333
nephroblastoma, 267
nephromegaly, 266
nephron, 261
nerve blocks, 356
nerve pathways, 137–38
nervous system, divisions, 130
nervous tissue, 50
neuritis, 143
neurogenic muscular disease, 113
neuroglia, 130
neurohypophysis, 301
    diseases, 305
    function, 302
neuron, 127–29
    pathways, 137
neurosis, 376
neurosurgery, 363
neutrophils, 194
nitrogenous byproducts, 260
nitrous oxide, 356
norepinephrine, 303
nose, 219
novocaine, 356
nuclear medicine, 353
nucleus, cell, 48
nupercaine, 356
nutritional deficiency anemia, 203
nyctalopia, 162
nystagmus, 162

oat cell carcinoma, 228
obsession, 377
obturator foramen, 108
occipital bone, 102
occipital region, 61
occlusion, 53
odontoblasts, 244
ointment, 319
olecranon, 95
olfactory sense, 163
oligodendroglia, 130

omentum, 244
oncofetal antigens, 338
oncology, 333
oocyte, 279
operating positions:
    Fowler's, 357
    jackknife, 358
    lateral, 357
    lithotomy, 357
    prone, 357
    Sim's, 357
    supine, 357
    Trendelenburg, 357
optic chiasm, 132
optic disc, 157
optic foramen, 102
optic nerve, 157
oral administration of medication,
    318
oral cavity, 61
orbital cavity, 61
orbital region, 61
order, in combining the elements of
    medical words, 7
order, in translating medical words,
    5
organ, 50
organelles, 48
organic brain syndrome:
    acute, 375
    chronic, 375
organic psychoses, 375
organ of Corti, 171
orthopedic surgery, 354
oscilloscope, 363
os coxae, 108
osmosis, 48, 191
ossicles of ear, 171
osteitis deformans, 112
osteitis fibrosa cystica, 112
osteoblast, 97
osteochondromas, 112
osteodystrophy, 112
osteogenic sarcoma, 112
osteoid osteoma, 112
osteoma, 112
osteomalacia, 112
osteomyelitis, 111
osteoporosis, 112
otitis, 172
otolaryngolic surgery, 354
otoliths, 172
otosclerosis, 173

oval window, 171
ovary, 279
    cancer, 287
ovulation, 279
ovum, 279
oxidants, 355
oxyhemoglobin, 192
oxyphils, 303
oxytocin, 302

Pacinian corpuscles, 77
palate, 240
palatine bone, 102
palliative, 354
palpation, 64
pancreas, 243, 303
    diseases of, 307
pancreozymin, 304
papillae of tongue, 163
papillary cystadenocarcinoma, 287
papillary ducts of nephron, 261
papillary layer of skin, 78
papilloma, 267
Pap smear, 337
papule, 81
paranoia, 377
parasympathetic division of the
    autonomic nervous system,
    141
parasympathicomimetic drugs, 303
parathyroid glands, 303
    diseases, 306
    oxyphil cells, 303
    principal cells, 303
parathyroid hormone, 303
parenteral administration of
    medication, 318
parietal bone, 102
Parkinson's disease, 143
parotid gland, 240
paroxysmal, 226
parturition, 282
patella, 108
patellar region, 61
patent diutus arteriosus, 200
pathology, 52
patterns of medical words, 6–7
pellagra, 323
pelvic cavity, 63
pelvic girdle, 108
pelvic inflammatory disease, 286

pemphigus, 82
penis, 279
peptic acid, 246
percussion, 222
pericardim, 183
pericarditis, 199
perichondrium, 100
perilymph, 171
perineal region, 61
perineum, 59
periosteum, 97
peripheral nervous system, 135–37
    cranial nerves, 135
        nerve classification, 135
        spinal nerves, 136
peripheral resistance, *see* blood
        pressure, 190
peristalsis, 240
peritoneum, 244
    diseases, 247
pernicious anemia, 203
peroneal bone, 95
pertussis, 226
petechiae, 81
Peyer's patches, 197
phagocytosis, 49, 194
phalanges, 108
    fingers, 108
    toes, 108
pharmacodynamics, 316
pharmacology, 315–32
    branches, 316
pharynx, 219, 240
phenols, 355
pheochromocytoma, 306
phimosis, 285
phobia, 377
phosphorus, 306
photofluorogram, 351
photoscan, 352
Physician's Desk Reference, 317
physiology, 52
pia mater, 141
pineal body, 304
pinna, 170
pinocytosis, 49, 265
pituitary gland, *see also* hypophysis,
        300
    hormones, 301–2
placenta, 187, 282
    tumors, 286
plantar region, 61
plasma, 191

plastic surgery, 354
platelets, 194
   plug, 195
pleura, 221
   diseases, 227
      parietal, 221
      visceral, 221
pleurisy, 227
plexus, 137
plural forms of medical words, 42–43
pneumoconioses, 227
pneumoencephalography, 351
pneumonia, 226
pneumotaxic center, 132
pneumothorax, 226
poliomyelitis, 143
polycythemia, 203
   vera, 203
polyp, 247
polypnea, 224
pons, 132
Pontocaine, 356
popliteal region, 61
portal system, 187
portal vein, 187
posterior, 63
potassium permanganate, 355
potentiation, drug, 317
precancerous disorders, 336
precocious puberty, 306
prefix, 1, 4, 25–35
pregnancy, 281–82
prepuce, 279
presbyacusia, 172
pressure points, 195
primary germ layers, 282
principal cells of parathyroid gland,
   303
procaine, 356
process, bone, 99
progesterone, 279, 302, 304
prognosis, 82
prolactin, 302
prolapse, 53
pronation, 63
prone position, 357
pronunciation of medical words,
   36–38
prostate gland, 279
   carcinoma, 285
   curettage, 285
   hyperplasia, 285
prostheses, 361

prostoglandins, 201
protein synthesis, 335
prothrombin, 195
protoplasm, 48
protraction, 64
proximal, 63
pruritus, 82
pseudohermaphroditism, 284
pseudohypertrophy, 113
psoriasis, 82
psychiatrist, 375
psychologist, 375
psychopathic personality, 377
psychosis, 375, 377
psychotherapy, 377
ptyalin, 240
pubic bone, 108
   region, 61
pulmonary abscesses, 226
pulmonary circulation, 183
pulmonary function tests, 223–24
   arterial blood gases, 223
   carbon monoxide technique, 223
   chest x ray, 224
   helium dilution technique, 223
   nitrogen washout technique, 223
   plethysmography, 224
   spirometry, 223
pulp, tooth, 244
pulse, 191
pupil, 157
purgatives, 321
Purkinje fibers, 185
purpura, 81
purulent, 52
pus, 194
pustule, 81
pyelogram, intravenous, 352
pyelonephritis:
   acute, 266
   chronic, 266
pyloric sphincter valve, 240
pyloroplasty, 246
pylorus, 240
pyuria, 265

quanine, 335

rachitis, 112

radiation, 350–52
   hard, 350
   ionization, 352
   seeds, 286, 353
   soft, 350
radioimmunoassy, 300
radioisotope therapy, 353
radiology, 350–52
radiolucent, 351
radiopaque, 351
radiotherapy, 352–53
radius, 108
rales, 222
rami, 137
ramification, 220
receptor organs, 157–73
reconstruction, 361
rectum, 244
red blood cells, 192–93
   formation, 192
   production, 193
red bone marrow, 97
red nucleus of mesencephalon, 132
reduction, 361
reflex arc, 141
reflexes, 138–41
refraction, 160
   medium, 160
regeneration, 53
regional anesthetics, 356
regurgitation of blood, 200
renal carcinoma, 267
renal corpuscle, 264
renal failure, 266
   acute, 266
   chronic, 266
renal pelvis, 261
renal tubules, 264
renin, 304
repair, surgical, 361
replacement, 53
replication, cell, 335
repression, 377
reproductive system, 273–98
   female, 279–83
   male, 277–79
   pathology, 284–88
resection, 361
respiration, 219
respiratory acidosis, 224
respiratory alkalosis, 225
respiratory cycle, 223
respiratory distress syndrome, 226

respiratory pigment, 192
respiratory system, 217–34
    anatomy, 219–22
    pathology, 224–28
respiratory tract cancer, 227–28
reticular layer of skin, 78
reticuloendothelial cells, 193
reticulum, endoplasmic, 48
retina, 157, 159
    rods and cones, 159–60
retraction, 64
retroperitoneal lymph nodes, 352
Rh factor, 196
rhabdomyoma, 113
rhabdomyosarcoma, 113
rheumatic carditis, 200
rheumatoid arthritis, 113
ribonucleic acid, *see* RNA, 48, 335
ribosome, 48
ribs, 107
    floating, 107
rickets, 112
ringworm, 82
RNA, 48, 335
    in cancer, 335
    messenger, 335
rods, of eye, 159–60
roentgens, *see* x rays, 350
rongeur, 361
root, tooth, 244
rotation, 63
Ruffini corpuscles, 77
rugae, 240

S-A node, 185
saccule, 172
sacral portion of vertebral column,
    105
sacrum, 94
sagittal suture, 102
saliva, 240
salivary glands, 240
salpingitis, 286
sarcoma, 334
scalp, 78
scalpel, 358
scapula, 108
scapular region, 61
scar, 81
schizophrenia, 375
    types, 375
scintiscan, 352

scissors, 358
sclera, 157
sclerosis, multiple, 142
scoliosis, 94
scotoma, 162
scotopsin, 160
scrotum, 277
sebaceous glands, 78
sebum, 78
secretin, 304
sedatives, 320
sedimentation rate of formed
    elements of blood, 192
seeds, radiation, 286, 353
semen, 279
semicircular canals, 172
seminal vesicles, 279
seminiferous tubules, 277
senile dementia, 375
sensory spots, 77
septa, 102, 200
septal cardiac defects, 200
sequestrum, 111
serial radiography, 351
serotonin, 304
serum, 195
sesamoid bones, 99
sex hormones, 277, 279
shin bone, 108
shingles, 143
short bones, 99
shortened forms, 41–42
shunt, 202, 361
sickle cell anemia, 203
side effects of drugs, 317
sight, 156
sigmoid colon, 244
silent letters, 40
silicosis, 227
Simmonds' disease, 305
simple instrument setup, 358
simple and radical excision, 287,
    361
Sim's position, 357
sinoatrial node, 185
sinus, 100
    paranasal, 219
skeletal muscle, 111
skeleton, axial, 100
skin, 76–92
    aging, 80
    anatomy, 78
    appendages, 78–79
    burns, 83

skin (*cont.*)
    cancers, 83–84
    clinical and pathological
        conditions, 81–84
    lesions, 81
small intestine, 242
smegma, 279
smell, sense, 163
smooth muscle, 110
snare, 361
sodium pentothal, 356
solutions, drugs, 318
somatotropin, 301
    hypersecretion, 305
    hyposecretion, 305
speculum, 361
spelling of medical words, 36–42
sperm, production, 277
spermatic cord, 279
spermatid, 277
spermatozoon, 277
sphenoid bone, 102
sphincter, 236
sphygmomanometer, 191
spina bifida, 143
spinal anesthetics, 356
spinal cavity, 61
spinal column, 102–5
spinal cord, 135
spinous process, 99
spirits, drugs, 318
spirochetes, 284
spirometry, 223
spleen, 197
sponges, 361
sprain, 112
sputum, 226
squamous cell carcinoma, 83
squamous epithelium, 49
staging of tumors, 335
stapes, 171
staphylococcus, 266
stem cells, 193
stereotactic surgery, 363
sternum, 107
stimulants, 319
stimulus, 127
stomach, 240
stones, urinary tract, 266
strabismus, 161
strata of skin, 78
stratified squamous epithelium, 49
stratum corneum, 78
stratum germinativum, 78

stratum granulosum, 78
stratum lucidum, 78
striations, 306
stripping, 362
stroma, 192
sty, 162
subarachnoid space, 141
subcutaneous injection, 318
subcutaneous tissue, 78
subdural hematoma, 143
sublimation, 378
sublingual glands, 240
submandibular glands, 240
subthalamus, 132
suction, 362
suffix, 4, 16–24
    compound, 16, 17–18
    simple, 16, 18–20
sulcus, 100
    bone, 100
    brain, 131
summation, 128
superego, 378
superficial, 63
superior, 63
supination, 63
supine, 357
suppression, 378
suppurative, 53
suprasternal notch, 64
surgery, 353–64
    branches, 354-55
    palliative, 354
surgery in cancer, 338
surface anatomy, 64
surgical instruments, 358
suture, 362
    classification, 362
    definition, 362
    materials, 362
suture, bones, 102
    coronal, 102
    lambdoidal, 102
    metopic, 102
    sagittal, 102
    squamous, 102
suture needles, 362
sweat, 80
sweat glands, 80
sympathetic division of the
    autonomic nervous system,
    141
sympathicomimetic, 303, 320
sympatholytic drugs, 320

symptoms, 52
synapse, 128
synarthrodial joint, 110
synchondrosis, 110
syncope, 143
syncytium, 111
syndesmosis, 110
syndrome, 52
synergism, 317
synovial fluid, 110
synovial membrane, 110
syphilis, 284
systemic circulation, 183
systole, 185
systolic pressure, 191

tablets, 318
tachycardia, 199
tachypnea, 224
tagging, radioactive, 353
talus bone, 108
target cells, 300
target tissue, 353
tarsals, 108
taste, sense, 163
tear duct, 159
tear gland, 159
tear sac, 159
technetium, 99, 352
teeth, 244
telangiectasia, 80
teletherapy, 353
template, 335
temporal bones, 102
tenaculum, 362
tendon, 110, 111
teratoma, 353
testes, 277
    carcinoma, 285
testosterone, 277, 302, 304
tetanization, 185
tetany, 306
tetracaine, 356, 357
tetralogy of Fallot, 200
thalamic syndrome, 143
thalamus, 132, 133
thalassemia, 203
thermodilution computer, 202
thermoregulation, 78
thigh bone, 108
thiopental, 356
thoracic cavity, 63

thoracic duct, 197
thoracic portion of vertebral
    column, 105
thoracic region, 61
thoracic surgery, 354
thoracic vertebrae, 105
thrombin, 195
thrombocyte, 192
thromboendarterectomy, 201
thrombophlebitis, 201
thrombus, 199
    cerebral, 142
    coronary, 199
thymine, 335
thymus gland, 197
thyroglobin, 302
thyroid gland, 302
    diseases, 305
    neoplasms, 305
thyrotropin, 302
thyroxin, 302
tibia, 108
tincture, 318
tinea, 82
tinnitus, 172
tissue, types, 49–50
TNM staging, 334
toe bones, 108
tolerance, drug, 317
tomograms, 351
tomography, 351
tongue, 163
tonsils, 197
topical administration of drugs, 319
toxic psychosis, 375
toxicity, drug, 317
toxicology, 316
tracer substances, 353
trachea, 219
trachoma, 162
tranquilizer, 320
transplantation, 362
transudation, 197
transverse colon, 244
transverse plane, 64
trauma, 53
treatment, 52
Trendelenburg position, 357
trephination, 362
trephine, 362
trichlorethane, 356
tricuspid valve, 184
triiodothyronine, 302
trocar, 362

trochanter, 100
trochlea, 100
trophoblast, 281
tropic hormones, 301
tubercle, bone, 100
tuberculosis, 227
tubules, 264
tumors, *see also* cancer, 333–47
    benign, 334
    grading, 335
    malignant, 334
    staging, 334–35
    treatment, 338–39
Turner's syndrome, 284
tympanic membrane, 171

ulcer, 246
    peptic, 246
ulna, 108
ultrasonic surgery, 363
umbilical:
    arteries, 187
    cord, 187
    region, 61
    vein, 187
United States Pharmacopeia, 317
upper GI series, 352
urea, 265
uremia, 266
ureter, 261
urethra, 262
uric acid, 265
urinary bladder, 262
    cancer, 267
urinary casts, 266
urinary disease, symptoms, 265–66
urinary system, 259–72
    anatomy, 260–64
    diseases, 265–67
    neoplasms, 267
urinary tract neoplasms, 267
urinary tract obstructions, 267
urinary tract stones, 266
urinary trigone, 262
urine:
    constituents, 265
    elimination, 262
    formation, 265

urogenital drugs, 322
urogenital surgery, 355
urticaria, 83
uterine tubes, 279
uterus, 280
    neoplasms, 286
utricle, 172

vagina, 280
    neoplasms, 286
vagotomy, 246
valve, heart:
    flap, 184
    mitral, 183
    semilunar, 184
varicose veins, 201
variocele, 285
varioles, 48
vascular drugs, 321
vas deferens, 279
vasoconstrictors, 321
vasodilators, 321
vasomotor:
    chemoreflexes, 191
    control mechanism, 190
    pressoreflexes, 190
vasopressin, 302
veins, 186
vena, cava:
    inferior, 187
    superior, 186
venostasis, 201
ventral, 63
ventricles:
    brain, 142
    heart, 183
ventriculography, 202
venules, 186
vermiform appendix, 244
vernix caseosa, 78
vertebra, structure, 105
vertebral arch, 105
vertebral body, 105
vertebral column, 102
vertigo, 173
vesicles, 81
vestibule, 172

villi:
    chorionic, 281
    intestinal, 242
viruses and cancer, 336
viscera, 63
vital signs, 52, 356
vitamins, 322–23
vitiligo, 80
vitreous chamber, 157
vitreous humor, 157
vocal mechanism, 224
volar region, 61
volvulus, 246
vomer, 102
Von Willebrand's syndrome, 203
vowel, combining, 3
vulva, 281
vulvovaginitis, 285

wheal, 81
wheezes, 222
white blood cells, *see also*
        leukocytes, 194–95
    formation, 194
    function, 194
    types, 194
white matter, brain, and spinal
        cord, 132, 135
whooping cough, 226
Wilm's tumor, 267
windpipe, 219
withdrawal, 378
wristbone, 108

xiphisternal junction, 66
xiphoid process, 107
x rays:
    hard and soft, 350
    production, 350
Xylocaine, 357

zygomatic bones, 102
zygote, 281